T0226898

Bovine Respiratory Disease

Editors

DOUGLAS L. STEP
AMELIA R. WOOLUMS

VETERINARY CLINICS
OF NORTH AMERICA:
FOOD ANIMAL PRACTICE

www.vetfood.theclinics.com

Consulting Editor
ROBERT A. SMITH

July 2020 • Volume 36 • Number 2

ELSEVIER

1600 John F. Kennedy Boulevard • Suite 1800 • Philadelphia, Pennsylvania, 19103-2899

http://www.vetfood.theclinics.com

VETERINARY CLINICS OF NORTH AMERICA: FOOD ANIMAL PRACTICE Volume 36, Number 2
July 2020 ISSN 0749-0720, ISBN-13: 978-0-323-76270-0

Editor: Colleen Dietzler
Developmental Editor: Nicole Congleton

Veterinary Clinics of North America: Food Animal Practice (ISSN 0749-0720) is published in March, July, and November by Elsevier Inc., 360 Park Avenue South, New York, NY 10010-1710. Subscription prices are $259.00 per year (domestic individuals), $456.00 per year (domestic institutions), $100.00 per year (domestic students/residents), $283.00 per year (Canadian individuals), $601.00 per year (Canadian institutions), $335.00 per year (international individuals), $601.00 per year (international institutions), $100.00 per year (Canadian students), and $165.00 (international students). To receive student/resident rate, orders must be accompanied by name of affiliated institution, date of term, and the signature of program/residency coordinator on institution letterhead. *Clinics* subscription prices. All prices are subject to change without notice. **POSTMASTER:** Send address changes to *Veterinary Clinics of North America: Food Animal Practice*, Elsevier Health Sciences Division, Subscription Customer Service, 3251 Riverport Lane, Maryland Heights, MO 63043. Customer Service (orders, claims, online, change of address): Elsevier Health Sciences Division, Subscription **Customer Service, 3251 Riverport Lane, Maryland Heights, MO 63043. Tel: 1-800-654-2452 (U.S. and Canada); 314-447-8871 (ouside U.S. and Canada). Fax: 314-447-8029. E-mail: journalscustomerservice-usa@elsevier.com (for print support); journalsonlinesupport-usa@elsevier.com (for online support).**

Reprints. For copies of 100 or more, of articles in this publication, please contact the Commercial Reprints Department, Elsevier Inc., 360 Park Avenue South, New York, NY 10010-1710. Tel.: 212-633-3874; Fax: 212-633-3820; E-mail: reprints@elsevier.com.

Veterinary Clinics of North America: Food Animal Practice is covered in *Current Contents/Agriculture, Biology and Environmental Sciences, MEDLINE/PubMed (Index Medicus), and Excerpta Medica.*

Contributors

CONSULTING EDITOR

ROBERT A. SMITH, DVM, MS
Diplomate, American Board of Veterinary Practitioners; Veterinary Research and Consulting Services, LLC, Greeley, Colorado, USA; Veterinary Research and Consulting Services, LLC, Stillwater, Oklahoma, USA

EDITORS

AMELIA R. WOOLUMS, DVM, MVSc, PhD
Professor, Department of Pathobiology and Population Medicine, College of Veterinary Medicine, Mississippi State University, Mississippi State, Mississippi, USA

DOUGLAS L. STEP, DVM
Diplomate, American College of Veterinary Internal Medicine; Professional Services Veterinarian, Boehringer Ingelheim Animal Health USA, Inc, Collinsville, Oklahoma, USA

AUTHORS

TREVOR W. ALEXANDER, PhD
Lethbridge Research and Development Center, Agriculture and Agri-Food Canada, Lethbridge, Alberta, Canada

SAMAT AMAT, MSc, PhD
Faculty of Veterinary Medicine, University of Calgary, Calgary, Alberta, Canada; Lethbridge Research and Development Center, Agriculture and Agri-Food Canada, Lethbridge, Alberta, Canada; Department of Agricultural, Food and Nutritional Science, University of Alberta, Edmonton, Alberta, Canada

LAURA L. BASSEL, DVM, MSc
Department of Pathobiology, Ontario Veterinary College, University of Guelph, Guelph, Ontario, Canada

CALVIN W. BOOKER, DVM, MVetSc
Managing Partner, Feedlot Health Management Services, Okotoks, Alberta, Canada

SÉBASTIEN BUCZINSKI, Dr Vét, MSc
Diplomate, American College of Veterinary Internal Medicine (Food Animal emphasis); Département des Sciences Cliniques, Faculté de Médecine Vétérinaire, Université de Montréal, St-Hyacinthe, Québec, Canada

JEFF L. CASWELL, DVM, DVSc, PhD
Department of Pathobiology, Ontario Veterinary College, University of Guelph, Guelph, Ontario, Canada

MANUEL F. CHAMORRO, DVM, MS, PhD
Diplomate, American College of Veterinary Internal Medicine; Assistant Professor of Food
Animal Medicine and Surgery, Department of Clinical Sciences, College of Veterinary
Medicine, Auburn University, Large Animal Teaching Hospital, Auburn, Alabama, USA

BRENT CREDILLE, DVM, PhD
Diplomate, American College of Veterinary Internal Medicine (Large Animal); Associate
Professor and Section Head, Food Animal Health and Management Program, Department
of Population Health, College of Veterinary Medicine, University of Georgia, Veterinary
Medical Center, Athens, Georgia, USA

TERRY J. ENGELKEN, DVM, MS
Associate Professor, Veterinary Diagnostic and Production Animal Medicine, College of
Veterinary Medicine, Iowa State University, Ames, Iowa, USA

T. ROBIN FALKNER, DVM
Elanco Animal Health, Greenfield, Indiana, USA

ROBERT W. FULTON, DVM, PhD
Diplomate, American College of Veterinary Microbiologists; Emeritus Regents Professor,
Department of Veterinary Pathobiology, College of Veterinary Medicine, Oklahoma State
University, Stillwater, Oklahoma, USA

JOHN T. GROVES, DVM
Livestock Veterinary Service, Eldon, Missouri, USA

CLINTON R. KREHBIEL, PhD, PAS
Marvel L. Baker Professor and Head, Department of Animal Science, University of
Nebraska-Lincoln, Lincoln, Nebraska, USA

BRIAN V. LUBBERS, DVM, PhD
Diplomate, American College of Veterinary Clinical Pharmacology; Associate Professor of
Food Animal Therapeutics, Clinical Sciences, College of Veterinary Medicine, Kansas
State University, Manhattan, Kansas, USA

JODI L. McGILL, MS, PhD
Assistant Professor, Department of Veterinary Microbiology and Preventative Medicine,
Iowa State University, Ames, Iowa, USA

CHRIS McMULLEN, BSc
Faculty of Veterinary Medicine, University of Calgary, Calgary, Alberta, Canada

THERESA L. OLLIVETT, DVM, PhD
Diplomate, American College of Veterinary Internal Medicine (Large Animal Internal
Medicine); Assistant Professor, Department of Medical Sciences, University of
Wisconsin-Madison School of Veterinary Medicine, Madison, Wisconsin, USA

ROBERTO A. PALOMARES, DVM, MS, PhD
Diplomate, American College of Theriogenologists; Associate Professor of Food Animal
Theriogenology, Department of Population Medicine, College of Veterinary Medicine,
University of Georgia, Athens, Georgia, USA

BART PARDON, DVM, PhD
Diplomate, European College of Bovine Health Management; Department of Large Animal
Internal Medicine, Faculty of Veterinary Medicine, Ghent University, Merelbeke, Belgium

DERRELL S. PEEL, PhD
Breedlove Professor of Agribusiness and Extension Livestock Marketing Specialist, Oklahoma State University, Stillwater, Oklahoma, USA

JOSE PEREZ-CASAL, PhD
Vaccine and Infectious Disease Organization – International Vaccine Centre (VIDO-InterVac), Saskatoon, Saskatchewan, Canada

JOHN T. RICHESON, PhD
Department of Agricultural Sciences, West Texas A&M University, Canyon, Texas, USA

RANDY E. SACCO, PhD
Microbiologist, Ruminant Diseases and Immunology Research Unit, Agricultural Research Services, USDA, Ames, Iowa, USA

RANDAL M. SHIRBROUN, DVM
Director, Ruminant Business Unit, Newport Laboratories, A Boehringer Ingelheim Animal Health Company, Worthington, Minnesota, USA

ROBERT A. SMITH, DVM, MS
Diplomate, American Board of Veterinary Practitioners; Veterinary Research and Consulting Services, LLC, Greeley, Colorado, USA; Veterinary Research and Consulting Services, LLC, Stillwater, Oklahoma, USA

EMILY SNYDER, DVM, MFAM
Graduate Assistant, Food Animal Health and Management Program, Department of Population Health, College of Veterinary Medicine, University of Georgia, Veterinary Medical Center, Athens, Georgia, USA

DOUGLAS L. STEP, DVM
Diplomate, American College of Veterinary Internal Medicine; Professional Services Veterinarian, Boehringer Ingelheim Animal Health USA, Inc, Collinsville, Oklahoma, USA

SAEID TABATABAEI, DVM, PhD
Department of Pathobiology, Ontario Veterinary College, University of Guelph, Guelph, Ontario, Canada

EDOUARD TIMSIT, DVM, PhD
Diplomate, European College of Bovine Health Management; Ceva Santé Animale, Libourne, France

AMELIA R. WOOLUMS, DVM, MVSc, PhD
Professor, Department of Pathobiology and Population Medicine, College of Veterinary Medicine, Mississippi State University, Mississippi State, Mississippi, USA

Contents

Histophilus somni is associated with several disease syndromes in cattle and plays an important role in the bovine respiratory disease complex. H somni isolates exhibit significant differences in terms of susceptibility to inactivation by normal serum corresponding to the general ability to cause clinical disease. Isolates possess a variety of virulence factors, and variation in virulence factor expression is well recognized and associated with antigenic differences. Sequencing of genes associated with known virulence factors has identified genetic variability between isolates. The antigenic and genomic differences represent significant challenges to the host immune system and are problematic for vaccine design.

The respiratory tract of cattle is colonized by complex bacterial ecosystems also known as bacterial microbiotas. These microbiotas evolve over time and are shaped by numerous factors, including maternal vaginal microbiota, environment, age, diet, parenteral antimicrobials, and stressful events. The resulting microbiota can be diverse and enriched with known beneficial bacteria that can provide colonization resistance against bacterial pathogens or, on the contrary, with opportunistic pathogens that can predispose cattle to respiratory disease. The respiratory microbiota can be modulated by nonantimicrobial approaches to promote health, creating new potential strategies for prevention and treatment of bovine respiratory disease.

Advances in viral detection in bovine respiratory disease (BRD) have resulted from advances in viral sequencing of respiratory tract samples. New viruses detected include influenza D virus, bovine coronavirus, bovine rhinitis A, bovine rhinitis B virus, and others. Serosurveys demonstrate widespread presence of some of these viruses in North American cattle. These viruses sometimes cause disease after animal challenge, and some have been found in BRD cases more frequently than in healthy cattle. Continued work is needed to develop reagents for identification of new viruses, to confirm their pathogenicity, and to determine whether vaccines have a place in their control.

Bovine respiratory disease (BRD) remains a leading cause of morbidity, mortality, and economic loss to the cattle industry. The continued high prevalence of the disease underlines a gap in understanding of the host immune response to respiratory infection. The host immune response is beneficial and detrimental, required for clearing the disease but often leading to tissue damage and long-term defects in lung function. This article highlights advancements made in understanding innate and adaptive immunity in BRD, factors that predispose animals to BRD, and novel intervention strategies that may lead to changes in the approach to treating and controlling BRD.

Laura L. Bassel, Saeid Tabatabaei, and Jeff L. Caswell

Calves vary considerably in their pathologic and clinical responses to infection of the lung with bacteria. The reasons may include resistance to infection because of pre-existing immunity, development of effective immune responses, or infection with a minimally virulent bacterial strain. However, studies of natural disease and of experimental infections indicate that some calves develop only mild lung lesions and minimal clinical signs despite substantial numbers of pathogenic bacteria in the lung. This may represent "tolerance" to pulmonary infection because these calves are able to control their inflammatory responses or protect the lung from damage, without necessarily eliminating bacterial infection. Conversely, risk factors might predispose to bovine respiratory disease by triggering a loss of tolerance that results in a harmful inflammatory and tissue-damaging response to infection.

Clinton R. Krehbiel

Bovine respiratory disease (BRD) complex remains one of the greatest challenges facing beef cattle producers, veterinarians, and feedlot managers. In receiving, stocker/backgrounding, and feedlot cattle, BRD has been associated with decreased dry matter intake and daily gain, resulting in economic losses during the feeding period. Inflammation associated with BRD has the potential to decrease carcass yield and quality. Newly received calves are at various risks to contract BRD. Proper nutrition for newly received calves is key to recovery from stress associated with weaning and transport. This article reviews nutrient impacts on BRD and BRD impacts on nutrient metabolism.

Terry J. Engelken

Confined cow-calf operations are a relatively new production model in the United States. As with any new technology, there will be a learning curve for producers and veterinarians as we attempt to optimize animal health and profitability. It is critical that cattle are managed properly in these units if disease issues are to be minimized. Allowing for adequate space in the pen and at the feed bunk is a critical factor affecting animal welfare, nutritional management, and disease transmission.

Bovine respiratory disease (BRD) is a leading cause of morbidity and mortality in young cattle. Housing factors that lead to poor ventilation and stagnant air are often considered the primary reasons for high levels of endemic disease. This article reviews the literature from the past 40 years in order to determine which housing factors have been associated with respiratory disease. Penning strategy and its affect on calf respiratory health were most commonly studied. The wide variation in disease definitions and quality of reporting make drawing conclusions from the available literature extraordinarily difficult.

Bovine respiratory disease (BRD) complex is a worldwide health problem in cattle and is a major reason for antimicrobial use in young cattle. Several challenges may explain why it is difficult to make progress in the management of this disease. This article defines the limitation of BRD complex nomenclature, which may not easily distinguish upper versus lower respiratory tract infection and infectious bronchopneumonia versus other types of respiratory diseases. It then discusses the obstacles to clinical diagnosis and reviews the current knowledge of readily available diagnostic test to reach a diagnosis of infectious bronchopneumonia.

When it is desired to identify infectious agents involved in an outbreak of bovine respiratory disease, a variety of possible sampling methods may be used. For field use, the deep nasopharyngeal swab, transtracheal wash, and nonendoscopic bronchoalveolar lavage are most feasible. At present, bacterial culture and polymerase chain reaction testing are most commonly used to identify infectious agents. Interpretation of test results can be challenging, particularly for opportunistic pathogens. Evidence-based guidelines for precise interpretation of microbiologic tests results are lacking; however, approaches that have been practically useful for the management of bovine respiratory disease outbreaks are presented.

This article provides insights into the management of bovine respiratory disease in high-risk cattle populations. Biocontainment strategies, records, procurement, transport, arrival/receiving management, vaccination, and treatment protocols are discussed from practical and systems-thinking perspectives regarding their impact on health in high-risk cattle.

Arrival management considerations, such as facilities, nutritional manage-ment, metaphylaxis, bovine viral diarrhea virus persistent infection testing, parasite control, and castration, are also addressed. Caretaker morale and job satisfaction are suggested as important factors to consider when man-aging high-risk cattle. The inter-relationships of variables within the system are explored as contributing causative factors to bovine respiratory dis-ease in high-risk cattle.

Vaccination of cattle against viral respiratory pathogens to minimize los-ses associated with bovine respiratory disease (BRD) is a common prac-tice among producers and veterinarians. Three different calf populations in which BRD is most prevalent (recently weaned beef calves, prewean-ing beef calves, and young dairy calves) are the principal focus of morbidity and mortality prevention through vaccination; however, the ev-idence of vaccination efficacy is inconsistent in the literature. This review addresses the evidence of efficacy of vaccination in the prevention or reduction of naturally occurring and experimentally induced BRD in each calf group.

Vaccination is the act of administering a vaccine, whereas immunization may occur if appropriate time is allowed for a competent host immune sys-tem to respond to the antigen contained in a vaccine. Timing is critical to ensure bovine respiratory disease (BRD) vaccine safety, efficacy, and effi-ciency. The current review provides temporal considerations of BRD vaccination within the North American beef production system with focus on vaccination timing in high-risk, newly received beef stocker and feedlot cattle.

Bovine respiratory disease (BRD) is often attributed to complex interac-tions between the host, pathogen, and the environment. Likewise, many BRD treatment failures result from interactions between the host, path-ogen, environment, drug, and drug administrator. Investigating and ad-dressing the underlying causes of BRD treatment failures can improve clinical outcomes and animal welfare of future cases, improve morale of employees, reduce direct costs of dealing with BRD treatment failures, refine antimicrobial prescribing practices, and advance antimicrobial stewardship. This article discusses these interactions and provides guid-ance to veterinary practitioners on evaluating the success of treatment protocols.

> Bovine respiratory disease (BRD) is a persistent negative economic impact on beef and dairy industries and the inability to show any progress in controlling BRD is a source of increasing frustration among animal health professionals and the industry. The complex economic structure of the cattle industry leads to market failures in which cow-calf producers do not have sufficient economic incentive to invest in improved BRD control. This leads to higher costs for stocker and feedlot sectors. An industry-wide comprehensive effort is needed to coordinate and motivate enhanced BRD control focusing on producing healthy calves with less morbidity rather than treatment.

VETERINARY CLINICS OF NORTH AMERICA: FOOD ANIMAL PRACTICE

FORTHCOMING ISSUES

November 2020
Toxicology
Steve Ensley and Timothy J. Evans, *Editors*

March 2021
Small Ruminants
Cynthia B. Wolf and Michelle Kutzler,
Editors

RECENT ISSUES

March 2020
Ruminant Parasitology
Ray M. Kaplan, *Editor*

November 2019
Ruminant Immunology
Christopher Chase, *Editor*

SERIES OF RELATED INTEREST

Veterinary Clinics of North America: Equine Practice

Preface

Bovine Respiratory Disease: What's New?

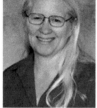

Amelia R. Woolums, DVM, MVSc, PhD   Douglas L. Step, DVM
Editors

Since the recognition of the importance of bovine respiratory disease (BRD) several decades ago, much effort has focused on improving our understanding of causes, designing preventive health programs, and developing treatment and control methods. Unfortunately, producers and veterinarians still must manage the production and economic risk of this disease. Given the importance of BRD for both beef and dairy cattle, the disease complex has been the focus of an issue of the *Veterinary Clinics of North America: Food Animal Practice* approximately every 10 years since the journal's inception. This frequency of issues on the topic may lead the reader to wonder how there can be anything new to say about BRD. Realizing this, we have asked our contributors to focus on information from the past 10 years, or to address topics that have not previously been investigated in-depth. Thanks to their efforts, we are able to present you with an issue that contains, we hazard to guess, something you haven't heard before, or perhaps something you haven't thought of. While you'll recognize the focus on the epidemiologic triad: cow, infectious agent, and environment/management, we think you will also appreciate some new or different perspectives that might even be considered a paradigm shift in the way we approach BRD diagnosis, attempt to control the interaction of cattle and the microbes in or around them, and care for cattle at different phases in the production and marketing chain.

One topic you might not expect that we felt merited public airing is the impact of market forces on decisions producers make regarding practices that can decrease BRD. Any producer or veterinarian should hope to see less BRD in the cattle they oversee, but some of us may have been a bit naïve in the degree to which we thought our research could improve cattle health when some producers actually have financial incentive to buy cattle at high risk for BRD. It is our hope that the information provided here will help people who care for cattle find new pathways to actually keep them healthier, whether these be microbiological, environmental, or economical.

Vet Clin Food Anim 36 (2020) xv–xvi
https://doi.org/10.1016/j.cvfa.2020.04.001
0749-0720/20/© 2020 Published by Elsevier Inc.

vetfood.theclinics.com

We offer heartfelt thanks to our colleagues, who have written the articles included here. They were all surely too busy to even open the e-mail containing our request for their participation, but nonetheless they have used their limited time to research and summarize a topic that, we hope, will provide the reader with information to use as a reference as well as to challenge some biases.

Amelia R. Woolums, DVM, MVSc, PhD
Department of Pathobiology and
Population Medicine
College of Veterinary Medicine
Mississippi State University
Mississippi State, MS 39762, USA

Douglas L. Step, DVM
Boehringer Ingelheim
Animal Health USA, Inc
12940 N 124th East Avenue
Collinsville, OK 74021, USA

E-mail addresses:
amelia.woolums@msstate.edu (A.R. Woolums)
dl.step@boehringer-ingelheim.com (D.L. Step)

Bovine Respiratory Disease

Looking Back and Looking Forward, What Do We See?

Robert A. Smith, MS, DVM[a], Douglas L. Step, DVM[b],
Amelia R. Woolums, DVM, MVSc, PhD[c],*

KEYWORDS

• BRD • Management • Virus • Bacteria • History • Future

KEY POINTS

- Changes in cattle feeding in the mid-twentieth century established practices such as long-distance transport and multisource comingling that are persistent risk factors for bovine respiratory disease (BRD).
- Research in the 1970s showed that respiratory viral infection followed by exposure to *Mannheimia haemolytica* led to fibrinous pneumonia, the hallmark of feedlot BRD.
- Despite much research, broadly focused surveys in the United States indicate that feedlot BRD morbidity has not decreased to an important degree over the past 45 years.
- Practices such as weaning, comingling, and on-arrival castration reliably increase BRD risk, but lack of incentives for small cow-calf operations to modify these practices leads to a persistent population of cattle at high risk for BRD.
- New technologies are in development that could bring "precision agriculture" approaches to improved BRD control; however, it will be necessary for producers to have incentive to use such practices if BRD morbidity and mortality are to be impacted.

INTRODUCTION

Bovine respiratory disease (BRD) continues to plague the cattle industry and is a major challenge for veterinarians as well as for beef and dairy producers. This topic dominates continuing education agendas at veterinary conferences and cattlemen's meetings alike. Hundreds of millions of dollars in research funds have been invested in studying factors that contribute to BRD, as well as its effect on longevity, performance,

[a] Veterinary Research and Consulting Services, LLC, 3404 Live Oak Lane, Stillwater, OK 74075, USA; [b] Boehringer Ingelheim Animal Health USA, Inc., 12940 North 124th East Avenue, Collinsville, OK 74021, USA; [c] Department of Pathobiology and Population Medicine, College of Veterinary Medicine, Mississippi State University, 240 Wise Center, Mississippi State, MS 39762, USA
* Corresponding author.
E-mail address: amelia.woolums@msstate.edu

Vet Clin Food Anim 36 (2020) 239–251
https://doi.org/10.1016/j.cvfa.2020.03.009
0749-0720/20/© 2020 Elsevier Inc. All rights reserved.

and carcass quality. Research topics span the spectrum of microbiology, pathophysiology, pharmacology, immune system responses, epidemiology, genetics, and husbandry practices. These specialty areas have influenced prevention, control, and treatment protocols for all phases of beef and dairy production.

Deaths owing to BRD, early marketing, reduced performance, and poorer carcass quality have a negative impact on sustainability within the cattle industry. Inputs such as forages, grain, supplements, water, and fossil fuels used to produce meat and milk are wasted when an animal dies or if performance is subpar. Often overlooked is the waste of resources invested in the dam; if her offspring does not complete the production cycle, resources invested in her during her pregnancy were for naught. Death loss is more costly than just the market value of the calf and cost of treatment.

The authors of this introductory article provide a brief review of BRD issues over the past few decades and venture into what BRD management might look like in the future. Because the authors are beef oriented, much of the emphasis in this article focuses on beef production rather than dairy. However, because BRD is the leading cause of mortality in postweaned dairy heifers,[1] and the second leading cause in preweaned dairy heifers,[1] the important effect of BRD on dairy calf and cow health and productivity is acknowledged.

TRANSFORMATION OF THE CATTLE FEEDING INDUSTRY

Before the 1960s, most cattle feeding was conducted in the Corn Belt, where corn production dominated. Beef packing plants were located primarily in or near river cities, close to population centers. Cattle feeding in the west, such as Texas, was underway, but generally these feedlots were located a long distance from packing houses.[2] Nonetheless, cattle feeding continued to grow in the southern Great Plains and High Plains, despite the challenges to market finished cattle. There were 15 sizable feedyards in Texas during the 1950s, and cattle feeding was also growing in Kansas, the Oklahoma Panhandle, and Colorado.[3]

In the 1960s and through the early 1970s, cattle feeding greatly expanded on the High Plains. Weather was more favorable for cattle feeding than in the Corn Belt, and it was cheaper to ship the corn to the cattle than cattle to the corn. At the same time, irrigation from plentiful wells provided water for grain production in the semiarid regions. Packing houses to the north were becoming antiquated, and packers quickly began movement west to build more efficient plants near the cattle.[3] Cattle, irrigation, grain, favorable weather, and packing plants were the perfect combination to support the cattle feeding industry. Although other prominent areas still fed significant numbers of cattle, the 1960s and 1970s were known to many as the Golden Age of Cattle Feeding on the High Plains.

As new technology was introduced into the feedlot industry, and universities geared up research and extension to support the industry, the size and number of feedlots continued to grow, and efficiencies were captured. The size and scale of feedlots attracted nutritionists, mostly with doctoral degrees, to support the industry, and veterinarians with interest and skills needed by feedlots developed health programs using some of the first "consulting veterinarian" models.

Prevention and treatment protocols were tailored for each feedlot, and by the early 1980s, descriptive statistics, computerized records, improved residue avoidance, and ongoing employee training were becoming the norm. Some of the early Beef Quality Assurance (BQA) programs were formalized in the 1980s, first centering on residue avoidance. BQA was in full swing by the early 1990s, providing guidance on such things as injection site lesion avoidance, cattle handling and stockmanship, antibiotic stewardship, and BQA certification, not only of individuals working with cattle, but also of BQA certification programs for feedlots, stocker, and cow-calf operations.[3] The dairy industry followed suit many years later with the BQA equivalent known as FARM: Farmers Assuring Responsible Management. In total, hundreds of thousands of people handling cattle are now BQA certified in various recognized programs.

Despite the research, education, and commitment of producers and veterinarians to manage BRD, it still plagues the industry today; in fact, death loss caused by BRD is no better, and by some measures is greater today than during the Golden Age of Cattle Feeding. The subsequent articles in this issue of *Veterinary Clinics of North America: Food Animal Practice* summarize recent information regarding the factors that contribute to BRD. It is hoped that the information will provide guidance to new practices and policies that actually decrease the prevalence of BRD before the end of the twenty-first century.

A BRIEF OVERVIEW OF BOVINE RESPIRATORY DISEASE OVER THE PAST 45 YEARS

History can be a measuring stick, a record of the past that provides information to make decisions for tomorrow. Although BRD is a challenge today as it was decades ago, extensive research has attempted to elucidate practices to reduce the impact of the disease on health and productivity. A 45-year timespan was selected because it covers the professional career of one of the authors (R.A.S.). Given the breadth of the subject, this review is necessarily selective, intended to provide historical context for some issues still relevant to BRD prevention and control today.

Viral-Bacterial Infection and Vaccination

A breakthrough in the understanding of feedlot BRD came when Canadian researchers reliably and repeatedly generated the typical pathology of fibrinous pneumonia with experimental aerosol challenge of recently weaned beef calves with bovine herpesvirus-1 (BHV-1) followed in 4 days or more by aerosol challenge with *Mannheimia* (formerly *Pasteurella*) *haemolytica*.[4] Primary challenge with parainfluenza type 3 virus (PI3V) followed by *M haemolytica* induced similar pathology; challenge with either virus or *M haemolytica* alone did not.[5] A series of experiments testing the effects of the duration of time between weaning and transport and challenge, or differences in ambient temperature and humidity at, or after, challenge, indicated that these factors were not as important as the time between the primary viral and secondary bacterial coinfection. Four days or more, but not less, between viral and bacterial exposure was required for challenged cattle to develop fibrinous lobar pneumonia.[4] The 4-day period was presumed to be the length of time required for virus-induced impairment of host defense mechanisms to increase susceptibility to bacterial infection. Experimental vaccination with some but not all BHV-1 or *M haemolytica* vaccines greatly mitigated disease owing to this challenge model,[6–8] leading to the belief that BRD could be eliminated or decreased substantially by proper vaccination. As a result of these findings, over the next 20 years intense research focus was applied to determine virulence mechanisms of BHV-1, *M haemolytica*, and other agents of BRD, and to develop and test vaccines to prevent infection and resulting disease.

During this time, bovine respiratory syncytial virus (BRSV) was recognized as a pathogen, and a vaccine was first developed and marketed in the 1980s; both intranasal and parenteral vaccines containing this agent are available today. Researchers conducted a systematic review comparing feedlot preventive health protocols using vaccines that included BRSV.[9] A Colorado study using more than 19,000 cattle compared combination modified live virus (MLV) BHV-1, BVDV, PI3V, and BRSV vaccine (4-way) with the same brand of vaccine without the BRSV (3-way). Respiratory mortality was low in both groups; however, the 4-way vaccine group experienced 0.3% respiratory mortality compared with 0.7% in steers in the 3-way vaccine group.[10] In contrast, a later large feedlot study in Colorado compared an MLV pentavalent vaccine (BHV-1, BVDV [types 1 and 2], PI3V, and BRSV) with a trivalent MLV vaccine produced by the same company. Mortality between vaccine treatment groups did not differ in this study,[11] similar to other studies evaluating the use of BRSV vaccine in feedlot cattle.[9]

Bovine viral diarrhea virus (BVDV) had been recognized as a pathogen since the 1940s, causing death primarily in cattle 6 months to 2 years of age.[12] A major step in understanding the manifestations of BVDV infections were research reports describing the mechanism for persistent infection (PI) with BVDV, thereby tying together fetal infection, immunotolerance, and mucosal disease.[13,14] Later, diagnostic tests with good sensitivity and specifically for detection of PI animals were developed that used testing of skin samples taken from the ear, making sample collection easy and simple.[15] Similar tests followed, along with more sophisticated diagnostics used by diagnostic laboratories.

With the recognition of genotype 2 BVDV, vaccine manufacturers incorporated both BVDV type 1 and BVDV type 2 into vaccines, and subgenotypes were described. The addition of type 2 BVDV antigen to vaccines broadened the spectrum of immunity against natural BVDV challenges. In addition to adding BVDV type 2 to commercial vaccines, control programs were developed as an additional step to control the disease, including identification and removal of PI cattle, biosecurity measures, and vaccination.[16,17]

Histophilus somni bacterins were introduced in the 1980s. In a metaanalysis of the effect of vaccination on the BRD complex, the investigators concluded that the risk of BRD was not affected by vaccination against this pathogen with currently available vaccines.[18] This finding was in agreement with an earlier systematic review that reported conflicting effects on morbidity and no significant effect on mortality among studies.[19]

Mannheimia is a major pathogen in the BRD complex. Various types of *M haemolytica* vaccines were brought to the market over the past few decades. It is important when reviewing literature to distinguish the type of vaccine studied, such as a traditional bacterin, live versus inactivated vaccine, toxoid, or bacterin-toxoid, and even the route of administration should be considered, as results for 1 type of vaccine may not be applicable to another type. A metaanalysis evaluating morbidity cumulative incidence and mortality relative risk in field trials of vaccines containing *M haemolytica* found a statistically significantly lower risk of morbidity but not mortality for feedlot cattle.[18] In 2 large-scale feedlot trials comparing vaccination with an *M haemolytica* toxoid to nonvaccinated controls, BRD mortality was reduced by 28% and 50%.[20,21] Vaccinates and controls were commingled within pens, and cattle were monitored until harvest.

Overall, the results of research since the 1970s to develop and test vaccines against specific BRD agents have been mixed. Although BRD vaccination decreases morbidity or mortality in some cases, in other cases it does not. Ultimately, the knowledge and tools gained have not been associated with a recognizable decrease in mortality because of BRD as reported by broadly focused epidemiologic investigations, such as the US Department of Agriculture (USDA) National Animal Health Monitoring System (NAHMS) surveys. A clue that BRD control would be complicated was provided by the first thorough epidemiologic investigations of BRD risks factors, the

Bruce County Beef Project.[22] In work contemporary with the early BHV-1/*M haemolytica* challenge studies, investigators found that administration of BRD vaccines to cattle within 2 weeks of arrival actually increased mortality risk. Commingling cattle, and introduction of silage in the first month after arrival, also increased mortality risk; when vaccination was delayed in cattle fed silage, mortality was ameliorated. These findings provided 1 example that the risk factors for feedlot BRD are complex, and evaluating control methods in isolation can provide a misleading picture.

Bovine Respiratory Disease and the Impact of Management Practices

Although much BRD research in the past 45 years focused on infectious agents and vaccines, some investigators evaluated the role of management, and the picture that emerged from that work was perhaps more clear. Numerous studies demonstrated that castration of bulls at arrival significantly increases their risk for BRD morbidity and mortality[23–25]; on-arrival castration is arguably the most evidence-based factor known to impact BRD. In a study designed to assess the effects of weaning in advance of marketing, single versus commingled source, and BRD vaccination, on health, performance, and costs over a 42-day backgrounding period, the effects of preweaning and the effects of not commingling had separate, significant beneficial impacts to decrease morbidity and total costs.[26] These results agreed with studies showing that preconditioning generally decreases BRD.[27,28]

Although purchase of preweaned, castrated, single-source calves may be the most reliable way to decrease BRD, the fact that many feedlots still purchase auction market–derived, freshly weaned bulls clearly indicates the uncomfortable truth that BRD prevention is not always prioritized. This point was succinctly described by Jim[29] at the 2009 BRD Symposium, when he said "…for a 500 pound animal costing $1/pound, for every cent reduction in purchase price, the feedlot can 'afford' an additional 1% death loss…the highest potential rate of return is often associated with 'high risk' BRD scenarios…." Put another way, producers in the various sectors of the cattle industry may simply not have proper economic incentives to invest in BRD control. This situation has been described as a type of market failure, a situation in which individual decisions do not lead to an optimal solution in the aggregate.[30] It may be that the most important cause of BRD is the lack of economic incentive to minimize it. The complicated, fragmented nature of the cattle industry also contributes, as was acknowledged in 1984,[31] and in 2019.[32]

Antimicrobial Use and Bovine Respiratory Disease

Until the late 1980s and early 1990s, antimicrobials used to control or treat BRD were quite antiquated by today's standards. Various single or combination therapies used to treat BRD included penicillin, oxytetracycline, sulfonamides, spectinomycin, erythromycin, and, regrettably, some use of parenteral aminoglycosides and chloramphenicol. The earliest new-generation antimicrobial labeled for treatment of BRD was ceftiofur sodium, introduced in 1988, followed by tilmicosin phosphate in 1992. Several new products followed, including different formulations of ceftiofur, enrofloxacin, florfenicol, danofloxacin, gamithromycin, tildipirosin, and tulathromycin. The introduction of these products virtually eliminated the need for extralabel use of antibiotics and untested combinations of antimicrobials.

Newer-generation antimicrobials changed protocols considerably. No longer did cattle with BRD have to receive daily treatments. Instead, there were choices that allowed single-injection therapy for BRD, and follow-up evaluation for treatment success after established posttreatment intervals. New-generation products, except for ceftiofur sodium and ceftiofur hydrochloride, were also labeled for control of BRD, which provided opportunities for better, and more proactive, management of BRD in high-risk cattle. Research consistently showed a reduction in morbidity and mortality in high-risk stocker and feeder cattle treated metaphylactically compared with controls, which also improved production efficiency and animal well-being. Florfenicol, gamithromycin, enrofloxacin, and tulathromycin were also labeled for treatment of *Mycoplasma bovis*. Despite the clear value of antimicrobial therapy for BRD treatment and control to date, recent identification of multidrug-resistant isolates of *M haemolytica*, *Pasteurella multocida*, and *H somni*[33,34] suggests that antimicrobials may not be the strongest tool for BRD control over the next 45 years.

The Contribution of Bovine Respiratory Disease to Feedlot Morbidity and Mortality

In the United States, the NAHMS periodically surveys feedlot operations regarding cattle health and management, using an approach designed and conducted to provide statistically valid inferences about the entire US cattle population. The 1999 NAHMS feedlot survey reported that 14.4% of placements were affected with BRD,[35] whereas the 2011 NAHMS feedlot survey found that 16.2% of placements were affected with BRD.[36]

The most objective measure of the deleterious effects of BRD is death loss. To the authors' knowledge, the routine and systematic collection and analysis of descriptive data in beef feedlots began in the late 1970s and early 1980s. Many of these benchmarks were and still are proprietary, but there are a few mortality summaries in the public domain.

In a 1988 report[37] describing morbidity and mortality in 11 beef feedlots over 1 year, the feedlots received 372,175 cattle, with 7% morbidity and 0.65% mortality. Respiratory disease (all forms) accounted for 65% of morbidity and 65% of the mortality. Respiratory diseases occurred throughout the feeding period; 27% of morbidity occurred after 45 days on feed (dof), as did 44% of morbidity. Bronchopneumonia was the most common cause of morbidity and mortality, 68% and 34%, respectively, of total respiratory cases with less than 45 dof. In cattle with more than 45 dof, pneumonia was the most common cause of morbidity, representing 23% of total respiratory cases. Death losses owing to pneumonia and chronic pneumonia in cattle with more than 45 dof represented 16% and 19% of the total death loss, respectably (**Table 1**).

Table 1				
Morbidity and mortality of respiratory diseases as percent of total respiratories from 1985				
	<45 d		**>45 d**	
	Morbidity	**Mortality**	**Morbidity**	**Mortality**
Respiratory (pneumonia)	68.1	34.2	23.2	16.0
Respiratory chronic	3.3	17.2	1.7	19.0
Diphtheria	0.5	0.1	1.0	0.1
Allergic pneumonia	0.2	2.4	0.3	6.9
Honker	0.4	0.3	1.3	2.8
TOTALS	72.5	54.2	27.5	44.8
Total number received	372,175			
Total hospital pulls	26,674 (7% of received)			
Total respiratory pulls	17,458 (65% of hospital pulls)			

From Edwards A. Diagnosis of respiratory disease in feedlot cattle occurring after being in feedlot for 45 days. *Bov. Pract.* 1988; 23:47-48; with permission.

This same author later summarized 9 years of feedlot death losses that occurred from 1986 through 1994.[38] A total of 5,972,825 cattle were received, with 7.8% morbidity and 0.86% mortality owing to all causes. Death owing to respiratory disease was 0.46% of cattle received during the 9-year period.

Death losses are also commonly reported as monthly death loss expressed as a percentage of average occupancy. Mortality data from 38,593,575 cattle were collected over a 3.5-year period from early 1990 through mid-1993.[39] Although variable from month to month, respiratory monthly death loss averaged 0.128% of occupancy and ranged from 0.072% to 0.234% based on month or year. Respiratory deaths represented 44.1% of the total death loss, whereas fatal digestive disease (ie, bloat, acidosis) was responsible for 25.9% of the total deaths. The remaining death losses were classified as "other."

Mortality from January 2005 through September of 2014 was summarized in a similar manner from more than 73 million steer and heifer feeder cattle.[40] Respiratory death loss averaged 0.091% of monthly occupancy from 2005 through 2007, 0.097% from 2008 through 2010, and 0.127% of monthly occupancy from 2011 through 2013. This death loss represents a 35% increase in monthly death loss during 2011 through 2013 compared with 2005 through 2010. Similarly, yearly mortality increased 27.6% in steers and 30.5% in heifers (1.41 vs 1.84% at close-out) between January 2005 and September 2014. This change represents an increase in respiratory death loss of 0.04% per year in steers, and 0.06% per year in heifers.[40] This finding is consistent with the increase in respiratory death loss of 0.05% per year in steers fed by a large cattle feeding company.[41] In a retrospective cohort study of 21.8 million cattle from 1994 to 1999, cattle entering the feedlot during 1999 had a significantly increased risk (relative risk, 1.46) of dying of respiratory disease compared with cattle that entered into the feedlot in 1994.[42]

The reason for the increases in death loss in feeder cattle over time is not clear. Published reports on death losses compare cattle fed in different years, breed types, origin, background, feeding systems, weather, and feedlot managers and employees, even within the same feedlot. Because of this variability, comparison of health trends across time, or between different reports by different authors, may lead to erroneous conclusions. Despite this, it must be acknowledged that trends point, at least, to no great decrease over the past 45 years in risk of death because of respiratory disease when cattle enter finishing feedlots. Mortality trends within the backgrounding and stocker operations are similar, but these production units are not studied as intensely as feedlots, and published data are lacking.

BOVINE RESPIRATORY DISEASE: WHERE ARE WE NOW?

It has become obvious that animal health products alone cannot prevent significant losses within the beef industry. In the face of 45 years of energetic administration of well-designed vaccines and antimicrobials, mortality has not decreased. However, maybe we should not be surprised that outsized attention to 1 component of a complex problem has not solved that problem. How much technology is the industry using? What proportion of the industry has adopted recommended animal husbandry practices, such as conducting routine surgical procedures early in life; maintaining adequate body condition scores in the cow-herd; proper supplementation with protein and trace minerals; low-stress marketing; preconditioning; adopting evidence-based health management programs; and low-stress cattle handling? What about the elephant in the room: if economic incentives to producers at various sectors in the cattle industry favor purchase of cattle at high risk for BRD, what technology or management can change that?

Challenges owing to BRD remain, despite decades of research, extension, "improved" health management tools, and diagnostics. Although the role of pathogens in BRD cannot be ignored, the authors suggest that it is time to increase focus on the host and environmental influences that contribute to this multifactorial complex. It is imperative that veterinarians and other animal health professionals continue to pursue answers to questions that remain. A growing world population, consumer demands for less antimicrobial use, public concerns over animal welfare, a declining agricultural land base, and narrow profit margins are just a few of the reasons that research into BRD management must continue.

BOVINE RESPIRATORY DISEASE: WHAT DOES THE FUTURE HOLD?
"Precision Agriculture" and Bovine Respiratory Disease Control

The term "precision agriculture," most often applied to crop production, refers to the practice of collecting data with a high degree of spatial or temporal resolution, then using the information to precisely target treatments or manipulations to areas most likely to benefit.[43] In the context of crop production, precision agriculture can decrease cost and negative environmental impacts of fertilizers, herbicides, and pesticides by precisely targeting their application. Although animal agriculture has lagged behind plant production in the use of precision agriculture methods, tools that should enable similarly precise management of animal health are beginning to appear.[44] In the future, BRD control could be substantially improved by precision agriculture practices. Such tools include methods to remotely detect sick cattle, to accurately and rapidly identify respiratory inflammation or infection, and to identify cattle likely to become sick, or stay healthy, based on their genetics, gene expression, normal flora, or metabolism.

To date, most sick cattle are identified by direct observation by a human. However, technology has been developed that allows identification of sick cattle before a human has noticed their signs of illness, through detection of changes in water or feed intake, movement, or physiologic status, such as body temperature.[45,46] In 1 study, remotely detected changes in feeding behavior identified cattle that were eventually treated for BRD 3 to 5 days sooner than pen checkers.[47] In other work, rumen temperature-sensing boluses identified episodes of fever that were undetected by pen checkers, with some episodes lasting up to 11 days.[48] Such technologies clearly have exciting potential to improve the speed and accuracy of BRD detection. At present, the cost of the required equipment and the complexity of required data analysis limit the widespread adoption of such methods.[45,47] However, given the rate at which technology can decrease in price and disseminate, it seems plausible that remote detection of sick cattle will be common practice in the coming decades.

Once sick cattle are identified, it is necessary to determine whether they actually have BRD. At present, BRD is most often identified based on clinical signs that lack sensitivity and specificity.[49] In fact, the entire concept of BRD held by veterinarians and producers may be limiting their ability to accurately diagnose it.[46] However, research is ongoing to refine BRD diagnosis through the use of imaging techniques, such as ultrasound,[50] computer-aided auscultation,[51] or assessment of compounds in exhaled breath[52,53] or blood.[54,55] It may in time be possible to use tests of compounds in breath, nasal secretions, or blood to precisely and accurately identify cattle with different types of respiratory disease. It may even be possible to predict which cattle will develop BRD, or resist BRD, based on their genetics or gene expression, before the cattle develop disease. For example, in a recent small study, evaluation of all messenger RNAs (the "transcriptome") in blood collected at arrival from high-risk stocker cattle revealed that cattle that were never identified to have signs of BRD had increased expression of genes related to production of "specific proresolving mediators", lipid molecules with anti-inflammatory effects, as compared with cattle that were eventually treated for BRD.[56] Although the results will need to be confirmed in larger studies, they suggested that modulation of inflammation may be a feature of cattle that stay healthy. Identification of substances that reliably predict BRD, or predict resistance to BRD, could allow more targeted management of cattle, potentially improving outcomes and decreasing use of antimicrobials. It may be possible to develop chute-side tests for such predictors of health or disease. The current availability of a test for BVDV infection that can be used cow-side and completed in 20 minutes (IDEXX SNAP BVDV Antigen Test; IDEXX Laboratories, Inc, Westbrook, ME, USA) demonstrates that it is possible for diagnostic technology to be developed that is convenient and rapid.

In addition to identifying or predicting cattle with BRD, it may ultimately be possible to prevent BRD by selecting cattle that either resist disease[57] or are tolerant to respiratory infection.[58] Genomic testing to support selection of cattle with a variety of traits is becoming commonplace,[59] although samples must be sent to a laboratory for evaluation. Given that it is now possible to sequence DNA in the field in locations as remote as Antarctica,[60] perhaps chute-side DNA sequencing will one day be applied to select cattle with genes for BRD resistance right on the farm.

Bovine Respiratory Disease Control: What Can Be Done, and What Will Be Done

Although the new technologies outlined above suggest intriguing possibilities for the future of BRD control, none address what may be the most important cause of BRD: lack of adequate incentive for producers to adopt methods to prevent BRD.[30] For many of these possibilities, the ultimate question may not be so much, "Is it possible?," as "Does it pay?" Perhaps the future of BRD control will be determined less by science and more by whether consumers begin to demand meat and milk from cattle that stay healthy.

SUMMARY

Changes in cattle feeding in the twentieth century led to increases in efficiency that have made beef readily and affordably available to people in North America and around the world. However, these practices were accompanied by recognition that BRD persists as the leading cause of illness and death in feedlot cattle. The failure of extensive research leading to the development of vaccines and pharmaceuticals to be accompanied by a clear-cut decrease in BRD suggests that management practices that increase risk of BRD must also be changed to effectively mitigate BRD risk. Until small operations that are the source of many cattle at high risk of BRD can realize financial returns to adopt preventive management practices, established and also new tools with potential to improve BRD are unlikely to have much effect. The status of BRD in feedlot cattle over the next 45 years may depend most on what producers hear from markets for their cattle.

DISCLOSURE

The authors have received financial support from veterinary biologics and pharmaceutical manufacturers for consulting and to conduct research to test the efficacy of products for BRD treatment, prevention, and control. Dr D.L. Step is employed by Boehringer Ingelheim Animal Health, a company that markets vaccines and antimicrobials for prevention, treatment, and control of BRD.

REFERENCES

1. USDA. Dairy 2014, "Health and management practices on U.S. dairy operations, 2014". Ft. Collins (CO): USDA-APHIS-VS-CEAH-NAHMS; 2018. #696.0218.
2. Ball CE. The finishing touch. Amarillo (TX): Trafton Printing; 1992. p. 1–46.
3. Beef quality assurance. 2020. Available at: http://bqa.org. Accessed April 28, 2020..
4. Jericho KWF, Langford EV. Pneumonia in calves produced with aerosols of bovine herpesvirus 1 and Pasteurella haemolytica. Can J Comp Med 1978;42:269–77.
5. Jericho KWF. Update on Pasteurellosis in young cattle. Can Vet J 1979;20:333–5.
6. Jericho KW, Yates WD, Babiuk LA. Bovine herpesvirus-1 vaccination against experimental bovine herpesvirus-1 and Pasteurella haemolytica respiratory tract infection: onset of protection. Am J Vet Res 1982;43:1776–80.
7. Darcel CL, Jericho KWF. Failure of a subunit bovine herpesvirius 1 vaccine to protect against experimental respiratory disease in calves. Can J Comp Med 1981; 45:87–91.
8. Jericho KW, Cho HJ, Kozub GC. Protective effect of inactivated Pasteurella haemolytica bacterin challenged in bovine herpesvirus-1 experimentally infected calves. Vaccine 1990;8:315–20.
9. Tripp HM, Step DL, Krehbiel CR, et al. Evaluation of outcomes in beef cattle comparing preventive health protocols utilizing viral respiratory vaccines. Bov Pract (Stillwater) 2013;47:59–64.
10. MacGregor S, Wray MI. The effect of bovine respiratory syncytial virus vaccination on health, feedlot performance, and carcass characteristics of feeder cattle. Bov Pract (Stillwater) 2004;38:162–70.
11. Bryant TC, Rogers KC, Stone ND, et al. Effect of viral respiratory vaccine treatment on performance, health and carcass traits of auction-origin feeder steers. Bov Pract (Stillwater) 2008;42:98–103.
12. Olafson P, McCallum AD, Fox FH. An apparently new transmissible disease of cattle. Cornell Vet 1946;36:205–13.
13. Ramsey FK, Chivers WH. Mucosal disease in cattle. North Am Vet 1953;34:629.
14. McClurkin AW, Littledyke ET, Cutlip RC, et al. Production of cattle immunotolerant to bovine viral diarrhea virus. Can J Comp Med 1984;48:156.
15. Njaa BL, Clark EG, Janzen E, et al. Diagnosis of persistent bovine viral diarrhea virus infection by immunohistochemical staining of formalin-fixed skin biopsy specimens. J Vet Diagn Invest 2000;12:393–9.
16. Fulton RW. Vaccines. In: Goyal SM, Ridpath JF, editors. Bovine viral diarrhea virus, diagnosis, management, and control. Ames (IO): Blackwell; 2005. p. 209–22.
17. Kelling CL, Grotelueschen DM, Smith DR, et al. Testing and management strategies for effective beef and dairy herd BVDV biosecurity programs. Bov Pract (Stillwater) 2000;34:13–22.
18. Larson RL, Step DL. Evidence-based effectiveness of vaccination against Mannheimia haemolytica, Pasteurella multocida, and Histophilus somni in feedlot cattle for mitigating the incidence and effect of bovine respiratory complex. Vet Clin North Am Food Anim Pract 2012;28:98–106.
19. Perino LJ, Hunsaker BD. A review of bovine respiratory disease vaccine field efficacy. Bov Pract (Stillwater) 1997;31:54–66.
20. Bryant TC, Nichols JR, Farmer TD, et al. Effect of tilmicosin alone or in combination with Mannheimia haemolytica toxoid administered at feedlot processing on morbidity and mortality of high-risk calves. Bov Pract (Stillwater) 2008;42:50–5.

21. Jim K, Guichon T, Shaw G. Protecting calves from pneumonic pasteurellosis. Vet Med 1988;83:1084–7.
22. Martin SW, Meek AH, Davis DG, et al. Factors associated with mortality and treatment costs in feedlot calves: the Bruce County Beef Project, years 1978, 1979, 1980. Can J Comp Med 1982;46:341–9.
23. Pinchak WE, Tolleson DR, McCloy M, et al. Morbidity effects on productivity and profitability of stocker cattle grazing in the Southern Plains. J Anim Sci 2004;82: 2773–9.
24. Richeson JT, Pinedo PJ, Kegley EB, et al. Association of hematologic variables and castration status at the time of arrival at a research facility with the risk of bovine respiratory disease in beef calves. J Am Vet Med Assoc 2013;243: 1035–41.
25. Coetzee JF, Edwards LN, Mosher RA, et al. Effect of oral meloxicam on health and performance of beef steers relative to bulls castrated on arrival at the feedlot. J Anim Sci 2012;90:1026–39.
26. Step DL, Krehbiel CR, DePra HA, et al. Effects of commingling beef calves from different sources and weaning protocols during a forty-two-day receiving period on performance and bovine respiratory disease. J Anim Sci 2008;86:3146–58.
27. Cole NA. Preconditioning calves for the feedlot. Vet Clin Food Anim 1985;1: 401–11.
28. Waggoner JW, Mathis CP, Löest CA, et al. Impact of preconditioning duration on feedlot performance, carcass characteristics and profitability of New Mexico Ranch to Rail steers. Proceedings, Western Section, American Society of Animal Science 2005;56:186–8.
29. Jim K. Impact of BRD from the perspective of the Canadian beef producer. Proceedings of the 2009 BRD Symposium. Colorado Springs, CO, August 5–6, 2009. p. 16-17.
30. Peel D. The effect of market forces on bovine respiratory disease. Vet Clin North Am Food Anim Pract 2020;36(2):497–508.
31. Horton D. Management, marketing, and medicine. Bovine Respiratory Disease, A Symposium. Proceedings of the North American Symposium on Bovine Respiratory Disease. Texas A&M University Press. September 7-9, 1984. p. 3–6.
32. Smith DR. Risk factors for bovine respiratory disease in beef cattle. Proceedings of the 2019 BRD Symposium. Denver, CO, August 7–8, 2019. p. 21–27.
33. Anholt RM, Klima C, Allan N, et al. Antimicrobial susceptibility of bacteria that cause bovine respiratory disease complex in Alberta, Canada. Front Vet Sci 2017;4:207.
34. Snyder E, Credille B. Mannheimia haemolytica and Pasteurella multocida: how are they changing in response to our efforts to control them? Vet Clin North Am Food Anim Pract 2020;36(2):253–68.
35. USDA. Feedlot 1999, "Treatment of respiratory disease in U.S. feedlots". Ft. Collins (CO): USDA-APHIS-VS-CEAH-NAHMS; 2001. #N347-1001.
36. USDA. Feedlot 2011, "Types and costs of respiratory disease in U.S. feedlots". Ft. Collins (CO): USDA-APHIS-VS-CEAH-NAHMS; 2013. #671-0513.
37. Edwards AJ. Diagnosis of respiratory disease in feedlot cattle occurring after being in feedlot for 45 days. Bov Pract (Stillwater) 1988;23:47–8.
38. Edwards A. Respiratory diseases of feedlot cattle in central USA. Bov Pract (Stillwater) 1996;30:5–7.
39. Vogel GL, Parrot C. Mortality survey in feedyards: the incidence of death from digestive, respiratory, and other causes in feedyards on the Great Plains. Compend Contin Educ Pract Vet 1994;16:227–34.

40. Vogel GL, Bokenkroger CD, Rutten-Ramos SC, et al. A retrospective evaluation of animal mortality in U.S. feedlots: rate timing, and cause of death. Bov Pract (Stillwater) 2015;49:113–23.
41. Engler M, Defoor P, King C, et al. The impact of bovine respiratory disease: the current feedlot experience. Proceedings of the 2014 BRD Symposium. Denver, CO, July 30–31, 2014. p. 12–13.
42. Lonergan GH, Dargatz DA, Morley PS, et al. Trends in mortality ratios among US feedlots. J Am Vet Med Assoc 2001;219:1122–7.
43. USDA NIFA. Precision, geospatial & sensor technologies programs. Available at: https://nifa.usda.gov/program/precision-geospatial-sensor-technologies-programs. Accessed March 11, 2020.
44. USDA NIFA. Precision agriculture in animal production. Available at: https://nifa.usda.gov/precision-agriculture-animal-production. Accessed March 11, 2020.
45. Wolfger B, Timsit E, White BJ, et al. A systematic review of bovine respiratory disease diagnosis focused on diagnostic confirmation, early detection, and prediction of unfavorable outcomes in feedlot cattle. Vet Clin Food Anim 2015;31:351–65.
46. Buczinski S, Pardon B. BRD diagnosis: what progress have we made in clinical diagnosis? Vet Clin North Am Food Anim Pract 2020;36(2):399–423.
47. Quimby WF, Sowell BF, Boman JGP, et al. Application of feeding behavior to predict morbidity of newly received calves in a commercial feedlot. Can J Anim Sci 2001;81:315–20.
48. Timsit E, Assié S, Quiniou R, et al. Early detection of bovine respiratory disease in young bulls using reticulo-rumen temperature boluses. Vet J 2011;190:136–42.
49. Timsit E, Dendukuri N, Schiller I, et al. Diagnostic accuracy of clinical illness for bovine respiratory disease (BRD) diagnosis in beef cattle placed in feedlots: a systematic literature review and hierarchical Bayesian latent-class meta-analysis. Prev Vet Med 2016;135:67–73.
50. Ollivett TL, Buczinski S. On-farm use of ultrasonography for bovine respiratory disease. Vet Clin Food Anim 2016;32:19–35.
51. Mang AV, Buczinski S, Booker CW, et al. Evaluation of a computer-aided lung auscultation system for diagnosis of bovine respiratory disease in feedlot cattle. J Vet Intern Med 2015;29:1112–6.
52. Burciaga-Robles LO, Holland BP, Step DL, et al. Evaluation of breath biomarkers and serum haptoglobin concentration for diagnosis of bovine respiratory disease in heifers newly arrived at a feedlot. Am J Vet Res 2009;70:1291–8.
53. Ellis CK, Stahl RS, Nol P, et al. A pilot study exploring the use of breath analysis to differentiate healthy cattle from cattle experimentally infected with Mycobacterium bovis. PLoS One 2014;9:e89290.
54. Blakebrough-Hall C, Dona A, D'occhio MJ, et al. Diagnosis of bovine respiratory disease in feedlot cattle using blood ^{1}H NMR metabolomics. Sci Rep 2020;10:115.
55. El-Deeb W, Elsohaby I, Fayez M, et al. Use of procalcitonin, neopterin, haptoglobin, serum amyloid A and proinflammatory cytokines in diagnosis and prognosis of bovine respiratory disease in feedlot calves under field conditions. Acta Trop 2020;204:105336.
56. Scott MA, Woolums AR, Swiderski CE, et al. Whole blood transcriptomic analysis of beef cattle at arrival identifies potential predictive molecules and mechanisms that indicate animals that naturally resist bovine respiratory disease. PLoS One 2020;15:e0227507.

57. Neupane M, Kiser JN, Seabury CM, et al. Genetic approaches to identify genomic regions associated with decreased susceptibility to bovine respiratory disease complex. Proc Am Assoc Bov Pract 2015;48:148–53.
58. Bassel LL, Tabatabaei S, Caswell JL. Host tolerance to infection with the bacteria that cause bovine respiratory disease. Vet Clin North Am Food Anim Pract 2020; 36(2):349–59.
59. Ishmael W. Genomic testing is growing up. BEEF. Available at: https://www.beefmagazine.com/genetics/genomic-testing-growing. Accessed March 14, 2020.
60. Johnson SS, Zaikova E, Goerlitz DS, et al. Real-time DNA sequencing in the Antarctic dry valleys using the Oxford Nanopore sequencer. J Biomol Tech 2017; 28:2–7.

Mannheimia haemolytica and *Pasteurella multocida* in Bovine Respiratory Disease

How Are They Changing in Response to Efforts to Control Them?

Emily Snyder, DVM, MFAM, Brent Credille, DVM, PhD*

KEYWORDS

- Bovine respiratory disease • Antimicrobial resistance
- Integrative conjugative element • *Mannheimia haemolytica* • *Pasteurella multocida*

KEY POINTS

- *Mannheimia haemolytica* and *Pasteurella multocida* often contribute to bovine respiratory disease (BRD) in North American cattle.
- *M haemolytica* and *P multocida* are facultative anaerobic, gram-negative coccobacilli that elaborate virulence factors, allowing them to evade clearance and activate inflammation.
- Extensively drug-resistant (XDR) strains of *M haemolytica* and *P multocida* are increasingly found in some cattle; these strains harbor integrative conjugative elements containing genes conferring resistance to up to 12 different antimicrobials.
- Few data regarding the impact of XDR strains on treatment outcomes are available, but clinical observations suggest that response to first treatment is decreasing, possibly because of resistance.
- Clinicians must consider the role of virulence factors and antimicrobial resistance in BRD caused by *M haemolytica* and *P multocida* when designing treatment and control programs.

INTRODUCTION

Bovine respiratory disease (BRD) is the most common and costly disease affecting beef cattle in North America and a significant contributor to morbidity and mortality in dairy calf populations.[1] Within feedlots, BRD is responsible for approximately 75% of all morbidity and 50% of all mortality. In stocker calves, BRD occurs at a

Food Animal Health and Management Program, Department of Population Health, College of Veterinary Medicine, University of Georgia, Veterinary Medical Center, 2200 College Station Road, Athens, GA 30602, USA
* Corresponding author.
E-mail address: bc24@uga.edu

Vet Clin Food Anim 36 (2020) 253–268
https://doi.org/10.1016/j.cvfa.2020.02.001
0749-0720/20/© 2020 Elsevier Inc. All rights reserved.

much greater frequency than is commonly seen in feedlot cattle and is estimated to be responsible for 90% of all morbidity and mortality in these operations. In dairy operations, BRD is estimated to affect more than 22% of all preweaned calves and is responsible for approximately 20% of all deaths that occur in this population of animals.[2] BRD is second only to neonatal calf diarrhea as the primary disease syndrome affecting these animals and is the leading cause of morbidity and mortality in postweaned dairy heifers.[2] Although multiple factors play a role in the development of BRD, bacteria, particularly *Mannheimia haemolytica* and *Pasteurella multocida*, are ultimately responsible for the clinical signs observed in affected cattle. These pathogens have adapted to colonize and persist on respiratory mucosal surfaces and evade host immune responses. Adaptive mechanisms include the expression of adhesins, elaboration and secretion of toxins and proteases, and formation of biofilms.[3] Antimicrobial resistance is an emerging issue in BRD pathogens and the isolation of extensively drug-resistant (XDR) strains of *M haemolytica* has become a more frequent occurrence.[4,5] This article reviews the literature on mechanisms of immune evasion and antimicrobial resistance in common BRD pathogens and discusses how these factors might affect current methods of disease control and, ultimately, the outcome of therapy in beef and dairy cattle diagnosed with BRD.

MANNHEIMIA HAEMOLYTICA AND *PASTEURELLA MULTOCIDA*: AN OVERVIEW

M haemolytica and *P multocida* are gram-negative facultative anaerobes that belong to the family Pasteurellaceae. Both organisms are coccobacilli that measure 0.2 μm by 2.0 μm and are usually oxidase positive, nitrate reducers, and carbohydrate fermenters, characteristics that distinguish this family of microorganisms from members of other families, particularly the Enterobacteriaceae. The organisms are commonly carried on the mucous membranes of the oropharynx in clinically healthy cattle. In general, clinical disease caused by these organisms in cattle results from a combination of stress, immunosuppression, and viral infection that ultimately leads to an overgrowth of the organisms in the lower airway of individual animals. There is mounting evidence to suggest that *M haemolytica*, at least, is transmitted contagiously and spreads from animal to animals within a population.[6,7]

P multocida is defined by 5 capsular serotypes (A, B, D, E, F) and 16 serotypes (1–16). In contrast, *M haemolytica* is defined by at least 12 capsular serotypes (1, 2, 5–9, 12–14, 16, and 17).[8] With both pathogens, the capsular serotypes are contributors to host specificity and pathogenicity. Despite the diversity of serotypes that exist, *M haemolytica* serotype A1 (>75% of cases) and *P multocida* serotype A3 (>30% of cases in beef and >60% of cases in dairy) are the serotypes most often associated with clinical disease.[8] It was recently shown that specific virulence determinants of *M haemolytica* serotype A1 facilitate invasion of bovine respiratory epithelial cells, allowing it to undergo uncontrolled replication and spread to adjacent cells.[9] Once inside the cells, the organism is able to cause extensive damage to the infected tissue. This same phenomenon was not seen with the serotypes considered to be commensals of the respiratory tract.[9]

In addition to the capsular types, both organisms are gram negative and are defined by the presence of lipopolysaccharide (LPS; endotoxin) in the outer cell wall. Endotoxin is a potent proinflammatory mediator that triggers the release of cytokines and stimulates an influx of inflammatory cells that contribute to disease pathogenesis.[8] Furthermore, endotoxin acts synergistically with *M haemolytica* leukotoxin to enhance pathogenicity.[8]

MECHANISMS OF IMMUNE EVASION AND VIRULENCE IN *MANNHEIMIA HAEMOLYTICA* AND *PASTEURELLA MULTOCIDA*

Many gram-negative pathogens have evolved mechanisms to colonize mucosal surfaces and augment the bacterial-host interaction. *M haemolytica* and *P multocida* are no different and, over the course of time, virulent strains have become known for the elaboration of a variety of factors that enable them to evade host immune responses or enhance clinical disease (**Table 1**).[3] This ability is important in that an understanding of the different virulence factors that contribute to disease pathogenesis might allow the development of control strategies centered on enhancing immunity to these compounds.

Both *M haemolytica* and *P multocida* produce a series of adhesins that allow epithelial cell attachment and prevent phagocytosis.[3] For example, the capsule of type A strains of *P multocida* is composed of hyaluronic acid, and this capsule enhances binding to respiratory epithelial cells and colonization of the lower airway. In addition, *M haemolytica* produces a fibrinogen binding protein that coats the bacterial cell, prevents binding of complement, and subsequently decreases opsonization.[3] It is also important to note that the capsule of other serotypes of these organisms is composed of substances very similar to host tissue components (eg, heparin, chondroitin) and this likely makes them poorly antigenic.

There are several other ways that these pathogens evade and manipulate the host immune system to their advantage. For example, *M haemolytica* elaborates a series of 2 immunoglobulin (Ig) A–specific proteases that cleave IgA and prevent it from binding to the pathogen.[10] The ultimate effect of these proteases is to prevent opsonization or complement-mediated killing. Furthermore, *M haemolytica* has the ability to form biofilms in the airway. Biofilm, an organized bacterial community encased in a polymer of polysaccharides, protein, and DNA, is a means by which bacteria adapt to living in potentially hostile environments.[11] It is likely that, in a healthy host, most *M haemolytica* exists in the oropharynx and tonsillar crypts in a biofilm. Within a biofilm, bacteria can be protected from exposure to antimicrobials and host immune responses. The minimum inhibitory concentration (MIC) of many antimicrobials against *M haemolytica* can increase from 8-fold to 16-fold when the organism is in a biofilm rather than in its planktonic state.[11] Furthermore, it has been shown that stress chemicals produced by

Table 1
Mechanisms of immune evasion and virulence factors in *Mannheimia haemolytica* and *Pasteurella multocida*

Factor	Origin	Mechanism	Immunogenicity
Capsule	Bacterial surface	Antiphagocytic	Poor
Leukotoxin	Secreted	Leukocyte necrosis	Strong
Lipopolysaccharide	Bacterial cell wall	Proinflammatory	Weak to moderate
IgA proteases	Secreted	Degradation of secretory IgA	Moderate
Biofilm formation	Bacteria	Evasion of protective responses	Poor
OmpP2	Bacterial membrane	Biofilm formation and cell adhesion	Weak

Abbreviation: IgA, immunoglobulin A.

the host (substance P, norepinephrine, epinephrine) allow the dispersal of biofilms, a factor that enables movement from the upper to the lower airway and links the association between stress and clinical BRD.[12]

Arguably the most important virulence factor associated with clinical disease is leukotoxin, a toxin elaborated by *M haemolytica*.[8,13] The importance of this toxin is shown by the fact that strains of *M haemolytica* that lack the gene for leukotoxin cause little, if any, damage relative to those with the leukotoxin gene. As a result, when designing a control program for *M haemolytica*, protection from the effects of leukotoxin has to be a primary consideration. Leukotoxin is in the repeat in toxin (RTX) family of toxins and is produced by all species of *Mannheimia* during the logarithmic phase of bacterial growth.[3,13] Leukotoxin interacts specifically with cluster of differentiation (CD) 18 on the surface of bovine neutrophils, macrophages, platelets, and lymphocytes. Once in contact with leukotoxin, neutrophils degranulate and release potent digestive enzymes into the surrounding tissue. In addition, leukotoxin stimulates the degranulation of tissue mast cells and the release of vasoactive mediators.[8] As stated previously, endotoxin and leukotoxin act synergistically. Endotoxin serves as a potent chemoattractant for neutrophils and other inflammatory cells into the airway. In addition, exposure to endotoxin upregulates the expression of CD18 on the surface of inflammatory cells. As a result, the presence of more cells with a greater affinity for leukotoxin creates the perfect scenario for severe clinical disease to occur (**Fig. 1**). The end result is the classic fibrinous pleuropneumonia often associated with *M haemolytica* (**Fig. 2**).

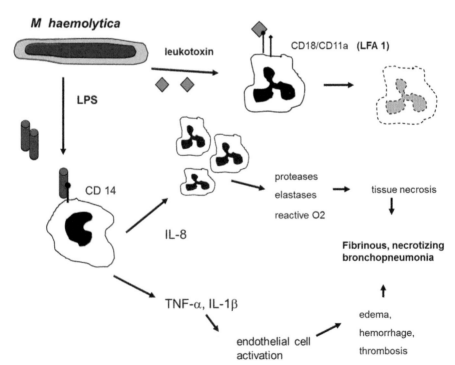

Fig. 1. Pathogenesis of *M haemolytica* leukotoxin and synergy with endotoxin. IL, interleukin; LFA, lymphocyte function-associated antigen; TNF, tumor necrosis factor. (*Courtesy of* A.Woolums, DVM, PhD, Starkville, MS.)

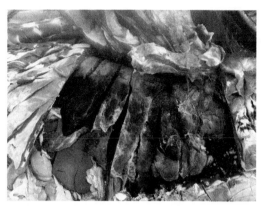

Fig. 2. Postmortem image of a feedlot steer with fibrinous pleuropneumonia associated with *M haemolytica*. (*Courtesy of* S. Crosby, DVM, Airdrie, Canada.)

ANTIMICROBIAL RESISTANCE IN *MANNHEIMIA HAEMOLYTICA* AND *PASTEURELLA MULTOCIDA*: RESISTANCE DEFINED

Veterinarians are most concerned about clinical resistance; they are interested in the probability that a specific antimicrobial will effectively treat an animal infected by a specific pathogen causing a particular disease.[14] The concept of clinical resistance is based on clinically derived breakpoints developed by the Clinical and Laboratory Standards Institute (CLSI) Veterinary Antimicrobial Susceptibility Testing Committee using the following criteria[14]:

1. Range of in vitro MICs of an antimicrobial for a representative population of a specific bacterial pathogen.
2. Pharmacokinetic/pharmacodynamic (PK/PD) parameters established from the relationship between drug concentration and microbial susceptibility.
3. Results of clinical trials in the target species.

For BRD pathogens, the CLSI has approved specific breakpoints for penicillin (broth dilution only), ceftiofur, danofloxacin, enrofloxacin, florfenicol, spectinomycin sulfate, tulathromycin, gamithromycin, tildipirosin, tetracycline (broth dilution only), and tilmicosin (**Table 2**). With these antimicrobial agents, a susceptible result indicates that the likelihood of treatment success is significantly greater than if the result indicated resistance. However, the relationship between antimicrobial susceptibility testing and clinical outcome is not perfect and these breakpoints apply only when the antimicrobial is used according to label directions and the susceptibility testing is performed using CLSI-approved methods and interpretive criteria. It is also important to realize that antimicrobial susceptibility testing does not guarantee a specific clinical result in an individual animal. Susceptibility breakpoints attempt to take an in vitro test result and extrapolate it to an in vivo response and, often, disease outcome is influenced by factors such as host immune status, variations in individual pharmacokinetic parameters, or increased disease severity/prolonged disease duration. For antimicrobials without CLSI-approved breakpoints, the interpretations have been adapted from interpretive criteria extrapolated from plasma and interstitial fluid in other species. Examples of this approach include penicillin G (disk diffusion), tetracycline (disk diffusion), potentiated sulfonamides, aminoglycosides, and erythromycin. For these antimicrobial agents, a susceptible result is better than a resistant one.

Table 2
Antimicrobial-pathogen combinations with Clinical and Laboratory Standards Institute–approved breakpoints for bovine respiratory disease

Antimicrobial	Pathogens
Ceftiofur	M haemolytica P multocida Histophilus somni
Danofloxacin	M haemolytica P multocida
Enrofloxacin	M haemolytica P multocida H somni
Florfenicol	M haemolytica P multocida H somni
Gamithromycin	M haemolytica P multocida H somni
Penicillin[a,b]	M haemolytica P multocida H somni
Spectinomycin	M haemolytica P multocida H somni
Tetracycline[b,c]	M haemolytica P multocida H somni
Tildipirosin	M haemolytica P multocida H somni
Tilmicosin	M haemolytica
Tulathromycin	M haemolytica P multocida H somni

[a] Only applies to the procaine penicillin G formulation used at 22,000 IU/kg intramuscularly (IM) every 24 hours.
[b] Approved breakpoints only valid for broth dilution.
[c] Derived from PK data of oxytetracycline at 20 mg/kg IM once and PD data.

However, there are no data available to correlate the results of susceptibility testing and expected outcome in cattle with BRD.

The second type of resistance is defined based on data surveilling changes in profiles of susceptibility distributions in wild-type populations of bacteria.[15] Rather than providing data correlated to clinical outcome, these epidemiologic cutoffs represent deviations of the MIC from the original bacterial population and can be used to indicate the appearance of resistance determinants. As a result, epidemiologic cutoffs might declare resistance at an MIC that is different (often lower) from a clinical breakpoint.[15] This article is most concerned about clinical resistance and this definition is used throughout. Also, although many of the studies mentioned herein might reference multiple antimicrobial drugs, only drugs for which the CLSI has established susceptibility breakpoints are discussed (see **Table 2**).

PREVALENCE AND PATTERNS OF RESISTANCE IN *MANNHEIMIA HAEMOLYTICA* AND *PASTEURELLA MULTOCIDA*

The earliest published MIC distributions for *M haemolytica* and *P multocida* established using modern diagnostic laboratory methodology and CLSI-approved breakpoints were derived from a survey of animals that died of BRD over the period from 1988 to 2002.[16] In this study, 461 *M haemolytica* and 318 *P multocida* isolates were submitted by numerous veterinary diagnostic laboratories across the United States and Canada (Pennsylvania, Wyoming, Iowa, Washington, California, Missouri, Nebraska, Oregon, Kansas, Arizona, Texas, South Dakota, Montana, Minnesota, Oklahoma, Colorado, Utah, Saskatchewan, Alberta, and Quebec) to a corporate pharmaceutical laboratory (Upjohn) for MIC determination. The results of this study are reported in **Table 3**. Note that the interpretive criteria for tilmicosin used in this study were not validated for either *M haemolytica* or *P multocida* and the prevalence of resistance to this drug would be dramatically decreased (>90% susceptible) using currently accepted criteria.

In another study, the susceptibility of 390 *M haemolytica* and 292 *P multocida* isolates obtained from the lungs of beef cattle that died of BRD and submitted to the Oklahoma Animal Disease Diagnostic Laboratory between 1994 and 2002 was investigated.[17] The susceptibility to tetracycline and spectinomycin varied over the course of the study period but was consistently low for each drug. In contrast, the susceptibility to ceftiofur and enrofloxacin remained high and relatively stable throughout the study (**Tables 4** and **5**).

Another large study evaluated the susceptibility of *M haemolytica* (n = 2977) and *P multocida* (n = 3291) isolates submitted to 24 diagnostic laboratories across the United States and Canada between 2000 and 2009.[18] The activity of ceftiofur against both pathogens remained consistent and high (100% susceptible) across all years evaluated. In addition, the susceptibility of the isolates to danofloxacin, enrofloxacin, and florfenicol remained stable over time. However, both isolates showed decreases in susceptibility to tilmicosin and tulathromycin over the years in which they were tested.[18]

A landmark study from Kansas State University evaluated the prevalence of multidrug antimicrobial resistance and antimicrobial coresistance patterns in *M haemolytica* isolated from the lungs of cattle with BRD over a 3-year period.[4] Between 2009

Table 3
Antimicrobial susceptibility of *Mannheimia haemolytica* isolates collected from the lungs of cattle that died of bovine respiratory disease

Organism	Isolates (N)	Antimicrobial	Susceptibility (%)
M haemolytica	461	Tilmicosin	69.1
		Ceftiofur	100
		Tetracycline	57
		Spectinomycin	83.5
P multocida	318	Tilmicosin	NA
		Ceftiofur	100
		Tetracycline	70.5
		Spectinomycin	83.3

Abbreviation: NA, not available.

Data from Watts JL, Yancey RJ, Jr., Salmon SA, et al. A 4-year survey of antimicrobial susceptibility trends for isolates from cattle with bovine respiratory disease in North America. Journal Clin Microbiol. 1994;32(3):725-731.

Table 4
Susceptibility of *Mannheimia haemolytica* obtained from the lungs of feedlot cattle from 1994 to 2002

Antimicrobial	Year								
	1994	1995	1996	1996	1998	1999	2000	2001	2002
Ceftiofur	97	98	100	100	98	100	98	96	97
Enrofloxacin	—	—	—	—	—	96	98	89	98
Florfenicol	—	—	100	96	98	97	96	87	90
Spectinomycin	65	49	71	53	55	63	45	29	51
Tilmicosin	90	78	93	83	80	74	85	71	79
Tetracycline	23	46	74	58	42	63	44	34	54

Data from Welsh RD, Dye LB, Payton ME, et al. Isolation and antimicrobial susceptibilities of bacterial pathogens from bovine pneumonia: 1994–2002. J Vet Diagn Invest. 2004;16(5):426-431.

and 2011, the proportion of isolates resistant to 5 or more antimicrobials increased from 5% to 35%. In addition, isolates resistant to either oxytetracycline or tilmicosin were significantly more likely to be resistant to at least 1 other antimicrobial class.

Several studies have investigated the prevalence of antimicrobial resistance in feedlot cattle between feedlot arrival and exit. In 1 study, samples obtained from 10% of animals from 30% of feedlot pens in 2 feedlots in southern Alberta were submitted for isolation and susceptibility testing of *M haemolytica*.[19] Swabs were collected from cattle at the time of feedlot entry and again within 30 days of feedlot exit. Over the course of the study, 409 *M haemolytica* isolates were obtained and resistance to all antimicrobials tested was low, ranging from 0.2% to 3.9%, with resistance to oxytetracycline being most common.[19] Note that many of the antimicrobials evaluated in that study do not have CLSI-established breakpoints for *M haemolytica* and BRD, making some of the conclusions from the study difficult to interpret.

In another study that sampled nearly 5500 cattle from 4 feedlots in Canada, deep nasopharyngeal (DNP) swabs were collected from enrolled animals at the time of arrival and again at a time point before feedlot exit.[20] In this study, susceptibility to 21 different antimicrobials was evaluated for 2989 individual *M haemolytica* isolates. Overall, resistance was rare, with 87% of isolates susceptible to all antimicrobials tested.[20] As with the aforementioned work, note that many of the antimicrobials

Table 5
Susceptibility of *Pasteurella multocida* obtained from the lungs of feedlot cattle from 1994 to 2002

Antimicrobial	Year								
	1994	1995	1996	1997	1998	1999	2000	2001	2002
Ceftiofur	98	100	100	100	95	100	99	96	100
Enrofloxacin	—	—	—	—	—	96	97	96	100
Florfenicol	—	—	100	100	100	97	86	88	96
Spectinomycin	34	63	33	63	46	63	31	42	47
Tetracycline	71	58	52	53	56	63	40	44	73

Data from Welsh RD, Dye LB, Payton ME, et al. Isolation and antimicrobial susceptibilities of bacterial pathogens from bovine pneumonia: 1994–2002. J Vet Diagn Invest. 2004;16(5):426-431.

evaluated did not have CLSI-established breakpoints for M haemolytica and BRD, making some of the conclusions difficult to interpret.

In a study from Canada evaluating resistance patterns in M haemolytica isolated from healthy cattle and cattle with BRD, a resistant phenotype was found in 18% of M haemolytica isolates tested.[21] Overall, resistance was more common in isolates collected from cattle with BRD (32%) than in isolates collected from healthy cattle (2%). Resistance to tetracycline was the most common phenotype observed and, in general, if an isolate was resistant to 1 drug it was also resistant to at least 1 other antimicrobial class.[21]

Work from our laboratory evaluating the prevalence of resistance in M haemolytica after metaphylaxis with the long-acting macrolide tulathromycin has yielded surprising results.[5] Lightweight, unweaned calves entering a stocker facility in northeast Georgia were given tulathromycin at the time of arrival to the facility to prevent BRD. DNP swabs were collected from each animal at arrival and again 10 to 14 days later. For all antimicrobials except ceftiofur, there was a significant increase in the proportion of isolates classified as intermediate or resistant at the time of second sampling compared with samples collected at arrival.[5] Of the 123 calves with M haemolytica cultured at the time of second sampling, 1 (0.8%) had only pansusceptible isolates, 30 (24.4%) had at least 1 isolate classified as intermediate or resistant to 2 antimicrobial classes (fluoroquinolones and macrolides), and 92 (74.8%) had at least 1 isolate classified as intermediate or resistant to 3 antimicrobial classes (fluoroquinolones and macrolides in addition to either phenicols or cephalosporins).[5] Additional work by our group evaluating efficacy and resistance in both enrofloxacin and tulathromycin in high-beef calves produced similar results.[7]

Similar work by researchers at Mississippi State University produced comparable results. DNP swabs were collected from calves at day 0 and then 7, 14, and 21 days after arrival processing and mass medication with tildipirosin.[22] Nearly 100% of M haemolytica isolates collected from calves at 7, 14, and 21 days after arrival processing and exposure to tildipirosin were classified as multidrug resistant (MDR) and were resistant to all drugs tested except ceftiofur.[22]

From what is presented earlier, it is clear that much of the work on resistance in BRD pathogens comes from stocker and feedlot populations. Comparatively little research on resistance has been performed in dairy cattle populations. Work from Switzerland evaluated the prevalence of resistance in M haemolytica and P multocida collected from calves in 52 dairy herds. M haemolytica isolates (n = 8) were consistently susceptible to tetracycline, enrofloxacin, penicillin, ceftiofur, spectinomycin, and florfenicol.[23] In contrast, P multocida isolates (n = 37) were consistently susceptible to enrofloxacin, ceftiofur, spectinomycin, and florfenicol but intermediate to tilmicosin and resistant to tetracycline.[23] More recent work evaluated the prevalence of resistance in M haemolytica and P multocida isolated from nasal swabs collected from calves in a feedlot and on a calf ranch in California.[24] M haemolytica and P multocida isolates were consistently susceptible to ceftiofur and enrofloxacin. With P multocida, most isolates were susceptible to penicillin and tulathromycin, whereas more than 50% of isolates were resistant to danofloxacin, 30% resistant to florfenicol, and greater than 90% resistant to tetracycline and tilmicosin.[24] In the case of M haemolytica, all isolates were susceptible to spectinomycin; 20% were resistant to danofloxacin, tulathromycin, and florfenicol; 30% resistant to tilmicosin; and 60% resistant to penicillin.[24]

Unpublished work from our laboratory evaluated the susceptibility of M haemolytica (n = 53) and P multocida (n = 175) isolates from nasal swabs, transtracheal washes, DNP swabs, and bronchoalveolar lavages collected from 100 dairy calves at the time of BRD diagnosis on a calf ranch in California. Most *P multocida* isolates (>90%) were susceptible to ampicillin, ceftiofur, penicillin, spectinomycin, and tulathromycin but resistant to enrofloxacin and florfenicol. In contrast, most *M haemolytica* isolates (>90%) were susceptible to ampicillin, ceftiofur, penicillin, and florfenicol; intermediate to enrofloxacin and spectinomycin; and resistant to tulathromycin (**Table 6**).

GENETIC MECHANISMS OF MULTIDRUG ANTIMICROBIAL RESISTANCE

The preceding discussion indicates that resistance in BRD pathogens, particularly *M haemolytica*, is increasing. It is also apparent that the isolation of XDR *M haemolytica* is becoming more common. Therefore, the question is how does resistance to multiple antimicrobials arise after exposure to only 1 drug? Often, it is horizontal gene transfer that drives this rapid increase in resistance. Horizontal gene transfer occurs in 3 different ways: (1) the acquisition of genes from so-called loose DNA in the environment via transformation, (2) the transfer of genetic material by a phage via transduction, or (3) via the acquisition of a mobile genetic element.[25,26] Although all 3 of these mechanisms can play a role in the acquisition of resistance, in *M haemolytica* and *P multocida* the primary driver for the increase in MDR strains seems to be the acquisition of a type of mobile genetic element called an integrative conjugative element (ICE).[27,28]

ICEs are mobile genetic elements that integrate into the host chromosome. They can then be propagated and passed on to progeny but can also excise themselves, replicate as a circular intermediate, and transfer to other neighboring cells via a type 4 secretion system to ultimately be integrated into the new host's chromosome.[26] Often, other cargo genes are carried along within the ICE, including antimicrobial resistance genes, and it is in this manner that multiple antimicrobial resistance genes are rapidly acquired by recipient cells with the transfer of an ICE.[29]

A large number of different ICEs have been documented in *M haemolytica* and other Pasteurellaceae associated with BRD. The first ICE identified in *P multocida* (ICE-*Pmu1*) carried genes conferring resistance to the tetracyclines, florfenicol, sulfonamides, spectinomycin, enrofloxacin, tilmicosin, and tulathromycin.[28] The first identified ICE in *M haemolytica* was ICE*Mh1*, which was discovered in *M haemolytica*

Table 6
Antimicrobial susceptibility of *Pasteurella multocida* (n = 175) and *Mannheimia haemolytica* (n = 53) isolated from preweaned dairy calves with bovine respiratory disease

	P multocida			M haemolytica		
Antimicrobial	MIC$_{50}$ (μg/mL)	MIC$_{90}$ (μg/mL)	Range (μg/mL)	MIC$_{50}$ (μg/mL)	MIC$_{90}$ (μg/mL)	Range (μg/mL)
Ampicillin	<0.25	<0.25	<0.25–16	<0.25	<0.25	<0.25
Ceftiofur	<0.25	<0.25	<0.25	<0.25	<0.25	<0.25
Penicillin	<0.12	.25	<0.12–8	<0.12	<0.12	<0.12–0.25
Enrofloxacin	>2	>2	<0.12 to >2	<0.12	1	<0.12–1
Florfenicol	8	8	<0.25–8	1	1	<0.25–8
Tulathromycin	4	8	<1–>64	4	>64	<1 to >64
Spectinomycin	16	16	8 to >64	64	>64	8 to >64

Abbreviations: MIC$_{50}$, MIC required to inhibit the growth of 50% of organisms; MIC$_{90}$; MIC required to inhibit the growth of 90% of organisms.

strain 42548.[30] This ICE was longer than ICEPmu1 but lacked some of the genes that conferred resistance to the same number of antimicrobials that *ICEPmu1* did.[30]

In 2014, an additional 25 ICEs from *M haemolytica*, *P multocida*, and *Histophilus somni* were characterized.[27] More recently, an additional 3 ICEs were identified in *M haemolytica* isolates collected from Georgia stocker cattle. These ICEs varied in length but share some homology with both ICEMh1 and ICEPMu1; the first one-quarter of ICEMh-UGA1 and ICEMh-UGA2 are similar to ICEMh1, whereas the remaining three-quarters are similar to ICEPmu1. In addition, these ICEs bear all of the same resistance genes present in ICEPmu1, with the exception of *floR*, the gene responsible for resistance to phenicols and that is absent from ICEMh-UGA2. Unlike the other 2 ICEs identified in the Georgia cattle, ICEMh-UGA3 only carries the *tetH/R* resistance gene complex that encodes for resistance to the tetracycline class of antimicrobials.

The resistance genes present in ICEs convey resistance to a large number of antimicrobials from a diverse array of antimicrobial classes. Among the β-lactam resistance genes, *blaOXA-2* seems to be the most common resistance gene carried by *M haemolytica* isolates, followed by *blaROB-1*, although that gene seems more likely to be carried on a plasmid independent of the ICE, much like the recently discovered *blaROB-2* gene.[6,27,31–33] All of these genes code for extended-spectrum β-lactamases and can have activity against not only the classic penicillins but also newer extended-spectrum cephalosporins.[34,35] All of these genes are known to convey resistance to both ampicillin and penicillin, and may increase the MIC of ceftiofur.[27,33] Nevertheless, the presence of these genes may not automatically result in resistance, because these genes have been known to develop point mutations that result in inactivation of the gene.[28,31]

Resistance to the phenicol class of antimicrobials in *M haemolytica* and *P multocida* is most often caused by the presence of the *floR* gene.[27,36] This gene encodes a drug efflux transporter that actively pumps phenicol antimicrobials out of the cell.[37] However, in some instances, *floR* does not confer complete resistance in *P multocida* and *M haemolytica*, but instead shifts the MIC into the intermediate range, perhaps because of reduced activity of the gene in these microbes.[38]

The most common genes encoding for resistance to the tetracyclines are the *tet* class of genes.[39] These genes code for an efflux pump that actively pumps tetracycline out of the bacterial cell.[40] In *M haemolytica* and *P multocida*, tetH, tetB, tetL, and tetG are some of the most common genes that code for this pump, and they can be found on both plasmids and within the bacterial chromosome.[39,41] However, only *tetH* has been noted in the ICEs found in *M haemolytica* and *P multocida*.[27,28,30] Within these ICEs, there is usually also a *tetR* gene present, sometimes in duplicate copies, which serves as a tetracycline concentration–sensitive transcriptional regulator of the *tet* genes.[27,28,30,42]

Macrolides are widely used in cattle at high risk of development of BRD.[43,44] The genes erm42, msrE, and mphE are the most common macrolide resistance genes observed in *M haemolytica* and *P multocida* ICEs, and all work in different ways to confer resistance to this class of antimicrobials. The mode of action of the *erm42* gene was recently elucidated by Desmolaize and colleagues,[45] who determined that this gene codes for a monomethyltransferase that adds a methyl group at nucleotide A2058 on the 23s ribosomal subunit, resulting in resistance to lincosamides, as well as low-level resistance in macrolides and streptogramins. The *msrE* gene codes for a macrolide efflux pump and confers resistance to 14-membered and 15-membered ring macrolides such as erythromycin, tulathromycin, and gamithromycin.[46] However, it does not confer resistance to macrolides with a 16-membered ring, such as tylosin, tilmicosin, and tildipirosin.[46] The *mphE* gene is a macrolide phosphotransferase and has a similar spectrum of activity to *msrE* with regard to the antimicrobials to which it conveys resistance.[46]

Sulfonamides have become less commonly used in cattle, because their effectiveness has decreased over time and newer antibiotics have become available.[47] The *sul1* and *sul2* genes are the primary genes associated with sulfonamide resistance in gram-negative bacteria.[47] Both of these genes act by encoding a drug-resistant dihydropteroate synthase. To date, only *sul2* has been found to be associated with an ICE in *M haemolytica* and *P multocida*.[19]

Other genes present in the ICE are *aadA25*, *aadB*, *strA* and *strB*, and *aphA1*, genes that encode for resistance to aminoglycosides. *aadA25* (*ant3''*) facilitates resistance to the aminocyclitol spectinomycin and the aminoglycoside streptomycin by coding for an aminoglycoside O-nucleotidyltransferase.[48,49] *aadB* (*ant2''*) also encodes an aminoglycoside O-nucleotidyltransferase but confers resistance to gentamicin, tobramycin, dibekacin, sisomicin, and kanamycin.[49] *strA* (aph3''), *strB* (*aph6*), and *aphA1* (*aph3'*) are resistance genes that encode for aminoglycoside O-phosphotransferases that modify and inactivate aminoglycosides.[49] Both *strA* and *strB* confer resistance to streptomycin, whereas *aphA1* confers resistance to kanamycin, neomycin, paromomycin, ribostamycin, and lividomycin.[49]

The elements responsible for the increase in prevalence of XDR in *M haemolytica* isolates can carry a wide array of genes that confer resistance to most of the antimicrobials currently in use for the prevention and treatment of BRD. It is important to understand that, with the nature of XDR in bovine respiratory pathogens, exposure to 1 antimicrobial no longer solely selects for resistance to that 1 antimicrobial. Resistance is now a multidrug phenomenon where exposure to 1 antimicrobial selects for resistance to multiple other related and unrelated antimicrobials. The other important thing to understand about resistance in BRD pathogens is that much of the increase in resistance is being driven by the amplification of XDR *M haemolytica* strains that carry ICEs.[6] What seems to be happening is that antimicrobial exposure is selecting for the amplification and propagation of XDR strains and, subsequently, for all of the genes and mutations carried in that strain's genome. Thus, if an animal is diagnosed with BRD and is treated with a specific antimicrobial, not only will that animal subsequently harbor isolates that are resistant to that antimicrobial but that animal will also carry isolates that are resistant to all of the other antimicrobials carried on the ICE because of the linkages between the different genes.[4,5,7] In addition, because XDR *M haemolytica* strains also contain mutations that confer resistance to fluoroquinolones, phenotypic resistance to this class of antimicrobial will be seen despite that gene/mutation not being carried on the ICE.[6,22] Importantly, there is emerging evidence to suggest that these strains might spread contagiously through the at-risk cattle population through calf-to-calf contact and exposure to contaminated environmental sources.[6,7,20] As a result, it is important to understand that XDR is not confined only to treated animals. Instead, it is possible to find XDR clones in animals that have been in contact with treated animals but never exposed to antimicrobials themselves.[20]

ANTIMICROBIAL RESISTANCE: IMPACT ON THERAPEUTIC OUTCOME

First treatment success, defined as the proportion of animals successfully responding to antimicrobial therapy at the time of first pull, has historically been high in most populations in cattle on feed. In general, a first treatment success risk of greater than 80% is considered acceptable. However, a recent retrospective study evaluating risk factors for treatment failure found that more than 30% of cattle failed to respond to first treatment.[50] High-risk calves showed a greater risk of treatment failure than low-risk calves.[50] However, little work has been done to evaluate the impact of antimicrobial resistance on clinical outcome in cattle with BRD. In the 1 published study that the authors are aware of, 62% of cattle infected with susceptible *M haemolytica* isolates (n = 688) responded to treatment with tilmicosin compared with 38% of animals (n = 6) with resistant isolates.[51]

SUMMARY

More so than ever, it is now critical that clinicians recognize the role of virulence factors and antimicrobial resistance in the pathogenesis of infection with *M haemolytica* and *P multocida* and consider these factors when designing disease treatment and control programs centered on these organisms. Despite the importance of BRD to the North American cattle industry, there are few well-designed studies that evaluate antimicrobial resistance in bacterial pathogens important to this disease syndrome. Most of the published literature includes diagnostic laboratory submissions obtained from dead cattle that have been treated multiple times with multiple different antimicrobials. Nevertheless, general trends suggest that a decrease in the susceptibility of *M haemolytica* has occurred over time. Recent work suggests that antimicrobial use practices that are common within certain cattle operations might be the primary factor driving selection of resistant clones. Placing a focus on animal husbandry, stress reduction, enhancing immune function, and antimicrobial stewardship will allow the successful control of the disease syndromes caused by these organisms moving forward.

DISCLOSURE

The authors have nothing to disclose.

REFERENCES

1. Magstadt DR, Schuler AM, Coetzee JF, et al. Treatment history and antimicrobial susceptibility results for *Mannheimia haemolytica, Pasteurella multocida,* and *Histophilus somni* isolates from bovine respiratory disease cases submitted to the Iowa State University Veterinary Diagnostic Laboratory from 2013 to 2015. J Vet Diagn Invest 2018;30(1):99–104.
2. Dubrovsky SA, Van Eenennaam AL, Aly SS, et al. Preweaning cost of bovine respiratory disease (BRD) and cost-benefit of implementation of preventative measures in calves on California dairies: The BRD 10K study. J Dairy Sci 2019; 103(2):1583–97.
3. Confer AW, Ayalew S. *Mannheimia haemolytica* in bovine respiratory disease: immunogens, potential immunogens, and vaccines. Anim Health Res Rev 2018; 19(2):79–99.
4. Lubbers BV, Hanzlicek GA. Antimicrobial multidrug resistance and coresistance patterns of *Mannheimia haemolytica* isolated from bovine respiratory disease cases–a three-year (2009-2011) retrospective analysis. J Vet Diagn Invest 2013;25(3):413–7.
5. Snyder E, Credille B, Berghaus R, et al. Prevalence of multi drug antimicrobial resistance in *Mannheimia haemolytica* isolated from high-risk stocker cattle at arrival and two weeks after processing. J Anim Sci 2017;95(3):1124–31.
6. Snyder ER, Alvarez-Narvaez S, Credille BC. Genetic characterization of susceptible and multi-drug resistant *Mannheimia haemolytica* isolated from high-risk

stocker calves prior to and after antimicrobial metaphylaxis. Vet Microbiol 2019; 235:110–7.

7. Crosby S, Credille B, Giguere S, et al. Comparative efficacy of enrofloxacin to that of tulathromycin for the control of bovine respiratory disease and prevalence of antimicrobial resistance in *Mannheimia haemolytica* in calves at high risk of developing bovine respiratory disease. J Anim Sci 2018;96(4):1259–67.

8. Confer A, Step DL. *Mannheimia haemolytica* and *Pasteurella multocida* induced bovine pneumonia. In: Rings MD, Anderson DE, editors. Current veterinary therapy: food animal practice. 5th edition. St Louis (MO): Saunders; 2009. p. 164–70.

9. Cozens D, Sutherland E, Lauder M, et al. Pathogenic *Mannheimia haemolytica* Invades Differentiated Bovine Airway Epithelial Cells. Infect Immun 2019;87(6) [pii: e00078-19].

10. Ayalew S, Murdock BK, Snider TA, et al. *Mannheimia haemolytica* IgA-specific proteases. Vet Microbiol 2019;239:108487.

11. Boukahil I, Czuprynski CJ. *Mannheimia haemolytica* biofilm formation on bovine respiratory epithelial cells. Vet Microbiol 2016;197:129–36.

12. Pillai DK, Cha E, Mosier D. Role of the stress-associated chemicals norepinephrine, epinephrine and substance P in dispersal of *Mannheimia haemolytica* from biofilms. Vet Microbiol 2018;215:11–7.

13. Zecchinon L, Fett T, Desmecht D. How *Mannheimia haemolytica* defeats host defence through a kiss of death mechanism. Vet Res 2005;36(2):133–56.

14. Apley MD. Susceptibility testing for bovine respiratory and enteric disease. Vet Clin North Am Food Anim Pract 2003;19(3):625–46.

15. Lubbers BV, Turnidge J. Antimicrobial susceptibility testing for bovine respiratory disease: getting more from diagnostic results. Vet J 2015;203(2):149–54.

16. Watts JL, Yancey RJ Jr, Salmon SA, et al. A 4-year survey of antimicrobial susceptibility trends for isolates from cattle with bovine respiratory disease in North America. J Clin Microbiol 1994;32(3):725–31.

17. Welsh RD, Dye LB, Payton ME, et al. Isolation and antimicrobial susceptibilities of bacterial pathogens from bovine pneumonia: 1994–2002. J Vet Diagn Invest 2004;16(5):426–31.

18. Portis E, Lindeman C, Johansen L, et al. A ten-year (2000-2009) study of antimicrobial susceptibility of bacteria that cause bovine respiratory disease complex– *Mannheimia haemolytica*, *Pasteurella multocida*, and *Histophilus somni*–in the United States and Canada. J Vet Diagn Invest 2012;24(5):932–44.

19. Klima CL, Alexander TW, Read RR, et al. Genetic characterization and antimicrobial susceptibility of *Mannheimia haemolytica* isolated from the nasopharynx of feedlot cattle. Vet Microbiol 2011;149(3–4):390–8.

20. Noyes NR, Benedict KM, Gow SP, et al. *Mannheimia haemolytica* in feedlot cattle: prevalence of recovery and associations with antimicrobial use, resistance, and health outcomes. J Vet Intern Med 2015;29(2):705–13.

21. Klima CL, Alexander TW, Hendrick S, et al. Characterization of *Mannheimia haemolytica* isolated from feedlot cattle that were healthy or treated for bovine respiratory disease. Can J Vet Res 2014;78(1):38–45.

22. Woolums AR, Karisch BB, Frye JG, et al. Multidrug resistant *Mannheimia haemolytica* isolated from high-risk beef stocker cattle after antimicrobial metaphylaxis and treatment for bovine respiratory disease. Vet Microbiol 2018;221:143–52.

23. Pipoz F, Perreten V, Meylan M. Bacterial resistance in bacteria isolated from the nasal cavity of Swiss dairy calves. Schweiz Arch Tierheilkd 2016;158(6):397–403.

24. Owen JR, Noyes N, Young AE, et al. Whole-Genome Sequencing and Concordance Between Antimicrobial Susceptibility Genotypes and Phenotypes of

Bacterial Isolates Associated with Bovine Respiratory Disease. G3 (Bethesda) 2017;7(9):3059–71.

25. Soucy SM, Huang J, Gogarten JP. Horizontal gene transfer: building the web of life. Nat Rev Genet 2015;16(8):472–82.

26. Johnson CM, Grossman AD. Integrative and Conjugative Elements (ICEs): What They Do and How They Work. Annu Rev Genet 2015;49:577–601.

27. Klima CL, Zaheer R, Cook SR, et al. Pathogens of bovine respiratory disease in North American feedlots conferring multidrug resistance via integrative conjugative elements. J Clin Microbiol 2014;52(2):438–48.

28. Michael GB, Kadlec K, Sweeney MT, et al. ICEPmu1, an integrative conjugative element (ICE) of *Pasteurella multocida*: analysis of the regions that comprise 12 antimicrobial resistance genes. J Antimicrob Chemother 2012;67(1):84–90.

29. Hall JPJ, Brockhurst MA, Harrison E. Sampling the mobile gene pool: innovation via horizontal gene transfer in bacteria. Philos Trans R Soc Lond B Biol Sci 2017; 372(1735) [pii:20160424].

30. Eidam C, Poehlein A, Leimbach A, et al. Analysis and comparative genomics of ICEMh1, a novel integrative and conjugative element (ICE) of *Mannheimia haemolytica*. J Antimicrob Chemother 2015;70(1):93–7.

31. Klima CL, Cook SR, Zaheer R, et al. Comparative Genomic Analysis of *Mannheimia haemolytica* from Bovine Sources. PLoS One 2016;11(2):e0149520.

32. Klima CL, Holman DB, Ralston BJ, et al. Lower Respiratory Tract Microbiome and Resistome of Bovine Respiratory Disease Mortalities. Microb Ecol 2019;78(2): 446–56.

33. Kadlec K, Watts JL, Schwarz S, et al. Plasmid-located extended-spectrum beta-lactamase gene blaROB-2 in *Mannheimia haemolytica*. J Antimicrob Chemother 2019;74(4):851–3.

34. Bush K. Proliferation and significance of clinically relevant beta-lactamases. Ann N Y Acad Sci 2013;1277:84–90.

35. Naas T, Oueslati S, Bonnin RA, et al. Beta-lactamase database (BLDB) – structure and function. J Enzyme Inhib Med Chem 2017;32(1):917–9.

36. Katsuda K, Kohmoto M, Mikami O, et al. Plasmid-mediated florfenicol resistance in *Mannheimia haemolytica* isolated from cattle. Vet Microbiol 2012;155(2–4): 444–7.

37. Braibant M, Chevalier J, Chaslus-Dancla E, et al. Structural and functional study of the phenicol-specific efflux pump FloR belonging to the major facilitator superfamily. Antimicrob Agents Chemother 2005;49(7):2965–71.

38. Michael GB, Kadlec K, Sweeney MT, et al. ICEPmu1, an integrative conjugative element (ICE) of *Pasteurella multocida*: structure and transfer. J Antimicrob Chemother 2012;67(1):91–100.

39. Kehrenberg C, Salmon SA, Watts JL, et al. Tetracycline resistance genes in isolates of *Pasteurella multocida, Mannheimia haemolytica, Mannheimia glucosida* and *Mannheimia varigena* from bovine and swine respiratory disease: intergeneric spread of the tet(H) plasmid pMHT1. J Antimicrob Chemother 2001;48(5): 631–40.

40. Roberts MC. Tetracycline resistance determinants: mechanisms of action, regulation of expression, genetic mobility, and distribution. FEMS Microbiol Rev 1996;19(1):1–24.

41. Kehrenberg C, Catry B, Haesebrouck F, et al. tet(L)-mediated tetracycline resistance in bovine *Mannheimia* and *Pasteurella* isolates. J Antimicrob Chemother 2005;56(2):403–6.

42. Moller TS, Overgaard M, Nielsen SS, et al. Relation between tetR and tetA expression in tetracycline resistant *Escherichia coli*. BMC Microbiol 2016;16:39.

43. Ives SE, Richeson JT. Use of Antimicrobial Metaphylaxis for the Control of Bovine Respiratory Disease in High-Risk Cattle. Vet Clin North Am Food Anim Pract 2015;31(3):341–50, v.

44. Booker CW, Abutarbush SM, Schunicht OC, et al. Evaluation of the efficacy of tulathromycin as a metaphylactic antimicrobial in feedlot calves. Vet Ther 2007; 8(3):183–200.

45. Desmolaize B, Rose S, Warrass R, et al. A novel Erm monomethyltransferase in antibiotic-resistant isolates of *Mannheimia haemolytica* and *Pasteurella multocida*. Mol Microbiol 2011;80(1):184–94.

46. Desmolaize B, Rose S, Wilhelm C, et al. Combinations of macrolide resistance determinants in field isolates of *Mannheimia haemolytica* and *Pasteurella multocida*. Antimicrob Agents Chemother 2011;55(9):4128–33.

47. Skold O. Resistance to trimethoprim and sulfonamides. Vet Res 2001;32(3–4): 261–73.

48. Schwarz S, Kehrenberg C, Salmon SA, et al. In vitro activities of spectinomycin and comparator agents against *Pasteurella multocida* and *Mannheimia haemolytica* from respiratory tract infections of cattle. J Antimicrob Chemother 2004;53(2): 379–82.

49. Ramirez MS, Tolmasky ME. Aminoglycoside modifying enzymes. Drug Resist Updat 2010;13(6):151–71.

50. Avra TD, Abell KM, Shane DD, et al. A retrospective analysis of risk factors associated with bovine respiratory disease treatment failure in feedlot cattle. J Anim Sci 2017;95(4):1521–7.

51. McClary DG, Loneragan GH, Shryock TR, et al. Relationship of *in vitro* minimum inhibitory concentrations of tilmicosin against *Mannheimia haemolytica* and *Pasteurella multocida* and *in vivo* tilmicosin treatment outcome among calves with signs of bovine respiratory disease. J Am Vet Med Assoc 2011;239(1):129–35.

Pathogenesis and Virulence of *Mycoplasma bovis*

Jose Perez-Casal, PhD

KEYWORDS

- *M bovis* • Virulence factors • Pathogenesis • Disease control

KEY POINTS

- *Mycoplasma bovis* is an important opportunistic pathogen associated with bovine respiratory disease.
- *M bovis* seems to be a primary pathogen of North American bison (*Bison bison*).
- The strategies that *M bovis* uses to evade the immune system of the host include the ability to penetrate and survive in numerous cells, including peripheral blood mononuclear cells, alveolar macrophages, erythrocytes, and epithelial cells.
- *M bovis* modulates the immune responses of the host by altering the expression of cytokines, inhibiting peripheral blood mononuclear cell proliferation, and reducing apoptosis of peripheral blood mononuclear cells, monocytes, and alveolar macrophages.

INTRODUCTION

The economic impact of bovine respiratory disease (BRD) in the US feedlot cattle industry has been estimated to be in the order of $23.60 per case or close to $55 million annually.[1] The costs associated include culling and death of animals, lack of performance, veterinary fees, antibiotic treatment, and other management costs. The current evidence indicates that young cattle are colonized early in life.[2] Transmission mostly occurs by aerosol and beef cattle do not usually show signs of disease, especially in cow–calf operations. In dairy cattle, *Mycoplasma bovis* can be transmitted by contaminated milk and by close contact, leading to the onset of respiratory disease. *M bovis* can be a primary pathogen, but it is usually a secondary pathogen.[3] *M bovis* disease is often seen in feedlot animals previously infected by other bacterial or viral pathogens such as *Mannheimia haemolytica*, *Pasteurella multocida*, *Histophilus somni*, bovine respiratory syncytial virus, parainfluenza type 3 virus, bovine viral diarrhea virus, and infectious bovine rhinotracheitis caused by bovine herpesvirus-1.[3] Stress owing to transportation, overcrowding, introduction of new animals to the herd, and weaning play an important role in the development of disease. Despite some outbreaks owing to the introduction of infected cattle, there are currently no

Vaccine and Infectious Disease Organization – International Vaccine Centre (VIDO-InterVac), 120 Veterinary Road, Saskatoon, Saskatchewan S7N 5E3, Canada
E-mail address: jose.perez-casal@usask.ca

restrictions on cattle movement related to *M bovis*; however, several countries are starting to demand that cattle be free of *M bovis* before shipment. This condition was notably true for New Zealand, were cattle importation was stopped in 2014 to prevent importation of *M bovis*. Despite this measure, *M bovis*–positive herds were identified, leading the New Zealand government to impose culling of all these herds, a measure aimed at removing the pathogen from the country (https://www.biosecurity.govt.nz/protection-and-response/mycoplasma-bovis/). In the European Union, *M bovis* was included in the European Union–funded Discontools project in their disease database (http://www.discontools.eu/Diseases/Detail/82;Ref.[4]).

THE PATHOGEN

Although *M bovis* is considered a secondary cattle pathogen, it can also be the primary cause of disease.[3,5,6] It colonizes the upper respiratory tract without effect on the health of young animals.[7,8] The stress caused by weaning, transport, and relocation to feedlots results in the lowering of immune responses. This colonization, together with contact with other bacterial and viral pathogens, results in the onset of BRD.[3] Recent studies on the bacterial population in the upper and lower respiratory tract of cattle indicate that *Mycoplasma dispar* is present in the upper respiratory tract of healthy animals. However, once BRD is present, *M bovis* is found in the lower respiratory tract of a higher proportions of cattle with disease than cattle without BRD.[9]

The occurrence of recent outbreaks prompted scientists to determine if a single or multiple clones or strains were responsible. Studies on cattle from different geographic areas of Switzerland revealed that herd-specific clones and not a particular strain or clone were responsible for the outbreaks.[10] In contrast, Australian researchers found a single *M bovis* strain circulating in the country.[11] The authors concluded that, despite the failure to eradicate the pathogen, efforts to prevent the introduction of multiple strains have been successful. A similar finding was reported from Austrian scientists, where a single and unique *M bovis* strain spread throughout the country by first causing an outbreak in 2007, crossing the species barrier to infect pigs to reemerge in dairy operations in 2009.[12] An analysis of 69 French isolates collected in the last 35 years led to the identification of 2 major clusters.[13] The first cluster showed more heterogeneity and included strains isolated before 2000. The second cluster, which included strains isolated after 2000, was more homogeneous; the authors suggested that this was due to the spread of a single clone resistant to many antibiotics.[13] In China, a study was conducted to determine the genetic distribution and similarity to strains from other countries. The results indicated that the vast majority (97%) of the strains were classified as belonging to the ST-10 profile.[14] The same study indicated that the ST-10 profile was present in strains from Australia and the United States, suggesting that this strain was introduced in China with imported cattle.

In the United Kingdom, 2 population clusters were identified. The CC1 cluster included most strains from the United Kingdom and Germany, whereas the CC2 cluster included strains from Australia and other European and Asian countries.[15] Similarly, a link between Australian and Israeli isolates was established, suggesting that *M bovis* was introduced into Israel with cattle imported from Australia.[16] Strains isolated from North American bison (*Bison bison*) were found to be genetically different than those obtained from cattle, suggesting that the recent outbreaks of *M bovis* disease in bison are due to the emergence of new variants.[17] To answer the question whether *M bovis* isolates could cause disease in North American bison, 4 *M bovis* bison isolates were used to challenge bison and cattle. The results showed the presence of disease in bison but not in cattle, despite the fact that the challenge strains were isolated from the lungs of both species.[6]

PUTATIVE VIRULENCE FACTORS

An analysis of the available genomic sequences of several *M bovis* isolates reveals the lack of canonical virulence factors, such as toxins and 2-component regulatory systems. The genome of *M bovis* encodes a family of variable surface proteins (Vsp) that may play a role in evading the host immune response. The Vsp on–off expression depends on high-frequency genomic rearrangements that may help the bacterium to evade the immune response of the host. Binding to serum or tissue matrix proteins by *M bovis* adhesins has been postulated to play a role in virulence. In vitro assays showed that the *M bovis* α-enolase and the fructose 1,6-biphosphate aldolase bind plasminogen,[18,19] whereas the methylenetetrahydrofolate-tRNA-(uracil-5-)-methyltransferase protein binds fibronectin.[20] All these proteins were shown to be expressed on the cell surface of *M bovis* and adherence to embryonic bovine lung cells in vitro was inhibited by antibodies against these proteins.

Surface proteins with nuclease activity have been isolated from *M bovis*. The Mun nuclease is reported to degrade neutrophil extracellular traps, a mechanism of defense by neutrophils composed of a web of nucleic acids and azurophilic granules that trap and kill the bacterium in the extracellular space.[21] Another nuclease, MBOV_RS02825, is reported to cause cytotoxicity when the purified protein is incubated with macrophages, resulting in the induction of apoptosis.[22]

The production of H_2O_2 by some mycoplasmas has been correlated with virulence. Examples include *Mycoplasma mycoides* subsp *mycoides*[23] and *Mycoplasma pneumoniae*.[24] Some *M bovis* isolates produce H_2O_2; however, the expression of H_2O_2 was not associated with the virulence of clinical strains.[25] Some *M bovis* isolates produce biofilms in response to harsh conditions, such as heat and drying. Biofilms are a complex matrix of extracellular polysaccharides and proteins that protect a pathogen from desiccation, changes in temperature and in some cases, antimicrobial activity.[26] The *M bovis* biofilm production is tied to the expression of certain Vsp; strains expressing VspF produced little biofilm as opposed to those expressing the VspO or VspB varieties.[27] However, despite a putative role of biofilms in antibiotic resistance, the minimum inhibitory concentration for several antibiotics did not change for *M bovis* evaluated in the presence of biofilms.[27]

The in vitro passage of isolates may decrease their virulence. A recent report describes the loss of a 14.2 kbp DNA region and several nonsense mutations in *M bovis* isolates that were passaged in vitro for several generations. The authors concluded that the strains became less virulent with more passages and that the loss of genes encoding proteins involved in sugar transport, sugar metabolism, production of H_2O_2, and the loss of putative lipoproteins may explain the decreased virulence.[28]

MECHANISMS OF IMMUNE SYSTEM EVASION

Numerous reports describe the ability of *M bovis* to evade and modulate the immune system of the host. Mechanisms include antigenic variation, inhibition of peripheral blood mononuclear cell (PBMC) proliferation; resistance to monocyte and macrophage phagocytosis; invasion of erythrocytes, PBMC, and epithelial cells; modulation of cytokine production; modulation of apoptosis; and interference with the programmed death ligand/programmed death (PD-1) PBMC activation cascade. As stated elsewhere in this article, *M bovis* encodes a family of surface-exposed Vsp proteins. Antigenic and genetic variation by high-frequency chromosomal rearrangements of the Vsp has been associated with virulence. This expression switch is not only observed in laboratory cultures, but also in vivo,[29] leading to the hypothesis that by the time the host mounts an immune response against a Vsp on the cell surface, other *M bovis* cells emerge expressing different Vsp and thus evading the immune response of the host.

Numerous laboratories have described the ability of *M bovis* to inhibit PBMC proliferative responses, resulting in abnormal function of these immune cells. Incubation of *M bovis* with PBMC from naïve or immunized animals results in lack of proliferation in response to the mitogen concanavalin A (ConA), which activates proliferation in normal lymphocytes (reviewed in Ref[30]). The *M bovis* factor(s) responsible for this effect remain unknown. These results conflict with the findings of Gondaira and colleagues.[31] In that study, the incubation of PBMC with different concentrations of *M bovis* resulted in significant PBMC proliferation in response to the mitogens ConA and phytohemagglutinin; however, these investigators did not evaluate the proliferative capacity of PBMC exposed to ConA or phytohemagglutinin alone. Thus, it is impossible to determine if, as seen before,[32] co-incubation with *M bovis* and ConA results in lower proliferation indexes compared with incubation with ConA alone. The discrepancies in PBMC proliferation between studies can be attributed to differences in the *M bovis* isolates used for stimulation, because differences were also detected between bovine and bison isolates.[33]

Another mechanism of inhibition of PBMC proliferation is the induction of expression of the PD ligand on tracheal, lung, and alveolar macrophage cells; and the PD-1 receptor on CD4$^+$ and CD8$^+$ cells.[34] This inhibition results in the impairment of the proliferative capacity of CD3$^+$ and CD8$^+$ cells, which means that these T cells cannot respond appropriately to activation stimuli, which is needed for normal clonal expansion during the immune response. A decrease in the clonal expansion of the cells together with immune exhaustion caused by the PD ligand/PD-1 interaction results in a reduction of cell-mediated immune responses, which may be needed to clear the infection. In the same study, the use of an antibody to block the PD-1 receptor partially restored proliferation in bovine PBMC,[34] proving the role of PD-1 activation on the *M bovis*-induced immune suppression.

To explain the lack of PBMC proliferation after these cells were incubated with *M bovis*, tests were carried out to determine if these cells could harbor the pathogen. In vitro assays confirmed the intracellular presence of *M bovis* in all bovine PBMC cell types and also in erythrocytes.[32] The intracellular presence of *M bovis* could also aid in the dissemination of the pathogen to other tissues of the host. The role of intracellular *M bovis* on bovine monocyte functions was investigated. The results indicated that expression of the proinflammatory interferon gamma and tumor necrosis factor alpha (TNF-α) cytokines were suppressed, whereas the anti-inflammatory IL-10 levels are increased.[35] Suppression of proinflammatory cytokines and activation of an anti-inflammatory cytokine could be related to persistence of *M bovis* infection owing to inadequate activation of inflammatory responses that lead to pathogen clearance. In addition, intracellular *M bovis* results in inhibition of monocyte apoptosis, which may help the bacterium to survive and to spread in these cells to other tissues of the host.

In experimental trials, cattle older than 6 months infected with *M bovis* do not present clinical signs of infection; however, *M bovis* can be isolated from lung tissue.[36] This raised the hypothesis that *M bovis* could avoid alveolar macrophage clearance by either being able to multiply inside the cells or by modulating macrophage responses that should lead to clearance of *M bovis*. *M bovis* isolates obtained from cattle and bison were incubated with alveolar macrophages from these 2 species. The results showed that some of the isolates were able to replicate, regardless of source of the strain or macrophage used.[33] As with bovine monocytes, intracellular *M bovis* causes inhibition of apoptosis of alveolar macrophages and a macrophage cell line.[33,37] Because apoptosis of infected cells can be 1 method of clearing infection, suppression of apoptosis by *M bovis* may be an important mechanism by which the bacteria persists in the host. In bovine neutrophils, *M bovis* increases apoptosis and expression of IL-12 and TNF-α and inhibits expression of nitrous oxide, but increases expression of elastase.[38] In addition, increased expression levels of CD46, CD86, and CD40 after incubation of neutrophils with *M bovis* suggests that the bacterium targets these upregulated receptors to aid its infectivity, survival, and spread.[38]

PATHOGENESIS

Several studies were designed to investigate the mechanism(s) of *M bovis*-induced pathogenesis by looking at PBMC, lungs, milk, and synovial tissue exposed to the pathogen. PBMC responses depended on whether the strains were isolated from a mastitis case, pneumonic calf, or from a fetus. The main host responses to *M bovis* infections are a stimulation of CD4$^+$ (T helper) cells, which activate adaptive immunity, and an enhancement of the B cell (antibody producing) response. The CD4$^+$, B cell, and an increased CD4:CD8 (T helper cell to T cytotoxic cell) ratio was most apparent in mastitic cows, whereas in the fetus a parallel CD4$^+$ and CD8$^+$ stimulation was observed.[39]

In vitro incubation of PBMC from naïve cows with *M bovis* at a multiplicity of infection of 1000 (ie, 1000 *M bovis* organisms per cell) significantly induced TNF-α, IL-12p40 (IL-12), and interferon-γ messenger RNA expression in PBMC.[31] Furthermore, culture supernatants of *M bovis* induced a significant increase in TNF-α, IL-6, and IL-10 messenger RNA expression in bovine PBMC, indicating that the products secreted or released by the bacteria could impact immune responses, without direct contact between immune cells and the bacteria. These increases were not detected after incubation at a lower multiplicity of infection of 10 *M bovis* organisms per cell, or 100 *M bovis* organisms per cell.[31] These results suggest that large numbers of live *M bovis* are required to induce an immune response in bovine PBMC. This result was confirmed by Valsala and colleagues,[40] where IL-6 was upregulated (by 9.32-fold at 24 hours) by live *M bovis*, whereas IL-1 and TNF-α levels were not altered at a multiplicity of infection of 1:10. Overall, these studies indicate that the number of *M bovis* present impacts the host immune response; this finding may explain in part why cattle resist disease owing to *M bovis* exposure in some situations but not in others.

In PBMC purified from animals injected with an experimental vaccine and challenged with *M bovis*, expression of IL-6, IL-10, IL-12, and IL-17a was detected in supernatants of PBMCs incubated with *M bovis* antigens[41] after challenge, although an expression of transforming growth factor beta (TGF-β) was detected by PBMC collected before the challenge. In another experimental trial, the levels of serum IL-1 increased and serum TGF-β decreased after challenge. After challenge, the levels of IL-1, IL-10, IL-12, TNF-α, and TGF-β increased after incubation with recall antigens.[42] Taken together, these studies provide information regarding the cytokines that are expressed by cattle before and after they have been vaccinated against *M bovis*. Because the pattern of cytokine expression is related to whether infection leads to recovery from infection, this research provides insight regarding the nature of protective immunity. More research will be needed to confirm the clinical relevance of these findings.

A recent trial described the response of cattle challenged with the virulent HB0801 and the attenuated HB0801-P150 strains of M bovis; outcomes were assessed after human killing at 60 days after infection.[43] The pathogenesis of HB0801 was predicted to be associated with enhanced T helper type-17 cells, whereas HB0801-P150–induced immunity with T helper type 1 response and expression of ubiquitination-associated enzymes. The results indicated that virulent and attenuated strains might be associated with biased differentiation of proinflammatory pathogenic T helper cell type 17 and protective T helper cell type 1 subsets, respectively.[43]

The mechanism of M bovis-induced pathogenesis was investigated in lungs of animals challenged with the bacterium. Colocalization of M bovis DNA, M bovis antigen, and macrophages expressing inducible nitric oxide synthase, nitrotyrosine, and manganese-dependent superoxide dismutase was observed. These findings suggest that the generation of reactive oxygen and nitrogen species is involved in the development of severe chronic lung damage in M bovis infection.[44] In calves with caseonecrotic pneumonia, necrotic foci were surrounded by epithelial cells resembling bronchial or bronchiolar epithelium.[45] M bovis Vsp antigens were constantly present in the cytoplasm of macrophages and were also present extracellularly at the periphery of necrotic foci. There was a considerable increase in numbers of IgG1- and IgG2-positive plasma cells with IgG1-containing plasma cells clearly predominated. Because these 2 subtypes of IgG differ in their efficacy for immune effects such as opsonization and neutralization, the predominance of IgG1 may be a clue as to why the cattle failed to clear M bovis and developed the caseonecrotic lesions. There were no differences between the number of CD4[+] and CD8[+] T cells between inoculated and control calves, supporting previous findings.[39]

The effects of M bovis in the mammary gland were examined. Milk concentrations of several cytokines, including cytokines indicating a T helper 1 and proinflammatory response (interferon-γ, IL-1β, IL-10, IL-12, TGF-α, and TNF-α), were elevated in response to infection over a period of several days, whereas increases in milk IL-8, a cytokine that strongly induces neutrophil influx, were of a more limited duration.[46] In another study, live M bovis triggered an immune response in primary bovine mammary epithelial cells, reflected by the upregulation of TNF-a, IL-1β, IL-6, IL-8, lactoferrin, toll-like receptor-2, RANTES, and serum amyloid A messenger RNA.[47] The presence of M bovis antigens in necrotic synovial tissue lesions was associated with expression of inducible nitric oxide synthase and nitrotyrosine by macrophages. The results suggest that nitritative injury is involved in the development of caseonecrotic joint lesions, as observed before for lung tissue.[44] Furthermore, expression of VspA, VspB, and VspC was also detected,[48] indicating persistence of M bovis protein expression in the affected joints.

THE PATH FORWARD

Despite significant progress in the identification of putative virulence factors, elucidating the outcome of host–pathogen interactions and testing of some experimental vaccines, M bovis continues to be a significant pathogen of beef and dairy cattle. The challenges remain many and are presented in a recent review by Calcutt and colleagues.[3] Owing to the limited host range of M bovis, cattle are the preferred animal model to test nonvirulent mutants and experimental vaccines; this process increases the cost and logistical constraints of needed research. Additional efforts should focus on the development of a small animal model for testing, which should help research to progress more quickly. More emphasis needs to be put on sequencing the genome of recent isolates and the application of in silico approaches to identify new targets for control. Examples of these approaches are the use of metabolomics combined with bioinformatics to investigate protein function,[49] kinome microarrays to determine host phosphorylation pathways modulated by *M bovis*,[35] reverse vaccinology to identify novel vaccine targets,[50,51] and synthetic biology[52] to determine the smallest genome of *M bovis* capable of causing disease.

ACKNOWLEDGMENTS

The author thanks present and past members of my laboratory: Ms Tracy Prysliak, Dr Harish Menghwar, Dr Musa Mulongo, Dr Jacques van der Merwe, Dr Sonja Mertins, Dr Steve Jimbo, Dr Teresia Maina, and Mr Kyle Clarke. The Saskatchewan Agriculture Development Fund (ADF), The Alberta Agriculture Research Institute (AARI), The Beef Cattle Research Council (BCRC), Alberta Livestock Industry Development Fund (ALIDF), Agriculture and Food Council of Alberta, Ontario Cattlemen's Association (OCA), Advancing Agriculture and Agri-Food (ACAAF) Program, and the Alberta Livestock and Meat Association (ALMA) have supported the research in my laboratory.

REFERENCES

1. Johnson KK, Pendell DL. Market impacts of reducing the prevalence of bovine respiratory disease in United States beef cattle feedlots. Front Vet Sci 2017;4:189.
2. Holman DB, Timsit E, Alexander TW. The nasopharyngeal microbiota of feedlot cattle. Sci Rep 2015;5:15557.
3. Calcutt MJ, Lysnyansky I, Sachse K, et al. Gap analysis of *Mycoplasma bovis* disease, diagnosis and control: an aid to identify future development requirements. Transbound Emerg Dis 2018;65(Suppl 1):91–109.
4. O'Brien D, Scudamore J, Charlier J, et al. DISCONTOOLS: a database to identify research gaps on vaccines, pharmaceuticals and diagnostics for the control of infectious diseases of animals. BMC Vet Res 2017;13(1):1.
5. Gille L, Pilo P, Valgaeren BR, et al. A new predilection site of *Mycoplasma bovis*: postsurgical seromas in beef cattle. Vet Microbiol 2016;186:67–70.
6. Register KB, Olsen SC, Sacco RE, et al. Relative virulence in bison and cattle of bison-associated genotypes of *Mycoplasma bovis*. Vet Microbiol 2018;222: 55–63.
7. Caswell JL, Bateman KG, Cai HY, et al. *Mycoplasma bovis* in respiratory disease of feedlot cattle. Vet Clin North Am Food Anim Pract 2010;26(2):365–79.
8. Nicholas RA. Bovine mycoplasmosis: silent and deadly. Vet Rec 2011;168(17): 459–62.
9. Timsit E, Workentine M, van der Meer F, et al. Distinct bacterial metacommunities inhabit the upper and lower respiratory tracts of healthy feedlot cattle and those diagnosed with bronchopneumonia. Vet Microbiol 2018;221:105–13.
10. Aebi M, Bodmer M, Frey J, et al. Herd-specific strains of *Mycoplasma bovis* in outbreaks of mycoplasmal mastitis and pneumonia. Vet Microbiol 2012; 157(3–4):363–8.
11. Parker AM, Shukla A, House JK, et al. Genetic characterization of Australian *Mycoplasma bovis* isolates through whole genome sequencing analysis. Vet Microbiol 2016;196:118–25.
12. Spergser J, Macher K, Kargl M, et al. Emergence, re-emergence, spread and host species crossing of *Mycoplasma bovis* in the Austrian Alps caused by a single endemic strain. Vet Microbiol 2013;164(3–4):299–306.

13. Becker CA, Thibault FM, Arcangioli MA, et al. Loss of diversity within *Mycoplasma bovis* isolates collected in France from bovines with respiratory diseases over the last 35 years. Infect Genet Evol 2015;33:118–26.

14. Menghwar H, He C, Zhang H, et al. Genotype distribution of Chinese *Mycoplasma bovis* isolates and their evolutionary relationship to strains from other countries. Microb Pathog 2017;111:108–17.

15. Rosales RS, Churchward CP, Schnee C, et al. Global multilocus sequence typing analysis of *Mycoplasma bovis* isolates reveals two main population clusters. J Clin Microbiol 2015;53(3):789–94.

16. Amram E, Freed M, Khateb N, et al. Multiple locus variable number tandem repeat analysis of *Mycoplasma bovis* isolated from local and imported cattle. Vet J 2013;197(2):286–90.

17. Register KB, Jelinski MD, Waldner M, et al. Comparison of multilocus sequence types found among North American isolates of *Mycoplasma bovis* from cattle, bison, and deer, 2007-2017. J Vet Diagn Invest 2019;31(6):899–904.

18. Gao X, Bao S, Xing X, et al. Fructose-1,6-bisphosphate aldolase of *Mycoplasma bovis* is a plasminogen-binding adhesin. Microb Pathog 2018;124:230–7.

19. Song Z, Li Y, Liu Y, et al. alpha-Enolase, an adhesion-related factor of *Mycoplasma bovis*. PLoS One 2012;7(6):e38836.

20. Guo Y, Zhu H, Wang J, et al. TrmFO, a Fibronectin-Binding Adhesin of *Mycoplasma bovis*. Int J Mol Sci 2017;18(8) [pii:E1732].

21. Mitiku F, Hartley CA, Sansom FM, et al. The major membrane nuclease MnuA degrades neutrophil extracellular traps induced by *Mycoplasma bovis*. Vet Microbiol 2018;218:13–9.

22. Zhang H, Zhao G, Guo Y, et al. *Mycoplasma bovis* MBOV_RS02825 encodes a secretory nuclease associated with cytotoxicity. Int J Mol Sci 2016;17(5) [pii: E628].

23. Pilo P, Frey J, Vilei EM. Molecular mechanisms of pathogenicity of *Mycoplasma mycoides subsp. mycoides* SC. Vet J 2007;174(3):513–21.

24. Schmidl SR, Otto A, Lluch-Senar M, et al. A trigger enzyme in *Mycoplasma pneumoniae*: impact of the glycerophosphodiesterase GlpQ on virulence and gene expression. PLoS Pathog 2011;7(9):e1002263.

25. Schott C, Cai H, Parker L, et al. Hydrogen peroxide production and free radical-mediated cell stress in *Mycoplasma bovis* pneumonia. J Comp Pathol 2014; 150(2–3):127–37.

26. Del Pozo JL. Biofilm-related disease. Expert Rev Anti Infect Ther 2018;16(1): 51–65.

27. McAuliffe L, Ellis RJ, Miles K, et al. Biofilm formation by mycoplasma species and its role in environmental persistence and survival. Microbiology 2006;152(Pt 4): 913–22.

28. Rasheed MA, Qi J, Zhu X, et al. Comparative Genomics of *Mycoplasma bovis* Strains Reveals That Decreased Virulence with Increasing Passages Might Correlate with Potential Virulence-Related Factors. Front Cell Infect Microbiol 2017; 7:177.

29. Buchenau I, Poumarat F, Le Grand D, et al. Expression of *Mycoplasma bovis* variable surface membrane proteins in the respiratory tract of calves after experimental infection with a clonal variant of *Mycoplasma bovis* type strain PG45. Res Vet Sci 2010;89(2):223–9.

30. Perez-Casal J, Prysliak T, Maina T, et al. Status of the development of a vaccine against *Mycoplasma bovis*. Vaccine 2017;35(22):2902–7.

31. Gondaira S, Higuchi H, Iwano H, et al. Cytokine mRNA profiling and the proliferative response of bovine peripheral blood mononuclear cells to *Mycoplasma bovis*. Vet Immunol Immunopathol 2015;165(1–2):45–53.

32. van der Merwe J, Prysliak T, Perez-Casal J. Invasion of bovine peripheral-blood mononuclear cells and erythrocytes by *Mycoplasma bovis*. Infect Immun 2010; 78(11):4570–8.

33. Suleman M, Prysliak T, Clarke K, et al. *Mycoplasma bovis* isolates recovered from cattle and bison (*Bison bison*) show differential in vitro effects on PBMC proliferation, alveolar macrophage apoptosis and invasion of epithelial and immune cells. Vet Microbiol 2016;186:28–36.

34. Suleman M, Cyprian FS, Jimbo S, et al. *Mycoplasma bovis*-Induced Inhibition of Bovine Peripheral Blood Mononuclear Cell Proliferation Is Ameliorated after Blocking the Immune-Inhibitory Programmed Death 1 Receptor. Infect Immun 2018;86(3) [pii:e00921-17].

35. Mulongo M, Prysliak T, Scruten E, et al. In vitro infection of bovine monocytes with *Mycoplasma bovis* delays apoptosis and suppresses production of gamma interferon and tumor necrosis factor alpha but not interleukin-10. Infect Immun 2014; 82(1):62–71.

36. Prysliak T, Van der Merwe J, Lawman Z, et al. Respiratory disease caused by *Mycoplasma bovis* is enhanced by exposure to Bovine Herpes Virus 1 (BHV-1) and not to Bovine Viral Diarrhoea Virus (BVDV) type 2. Can Vet J 2011;52:1195–202.

37. Maina T, Prysliak T, Perez-Casal J. *Mycoplasma bovis* delay in apoptosis of macrophages is accompanied by increased expression of anti-apoptotic genes, reduced cytochrome C translocation and inhibition of DNA fragmentation. Vet Immunol Immunopathol 2019;208:16–24.

38. Jimbo S, Suleman M, Maina T, et al. Effect of *Mycoplasma bovis* on bovine neutrophils. Vet Immunol Immunopathol 2017;188:27–33.

39. Dudek K, Bednarek D, Ayling RD, et al. An experimental vaccine composed of two adjuvants gives protection against *Mycoplasma bovis* in calves. Vaccine 2016;34(27):3051–8.

40. Valsala R, Rana R, Remesh AT, et al. Effect of *Mycoplasma bovis* on production of pro-inflammatory cytokines by peripheral blood mononuclear cells. Adv Anim Vet Sci 2017;5(10):400–4.

41. Prysliak T, Maina T, Perez-Casal J. Th-17 cell mediated immune responses to *Mycoplasma bovis* proteins formulated with Montanide ISA61 VG and curdlan are not sufficient for protection against an experimental challenge with *Mycoplasma bovis*. Vet Immunol Immunopathol 2018;197:7–14.

42. Prysliak T, Maina T, Yu L, et al. Induction of a balanced IgG1/IgG2 immune response to an experimental challenge with *Mycoplasma bovis* antigens following a vaccine composed of Emulsigen, IDR peptide1002, and poly I:C. Vaccine 2017;35(48 Pt B):6604–10.

43. Chao J, Han X, Liu K, et al. Calves Infected with Virulent and Attenuated *Mycoplasma bovis* Strains Have Upregulated Th17 Inflammatory and Th1 Protective Responses, Respectively. Genes (Basel) 2019;10(9) [pii:E656].

44. Hermeyer K, Jacobsen B, Spergser J, et al. Detection of *Mycoplasma bovis* by in-situ hybridization and expression of inducible nitric oxide synthase, nitrotyrosine and manganese superoxide dismutase in the lungs of experimentally-infected calves. J Comp Pathol 2011;145(2–3):240–50.

45. Hermeyer K, Buchenau I, Thomasmeyer A, et al. Chronic pneumonia in calves after experimental infection with *Mycoplasma bovis* strain 1067: characterization of

lung pathology, persistence of variable surface protein antigens and local immune response. Acta Vet Scand 2012;54(1):9.

46. Kauf AC, Rosenbusch RF, Paape MJ, et al. Innate immune response to intramammary *Mycoplasma bovis* infection. J Dairy Sci 2007;90(7):3336–48.

47. Zbinden C, Pilo P, Frey J, et al. The immune response of bovine mammary epithelial cells to live or heat-inactivated *Mycoplasma bovis*. Vet Microbiol 2015; 179(3–4):336–40.

48. Devi VR, Poumarat F, Le Grand D, et al. Histopathological findings, phenotyping of inflammatory cells, and expression of markers of nitritative injury in joint tissue samples from calves after vaccination and intraarticular challenge with *Mycoplasma bovis* strain 1067. Acta Vet Scand 2014;56(1):45.

49. Masukagami Y, De Souza DP, Dayalan S, et al. Comparative metabolomics of *Mycoplasma bovis* and *Mycoplasma gallisepticum* reveals fundamental differences in active metabolic pathways and suggests novel gene annotations. mSystems 2017;2(5) [pii:e00055-17].

50. Nkando I, Perez-Casal J, Mwirigi M, et al. Recombinant *Mycoplasma mycoides* proteins elicit protective immune responses against contagious bovine pleuropneumonia. Vet Immunol Immunopathol 2016;171:103–14.

51. Perez-Casal J, Prysliak T, Maina T, et al. Analysis of immune responses to recombinant proteins from strains of *Mycoplasma mycoides* subsp. *mycoides*, the causative agent of contagious bovine pleuropneumonia. Vet Immunol Immunopathol 2015;168(1–2):103–10.

52. Gibson DG, Glass JI, Lartigue C, et al. Creation of a bacterial cell controlled by a chemically synthesized genome. Science 2010;329(5987):52–6.

Histophilus somni
Antigenic and Genomic Changes Relevant to Bovine Respiratory Disease

Randal M. Shirbroun, DVM

KEYWORDS

- Virulence factor • Phase variation • Serum resistance • Lipooligosaccharide
- Immunoglobulin-binding protein • Immune evasion • Whole-genome sequencing

KEY POINTS

- *Histophilus somni* is associated with various bovine disease syndromes. It is an important causative agent in the bovine respiratory disease (BRD) complex.
- *H somni* isolates may express a variety of virulence factors, some of which are involved with evasion of the host immune response.
- Some isolates are susceptible to inactivation by normal bovine serum whereas others are not, suggestive of strain variation.
- Significant antigenic variation between some isolates has been identified.
- Studies to evaluate the *H somni* genome have revealed significant genetic differences, some of which are associated with presence or absence of virulence factors.

INTRODUCTION

The bovine respiratory disease (BRD) complex has been associated with several infectious organisms, including bacteria, mycoplasmas, and viruses. *Histophilus somni* is 1 of the bacteria commonly isolated from cases of BRD as well as other disease syndromes in domestic cattle. In addition to respiratory disease, *H somni* is associated with thrombotic meningoencephalitis, septicemia, myocarditis, arthritis, and reproductive failure.[1] *H somni* also is the causative agent for respiratory disease in sheep, bison, and bighorn sheep.[2]

CLINICAL DISEASE

BRD has been a persistent problem for the cattle industry for decades. Although management deficiencies or challenges may play a role in the incidence and severity, BRD can be a significant issue even in well-managed cattle operations.[3] It is a major cause

Ruminant Business Unit, Newport Laboratories, A Boehringer Ingelheim Animal Health Company, 1520 Prairie Drive, Worthington, MN 56187, USA
E-mail address: rshirbroun@newportlabs.com

Vet Clin Food Anim 36 (2020) 279–295
https://doi.org/10.1016/j.cvfa.2020.02.003
0749-0720/20/© 2020 Elsevier Inc. All rights reserved.

of economic loss for cattle operations across North America. Despite advances in biologicals and antibacterial pharmaceuticals, the bacterial components of BRD, including *H somni*, continue to cause severe health disease problems with a significant economic impact.[4]

H somni commonly is isolated in pure culture from pneumonic lungs.[5] Typically, respiratory infections involve more than 1 organism, and *H somni* often is found in conjunction with other BRD pathogens. Fulton[6] isolated *H somni* from 10% of the lungs from animals that died due to BRD in a study in 2002 to 2003. *H somni* infection of the respiratory tract has been associated with bovine respiratory syncytial virus (BRSV), with the coinfection demonstrating a synergistic effect in pulmonary alveoli.[7,8] Infection by both BRSV and *H somni* resulted in the most severe disease as well as the highest serum IgE antibody responses to *H somni* compared with other coinfections.[9] Duration of pneumonia and persistence of *H somni* in the lungs also were greatest in calves that were concurrently infected with BRSV.

BRD associated with *H somni* infection results in pleuropneumonia. Clinical signs include dyspnea, persistent fever, and eventually death in many cases. Affected groups of cattle also may exhibit other syndromes due to *H somni* infection, such as myocarditis and thrombotic meningoencephalitis, both of which may result in sudden death.[10] *H somni* has been isolated from many different tissues in association with a variety of disease syndromes. In addition, it also has been recovered from tissues for which there is no apparent pathology. This article focuses on the respiratory form of disease due to *H somni,* although many of the antigenic and genomic aspects of the organism apply regardless of what tissues or body systems are infected.

The association of *H somni*, at that time identified as *Haemophilus somnus*, with severe fibrinous pleuritis was noted as early as the late 1960s.[11] In the late 1980s, it was noted that the respiratory form of hemophilosis was increasing in frequency and severity, recognized as causing disease in both the upper and lower respiratory tract.[5] Harris and Janzen[5] noted that exposure to the organism was widespread, with up to 25% of cattle being seropositive but as high as 50% to 100% on some premises. The incidence of feedlot disease due to infection by *H somni* has been estimated at 50% to 60%.[12] Traditionally, BRD due to *H somni* has been associated with cattle in feedlots in Canada and the Northern Plains of the United States; however, in the past decade it has been identified frequently in calves coming out of the southeastern and northeastern parts of the United States.[13] It is being identified in all ages of beef cattle as well as dairy breeds.

Although vaccination against *H somni* using commercial whole-cell bacterins has been practiced for several decades, effective protection in vaccinated animals has been inconsistent and generally elusive. As a result, the *H somni* component of the BRD complex continues to produce detrimental effects in cattle.[3,10] In addition to commercial bacterins, autogenous bacterins manufactured from field isolates have been utilized in preventive health programs.

ORGANISM

The organism now known as *H somni* was first isolated in 1956, associated with what was then described as infectious embolic meningoencephalitis.[1,14] The bacteria is a small, gram-negative non–spore-forming, pleomorphic bacillus, a member of the Pasteurellaceae family,[14,15] but does not express flagella or have a polysaccharide capsule.[16] At that time it was identified as a *Haemophilus*-like organism despite the fact that it was not accurate taxonomically. Unlike other members of the genus, it does not require the special growth factor X or V nor does it satellite around

Staphylococcus spp streak nurse colony.[17] *Haemophilus somnus* was proposed as the name for the organism in 1969, even though it did not truly fit the requirements of the genus. Similar organisms isolated from sheep were identified as *Haemophilus ovis* and *Haemophilus agni*.

Further analyses, including phylogenetic analysis of 16s rDNA and rpoB sequences, indicated a significant difference from *Haemophilus influenzae*, the type species of the genus.[18] Those results, as well as recognition of the lack of the requirement for growth factors, resulted in a nomenclature change to *H somni*, which also includes the bacteria previously identified as *Haemophilus ovis* and *Haemophilus agni*. It now represents a novel genus within the family Pasteurellaceae with only 1 species.[17]

H somni is considered a commensal bacteria that can be an opportunistic pathogen, complicating viral infections and increasing the severity of infection by other bacteria.[17] Depending on the situation, a single strain may be a commensal or pathogenic[19] The organism may penetrate mucosal surfaces and become septicemic, colonizing a variety of tissues.

H somni was once was considered a facultative intracellular pathogen based on studies that indicated that opsonized *H somni* was ingested, but not killed, by bovine macrophages or monocytes, apparently inhibiting phagocyte function.[5,20] It also was suggested that intracellular survival may be an important virulence factor in the dissemination of infection within the host.[17] This presumed survival of phagocytosis not only led to a mischaracterization of the organism as an intracellular pathogen but also implied that cell-mediated immunity would be a more important component in providing protection.[21]

Eventually it was determined that *H somni* does not live for extended periods of time in macrophages, but in fact the bacteria kills the cell. It now is considered an extracellular pathogen based on its limited survival in phagocytes before killing them.[2] As a result, humoral immunity would be considered important to protection. The apparent value of humoral immunity has been demonstrated by use of maternal serum to provide effective passive protection.[22–24] Further studies indicated that IgG2 is specifically involved with protection against *H somni*.[2] Isolates typically were classified according to their susceptibility to inactivation by normal bovine serum as serum sensitive or serum resistant.

The organism appears to persist longer in the lower respiratory tract than the upper tract. In 1 study, the clinical pneumonia resulting from infection lasted for less than a week, but *H somni* could be recovered for several weeks after resolution of the pneumonia.[25]

VIRULENCE FACTORS: CURRENT UNDERSTANDING AND CLINICAL SIGNIFICANCE

H somni has a wide array of virulence factors that contribute to its ability to cause disease as well as evade the host immune system. It does not have a capsule but it is a formidable organism with some novel characteristics.

Adherence

H somni has the ability to colonize the mucosal membrane surface by attaching to cells.[17,26] Based on work with *Haemophilus influenzae*, it is likely that nonpilus adhesions are involved primarily in adhesion to mucosal surfaces.[27] A bacterial surface protein, identified as p76, may be involved.[28]

Surface Protein Antigens

The outer membrane proteins (OMPs) are important from an immunologic perspective due to their location and potential accessibility to host defenses.[29] Multiple studies have identified several OMPs of differing molecular weight and varying significance immunologically.[22] Studies utilizing antisera recognized 2 OMPs of primary importance immunologically: 40 kDa (40 kDa) and 78 kDa (78 kDa). Of these, it was determined that the antibodies to the 40-kDa antigen provided protection against pneumonia but antibodies specific to the 78-kDa OMP were not protective.[24] The 40-kDa OMP is surface exposed and it has been shown that bovine antibodies specific for it provide passive protection against pneumonia.[23] The 40-kDa OMP is considered one of the most critical antigenic proteins for H somni.[2]

There also is a 41-kDa major OMP (MOMP) that is strain variable[30] but it is not well recognized by bovine IgG.[2] The MOMP of H somni, unlike other gram-negative pathogens, does not stimulate a significant protective immune response; however, IgE antibodies react strongly with the MOMP of virulent isolates. This characteristic may be related to the anaphylactoid reactions associated with some whole-cell bacterins.[31]

Iron Uptake

H somni utilizes transferrin-binding proteins to acquire iron from bovine transferrin. These proteins are on the outer membrane of the organism and appear to differ between strains. The ability of these iron-regulated OMPs to obtain iron is specific to bovine transferrin and this was assumed to explain the host species specificity of H somni. Sheep (domestic and bighorn) and bison, however, also experience respiratory disease associated with H somni.[32] No mutants lacking transferrin-binding proteins have been reported.[33]

Histamine Production

In vitro growth of H somni, in both broth and on agar plates, results in the production of histamine. The mechanism is not well understood, but the ability of the bacteria to produce this mediator may contribute to a direct inflammatory response during in vivo infection by H somni.[33]

Biofilm

Some bacteria, including H somni, can form large colonies in vivo that are covered by a biofilm, essentially a matrix, or mat, of extracellular polymeric material that aids in persistence of the bacteria and resistance to host defense.[34] Clinical isolates have demonstrated greater and more organized biofilm formation than that from isolates from the healthy prepuce of bulls,[23] suggesting a correlation with virulence. Biofilm formation may be a more common occurrence in the myocardial form of the H somni disease complex than in BRD. The biofilm may play a significant role in shielding the organism from the host immune response and potentially therapeutic antimicrobials.[35,36] Some studies have demonstrated that Pasteurella multocida and H somni grow equally well in a biofilm suggestive of a possible symbiotic relationship,[37] potentially important in BRD.

Lipooligosaccharides

Lipooligosaccharides (LOSs) are an important virulence factor for H somni. They lack the long, repeated polysaccharide side chains typical of the lipopolysaccharides of gram-negative enteric bacteria, thus the difference in terminology.[32] LOSs induce apoptosis of bovine endothelial cells in vitro; this effect is likely to contribute to vasculitis in vivo. Bacterial induction of apoptosis appears to be important in evasion of destruction by host neutrophils.[17,33]

The LOSs of H somni are subject to sialylation, whereby the LOSs incorporate neuraminic acid. This is presumed an important host defense evasion technique, blocking the binding of antibodies, enabling an escape from phagocytosis. Siddaramppa and Inzana[33] demonstrated that sialylation of the LOSs interferes with the binding of the bacteria by antibodies. This results in resistance to immunoglobulins in normal bovine serum. This effect may be associated with a form of antigenic mimicry of the host cells.[19]

Immunoglobulin-Binding Proteins

Corbeil and others[38] demonstrated the existence of immunoglobulin-binding proteins (IgBPs), initially called Fc receptors. They later were determined to form fibrils on the *H somni* cellular surface and are secreted and associated with the outer surface of the bacteria via a known pathway.[8] These fibrils are easily shed from the outer surface of the bacteria.[39]

These fibrillar proteins have the ability to bind with immunoglobulins and may be cytotoxic for macrophages. This essentially assists the organism in evading the host's immune response by providing a shield against recognition and inactivation by the cells of the immune system. This immune evasion capability may contribute to the organism's virulence and resistance to phagocytic killing.[2] It has been shown that there are 2 different types of IgBPs with varying affinity for the Fc region of bovine immunoglobulins. IgBPA is a high-molecular-weight (HMW) protein, 120 kDa, with a strong affinity specifically for IgG2 whereas IgBP (p76) is a 76-kDa protein with less affinity for several classes of immunoglobulins.[35] Later work indicated that the IgBP (p76) is surface exposed and functionally related to the larger IgBPs but is not shed.[34] This protein binds IgG2 and is associated with serum resistance but is not present in serum-sensitive strains. It has been suggested that this protein may have a blocking effect on the binding of antibodies to *H somni*.[33]

Antibacterial Resistance

H somni traditionally has exhibited susceptibility to a wide variety of antimicrobial agents. Many diagnostic laboratories, however, have recognized a trend of increasing antimicrobial resistance based on in vitro testing. This evolving pattern and the potential causes and genetic markers are an area of ongoing research.[40] In addition, the ability to form biofilms in some tissues of the host, may contribute to possible decreased in vivo efficacy of antimicrobials against some of the *H somni* disease syndromes.[33]

Stimulation of IgE Response

H somni has been shown to stimulate a significant IgE response in the host and this appears important in BRD.[31] The IgE antibodies seem to react notably with the 41-kDa MOMP of virulent strains whereas the IgG antibodies react primarily with the 40-kDa OMP as well as IgBPs.[41] The IgE response may account for increased severity in clinical signs of *H somni*–associated BRD and also may be involved with some adverse reactions associated with vaccination.

VARIATION IN VIRULENCE

H somni had been thought to have limited antigenic diversity due to early serologic studies indicating a high degree of homology.[42] In the 1980s, it was noted that there was no apparent strain variation, as indicated by serology and early electrophoresis; however, there was evidence to suggest difference in virulence between some isolates, with recognition of apparently avirulent and virulent strains.[5]

Since the 1980s, studies indicated variation between isolates in the susceptibility or resistance to normal bovine serum and this method was used to characterize isolates, as previously indicated. Some *H somni* isolates, identified as serum sensitive, were subject to inactivation by normal bovine serum. Other isolates, appropriately termed, serum resistant, however, were not affected by the serum. Some preputial isolates, considered avirulent, typically are serum sensitive, whereas most isolates associated with clinical disease are identified as serum resistant.[26] Specific reference isolates have been well recognized as representatives of these 2 groups and used for comparison purposes in many studies. Strain 2336 is a classic pneumonic isolate, demonstrating a high level of virulence, whereas strain 129Pt is a normal, avirulent isolate initially isolated as a commensal from the prepuce. IgBPs are absent in some isolates, which tend to be serum sensitive, whereas serum-resistant isolates usually possess IgBPs. Although there are exceptions to this generalization,[26,43] it does appear that IgBPs are strongly correlated to serum resistance.[2]

It was suggested that serum-susceptible strains from carriers might deserve further investigation as possible vaccine seed candidates, but the serum-resistant strains from carriers most likely are pathogenic.[26] Subsequent work with convalescent serum, evaluating the ability to passively protect calves against pneumonia associated with *H somni*, suggested that the bacterial surface antigens, accessible to antibodies, may be candidates as antigens for a subunit vaccine.[23]

ANTIGENIC VARIATION

Differences in the composition of LOSs and protein surface antigens have been noted between preputial and clinical isolates[25] Inzana and associates[30] demonstrated that the LOS electrophoretic profile for isolates associated with disease indicated major changes during subculturing but no changes were noted with the profiles for the commensal isolates. That is suggestive of antigenic variation due to repeated in vitro passages and potential loss of virulence.

Other studies have shown that the LOS exhibits considerable variability and might undergo phase variation,[17,42] whereas some have described antigenic variation associated with *H somni* LOSs in the face of an immune response.[21,30] This antigenic variation was demonstrated by using monoclonal antibodies to various LOS epitopes.[42] This information is important because it suggests that *H somni* LOS antigenic changes associated with phase variation may facilitate evasion of the host immune response by avoiding recognition.[30] This variation in LOS appears associated with the outer core phosphorylcholine (ChoP) because the inner core epitopes are thought to be well conserved.[19] Howard and colleagues[42] concluded that the high degree of random, phase-variable antigenic heterogeneity exhibited by *H somnus* "must be considered in the design of vaccines and diagnostic tests." These LOS changes probably are related to sialylation.

Some studies have focused on the role of ChoP in colonization and pathogenesis of *H somni*. Sialylation associated with phase variation appears to affect the expression of ChoP on the LOS. Expression of ChoP contributed to colonization of the respiratory tract, whereas phase variable loss of ChoP expression is associated with systemic survival and dissemination.[36] There is a direct relationship between sialylation and virulence, with most clinical (pathogenic) isolates capable of sialylation and commensals, for example, classic preputial isolates, not possessing that trait.[33]

Some isolates possess IgBPs whereas some, typically avirulent strains, do not. Similarly, not all OMPs are possessed by all *H somni* isolates. As discussed previously, some isolates, for example, strain 129Pt, do not have a 41-kDa MOMP.[38] These findings may be of interest in the future development of vaccines. Studies have been conducted to assess the relationship of the 76-kDa IgBP (p76) to the HMW IgBPs. It was concluded that both p76 and the HMW IgBPs play a role in the virulence of H somni[28]

Immune reactivity to both surface and shed fibrils of IgBPs has been observed. Researchers demonstrated a difference in the serologic response of cattle exposed to H somni, compared with other respiratory bacterial pathogens, to a purified IgBP.[44] Convalescent serum from calves recovered from H somni pneumonia neutralize live H somni or concentrated supernatant from bacteria grown in vitro as do antibodies specific to IgBPA.[21] Both p76 and HMW IgBP types are expressed by serum-resistant strains and in 1 study it was noted that all 60 serum-resistant pathogenic strains expressed IgBPs; however, the 4 serum-sensitive preputial strains did not.[36]

In studies of antibody responses to H somni, IgG2 appears more protective against H somni infection than IgG1.[24,38] This difference was confirmed in a study using anti-serum specific to the 40-kDa OMP.[45] Disease severity in challenged calves is inversely proportional to IgG2 antibody levels to H somni.[46]

The 40-K and 78-K OMP antigens appear well conserved among H somni isolates. Even though the MOMP is conserved in isolates associated with disease, some antigenic variation exists. The MOMP may be limited in stimulating an immune response to most disease isolates and may be involved in evading host immune response.[29] It appears that MOMP evades host defenses by both antigenic variation and lack of stimulating responses, perhaps due to limited exposure by being covered by IgBP fibrils. Antibodies to the 40-K OMP provide protection but those to the 78-K MOMP do not, leading to the conclusion that antibody specificity is crucial to protection.[21]

Phase variation associated with the OMP antigens is important. This antigenic variation helps H somni to evade host defenses in the face of an immune response. Phase variation of the OMPs, associated with antigenic variation, also presumably would decrease their value in stimulating a widely protective host response.[42]

GENOMIC VARIATION

Phenotypic variation among H somni isolates was not well recognized until more specific typing techniques evolved. The traditional serotyping methods did not have the specificity required to recognize antigenic differences effectively.[42] In the 1970s, Garcia-Delgado and colleagues[47] compared different H somni isolates and recognized some apparent strain variation using traditional serologically based phenotyping methods. Serology lacked the discriminatory power, however, of later molecular biology-based methodologies, sometimes referred to as DNA fingerprinting or genotyping. Eventually, genetic variation of H somni, then identified as Haemophilus somnus, was recognized using molecular biology.

Three early genotyping or gene sequencing methods used to differentiate H somni isolates included enterobacterial repetitive intergenic consensus (ERIC)–based polymerase chain reaction (PCR), repetitive extragenic palindromic (REP) element–based PCR, and PCR ribotyping. Although all 3 techniques demonstrated variability between isolates, REP-PCR and ERIC-PCR yielded more complex banding patterns with increased discrimination between strains.[48,49] These pioneering PCR typing methodologies have been replaced by newer, more sophisticated sequencing technologies, including multilocus sequence typing (MLST) and whole-genome sequencing (WGS).

WGS of virulent pneumonic isolate strain 2336 and avirulent preputial isolate strain 129Pt indicated significant genomic divergence between these 2 reference isolates.[19] There are similarities as well as differences in the genetic sequences and both appear to have undergone multiple deletions, insertions, and rearrangements. It was noted that many genes that are present in strain 2336, but absent in strain 129Pt, code for various virulence factors, including IgBPs. Kolander and Lawrence noted similar results in a 2013 study, in which they evaluated genomic variation between *H somni* field isolates and reference isolates, both virulent and avirulent, using WGS (Kolander T, Lawrence P. Comparative genomic analysis of virulent and avirulent *H somni* isolates. Unpublished Newport Laboratories Research Report – 14 Oct 2013). They sequenced isolates that expressed varying degrees of virulence in mice and cattle. One particularly virulent isolate in the study, strain TK #21, proved an excellent challenge strain, leading to experimentally induced disease typical of challenge strains in the literature: 2336 and HS91. Strain TK #21 was more virulent in mice than the standard 2336 reference strain.

Three genes, a hemagglutinin OMP, a glycoside hydrolase family protein, and a lipoprotein, present in strain TK #21, were found missing in an avirulent field strain, TK #4 (Kolander T, Lawrence P. Comparative genomic analysis of virulent and avirulent *H somni* isolates. Unpublished Newport Laboratories Research Report – 14 Oct 2013). Although strain TK #4 lacked the genes to be virulent, it was still capable of stimulating an adequate immune response. Some of the missing genes are those thought to be involved in host evasion. As Kolander and Lawrence stated, "PCR testing of the avirulent wild type did not reveal any missing virulence factors when attempts were made to amplify specifically-identified genes. A different avirulent isolate did not result in protective immunity to challenge (Kolander T, Lawrence P. Comparative genomic analysis of virulent and avirulent *H somni* isolates. Unpublished Newport Laboratories Research Report – 14 Oct 2013)." The Kolander and Lawrence study concluded that the genotype of strain TK #4 contributed to its avirulent phenotype. The data suggest that a combination of several genes may be required to make an isolate an effective vaccine or challenge candidate, and the loss of only a few genes can result in significant phenotypic changes, including attenuation of virulence (Kolander T, Lawrence P. Comparative genomic analysis of virulent and avirulent *H somni* isolates. Unpublished Newport Laboratories Research Report – 14 Oct 2013).

All of the recent field isolates in the Kolander and Lawrence study were somewhat similar genotypically, but they were all notably different from the older 2336 and HS91 reference strains, suggesting that the *H somni* population is evolving over time. The newer field isolates from 2012 and 2013 lacked 211 to 316 genes compared with the 2336 reference, isolated in 1985. This also suggests that the generally accepted challenge strain 2336 may no longer be relevant to the *H somni* gene pools currently faced by cattle. Strain HS91, an isolate from 1991, lacked only 15 genes compared with 2336. Because the more recent field isolates were from several different states, it suggests that the genetic drift is a phenomenon occurring nationally with no detectable geographic pattern. Based on the genetic drift observed, the researchers suggested that the vaccine industry needs to evolve in order to maintain relevant vaccines (Kolander T, Lawrence P. Comparative genomic analysis of virulent and avirulent *H somni* isolates. Unpublished Newport Laboratories Research Report – 14 Oct 2013).

Sandal and Inzana[19] used WGS of the pathogenic *H somni* reference strain 2336 to identify several genes associated with recognized virulence factors, including IgBPs, OMPs, LOSs, and iron transport, thus related to the virulence of the organism. A study to compare the genomes of isolates from the 1980s with more recent isolates from

2012 to 2013 suggested there were significant genetic differences in various genes between the old and new isolates.[35] The researchers expressed the concern that these apparent genetic shifts could have significant impact on the effectiveness of bacterins because they all contain seed isolates from the 1970s.

A more recent WGS study by Wiener and Lawrence[50] compared 30 recent field isolates with the well-known historical reference strains, 129PT, HS91, and 2336 (**Table 1**). The validity of their comparative mapping technique was confirmed by comparison with the reference database for strain 2336 (99.67% identical to the National Center for Biotechnology Information reference genome). The newer isolates were only 82% identical to the historical isolates at the whole-genome level. When the genes specifically associated with known virulence factors were evaluated, the 129PT commensal, nonpathogenic historical reference strain lacked many virulence-associated genes compared with the 2336 virulent strain. The commensal strain also lacked more genes associated with virulence than any of the field isolates evaluated (**Table 2**).[50] The data from this study indicate that a combination of several genes is required to make an effective vaccine seed or a challenge isolate and the loss of just a few select genes \ produce significant attenuation effectively resulting in avirulence. Based on the gene changes noted between all the historical isolates and the contemporary isolates, it also was concluded that the *H somni* population is exhibiting genetic drift.[50] This is problematic for the development of effective vaccines that will be universally effective and emphasizes the concern about using vaccine seeds that are several decades old.

One veterinary diagnostic laboratory has developed a MLST technique to assess *H somni* isolates from diagnostic submissions for routine diagnostic use and reporting to submitting practitioners. This method utilizes published data to evaluate nucleotide sequence differences at 7 specific genes, most of which are associated with recognized virulence factors, including IgBPs and OMPs. In addition, gapDH is used as an internal control.[19] This technology allows for characterization of diagnostic isolates submitted from individual veterinary clinics to facilitate comparison for possible strain variation and selection as seeds for bacterin production.

The MLST method also was used to compare multiple contemporary isolates from across the United States for apparent genetic differences at the targeted genes to identify genetic differences. The concatenated dendrogram shown in **Fig. 1** demonstrates that MLST placed the isolates into discrete clusters or clades with genetic distances of 0.7% or more from other clades, which indicates the significant variability of nucleotide sequences at those important genes. There were no significant geographic patterns of distribution. Two large, distinct clades are shown, each containing many isolates that essentially have identical nucleotide sequences at the targeted genes within the clade. The 2 clades differ from each other by approximately 1.2%. There also are several small isolated clusters of just 2 or 3 unique strains and, in 1 case, only 1 isolate. These differences demonstrate the variability of the genomes of contemporary isolates.

The variation in nucleotide sequences of genes coding for known virulence factors is consistent with previously identified antigenic differences. Sequencing technology has advanced rapidly and now can provide more refined and robust results with greater resolution. The genomic testing has become much less expensive and is more feasible to run on a routine basis. Thus, gene sequencing represents a quick and effective methodology of assessing the genomes of *H somni* isolates for the presence, or absence, of virulence factors. Sequencing also allows the comparison of isolates for differences that may be related to antigenic differences, which may affect a host's ability to mount an immune response to different field isolates. Those

Table 1
Histophilus somni isolates evaluated by whole-genome sequencing, including reference isolates and field isolates

Gene Table ID	Date Isolated	Tissue of Origin	Geographic Location	Pathogenic
NPL1	2-May-16	Lung	Ohio	Yes
NPL2	23-May-16	Lung	Iowa	Yes
NPL3	25-May-16	Lung	Ohio	Yes
NPL4	31-May-16	Lung	Ohio	Yes
NPL5	23-Aug-16	Lung	Indiana	n/a
NPL6	1-Nov-16	Heart	Oklahoma	Yes
NPL7	1-Nov-16	Lung	Oklahoma	Yes
NPL8	8-Nov-16	Lung	Oklahoma	Yes
NPL9	22-Dec-16	Lung (central nervous system signs)	Oklahoma	Yes
NPL10	29-Dec-16	Lung	Oklahoma	Yes
NPL11	7-Feb-17	Lung	Iowa	Yes
NPL12	25-Jul-17	Lung	Iowa	Yes
NPL13	13-Sep-17	Pharyngeal swab	Tennessee	Yes
NPL14	4-Oct-17	Lung	Indiana	Yes
NPL15	4-Oct-17	Lung	Indiana	Yes
NPL16	4-Oct-17	Lung	Indiana	Yes
NPL17	10-Oct-17	Lung	Minnesota	Yes
NPL18	3-Nov-17	Lung	Nebraska	Yes
NPL19	19-Nov-17	Lung	Kansas	Yes
NPL20	18-Dec-17	Trachea	Iowa	Yes
NPL21	18-Dec-17	Lung	Nebraska	Yes
NPL22	20-Dec-17	Lung	Iowa	Yes
NPL24	8-Jan-18	Lung	Minnesota	Yes
NPL25	9-Jan-18	Lung	Indiana	Yes
NPL26	12-Jan-18	Lung	Minnesota	Yes
NPL27	18-Jan-18	Lung	South Dakota	Yes
NPL29	13-Feb-18	Lung	South Dakota	Yes
NPL30	23-Feb-18	Heart valve	Texas	Yes
NPL23	28-Dec-17	Lung	Nebraska	Yes
NPL28	5-Feb-18	Nasal swab	Kansas	Yes
NPL31	17-Aug-11	Lung	Minnesota	Yes
NPL33 (HS91 mutant)	1991	Lung		No
NPL34	6-Dec-11	Lung	Kansas	Yes
NPL35	11-Jan-12	Brain	South Dakota	Yes
NPL36	17-Jan-12	Lung	Texas	Yes
NPL37	14-Dec-11	Lung	Idaho	Yes
NPL38	23-Jul-12	Lung	Minnesota	Yes
NPL39 (HS91 mutant)	1991	Lung		No

Courtesy of Newport Laboratories, a Boehringer Ingelheim company, Worthington, MN.

Table 2
Whole-genome sequencing comparison of various *Histophilus somni* isolates showing the number of gene differences

Isolate	Year Isolated	Alignment Rate to 2336 (%)	Genes Present in Comparison to 2236	Genes Absent in Comparison to 2336
2336 (ref pathogen)	1985	99.66	2065	0
129Pt (commensal)	1991	87.82	1616	449
Hs91 (ref pathogen)	1991	99.70	2065	0
NPL33	1991	97.74	1964	101
NPL39	1991	96.86	1965	100
NPL31	2011	92.05	1771	294
NPL34	2011	*88.25*	1856	209
NPL37	2011	91.21	1771	294
NPL35	2012	*83.73*	1871	194
NPL36	2012	*83.23*	1873	192
NPL38	2012	96.03	1874	191
NPL1	2016	90.55	1794	271
NPL2	2016	91.00	1871	194
NPL3	2016	90.49	1804	261
NPL4	2016	90.50	1803	262
NPL5	2016	92.68	1803	262
NPL6	2016	91.08	1788	277
NPL7	2016	91.13	1822	243
NPL8	2016	90.15	1791	274
NPL9	2016	91.81	1769	296
NPL10	2017	*89.72*	1866	199
NPL11	2017	91.52	1763	302
NPL12	2017	*89.28*	1858	207
NPL13	2017	92.41	1708	357
NPL14	2017	90.00	1864	201
NPL15	2017	90.88	1864	201
NPL16	2017	91.30	1763	302
NPL17	2017	*89.02*	1830	235
NPL18	2017	*89.44*	1858	207
NPL19	2017	*87.36*	1767	298
NPL20	2017	92.20	1698	367
NPL21	2017	92.09	1744	321
NPL22	2017	90.94	1853	212
NPL23	2017	*89.00*	1858	207
NPL24	2018	*89.65*	1868	197
NPL25	2018	90.19	1863	202
NPL26	2018	*88.93*	1855	210
NPL27	2018	91.76	1764	301
NPL28	2018	90.62	1765	300
NPL29	2018	90.80	1776	289
NPL30	2018	89.66	1867	198

Courtesy of Newport Laboratories, a Boehringer Ingelheim company, Worthington, MN.

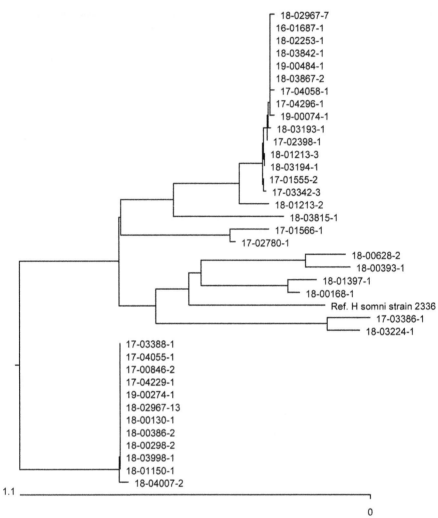

Fig. 1. A concatenated dendrogram from an MLST comparing clinical field *H somni* isolates from across the United States. The scale indicates the percentage of nucleotide sequence differences at the targeted genes. (*Courtesy of* Newport Laboratories, a Boehringer Ingelheim company, Worthington, MN.)

differences identified by gene sequencing technologies also should be considered when selecting seed isolates for vaccines. Field trials of vaccines developed using information gained from sequencing technology are necessary to confirm the practical impact of these findings.

VACCINATION

Killed, whole-cell bacterins have been used for many years to help prevent the *H somni* component of BRD as well as other syndromes, with varying degrees of perceived efficacy.[12] There also have been concerns with adverse effects associated with vaccination with these products.[31] The adverse effects associated with some commercial bacterins may be due to the stimulation of an IgE response involving the 41-kDa MOMP associated with clinical isolates. There currently are 25 US Department of Agriculture commercial *H somni* bacterin licenses held by 9 firms. Many of these products no longer are manufactured. It has been estimated that 69.7% of all large US feedlots currently use *H somni* bacterins.[51] The seed isolates for most of these bacterins were first isolated in the 1970s and because all of the commercial bacterins were licensed before 1985, they are not subject to efficacy testing requirements.[51]

Potential phase-related antigenic heterogeneity of *H somni* is a crucial factor when considering the design of bacterins.[42] In addition, innate antigenic variation between different clinical isolates may make universal vaccine coverage problematic. Some strains, for example, 129Pt, which is from an avirulent carrier, do not possess an intact MOMP but do have the protective 40-kDa OMP to stimulate an IgG response. Those strains might be considered for bacterin seeds to reduce adverse effects.[38] Strain 129Pt, however, does not possess IgBPs, which also are important for protective IgG response. Another factor that complicates the selection of strains for bacterin development is that IgBPs also contribute to the IgE reaction, which likely contributes to adverse reactions.

SUMMARY

H somni is related to a variety of disease syndromes in cattle and plays a significant role in the BRD complex. Although the organism can be an opportunistic pathogen, some isolates are avirulent commensals. Significant research has been conducted to discover the contributing factors that allow some strains to cause disease. *H somni* possesses a wide array of virulence factors, but not all strains exhibit them. Some of these virulence factors are related to the ability to cause disease, such as the stimulation of the host IgE response. In addition, the organism has demonstrated an impressive ability to evade the immune response of the host, primarily due to the function of some of the recognized virulence factors, notably IgBPs that form fibrils on the outer membrane and may be shed. The result is a shielding effect, protecting the actual organism from inactivation by antibodies.

For decades some *H somni* isolates have been categorized as serum sensitive whereas others are serum resistant, based on the ability of normal bovine serum to inactive the organism. The serum-resistant strains tend to be clinically significant whereas commensal, avirulent strains are serum sensitive. The inherent resistance to normal serum antibodies most likely is due to immune evasion.

Many studies have identified antigenic differences between various isolates. Innate antigenic differences between strains represent a challenge to the host immune system due to the specificity of antibody response. Phase variation, related to differences in the chemical structure of the outer membrane LOSs due to sialylation, is another important factor, confounding the ability of the host immune response to react appropriately. Both antigenic variation between isolates and genomic variability correlating to that antigenic variation have been recognized by various researchers in the evaluation of difference between *H somni* isolates. Improved and less expensive gene sequencing techniques provide a quick and effective method of evaluating field isolates.

Evaluation of the WGSs of isolates, with emphasis on those specific genes associated with known virulence factors, has revealed significant differences between contemporary isolates. Evidence also has indicated genetic drift within *H somni* over the past several decades. In addition, genomic analysis utilizing WGS-based MLST to assess variation of targeted genes associated with known virulence factors represents an effective manner of characterizing isolates for potential virulence. This methodology is used routinely to compare field isolates and select appropriate vaccine seeds for autogenous bacterins.

H somni strain differences and phase variations are problematic not only for the host immune system but also for the design of effective vaccines for BRD preventive health programs. The use of commercial whole-cell bacterins to prevent *H somni*–associated respiratory disease has been met with mixed results. Further studies may provide feasible pathways to better address *H somni*–associated BRD through the development of more effective vaccines and preventive health strategies.

DISCLOSURE

The author is employed by Newport Laboratories, owned by Boehringer Ingelheim. Newport Laboratories operates a private veterinary diagnostic laboratory and autogenous biologic manufacturing facility utilizing some of the technologies described in this article.

REFERENCES

1. Brown WW, Griner LA, Jensen R. Infectious embolic meningoencephalitis in cattle. J Am Vet Med Assoc 1956;129:417–21. Available at: https://europepmc.org/abstract/med/13366849.
2. Corbeil LB. *Histophilus somni* host-parasite relationships. Anim Health Res Rev 2008;8(2):141–60. Available at: https://www.researchgate.net/publication/5633891_Histophilus_somni_host-parasite_relationships.
3. Guzman-Brambila C, Rojas-Mayorquin AE, Flores-Samaniego BF, et al. Two outer membrane lipoproteins from *Histophilus somni* are immunogenic in rabbits and sheep and induce protection against bacterial challenge in mice. Clin Vaccine Immunol 2012;19(11):1826–32. Available at: https://www.ncbi.nlm.nih.gov/pmc/articles/PMC3491538/.
4. Griffin D. Bovine pasteurellosis and other bacterial infections of the respiratory tract. Vet Clin North Am Food Anim Pract 2010;26:57–71. Available at: https://www.vetfood.theclinics.com/article/S0749-0720(09)00108-X/fulltext.
5. Harris FW, Janzen ED. The *Haemophilus somnus* disease complex (Hemophilosis): a review. Can Vet J 1989;30:816–22. Available at: https://www.ncbi.nlm.nih.gov/pmc/articles/PMC1681297/pdf/canvetj00563-0050.pdf.
6. Fulton R. Respiratory disease in cattle: isolation of infectious agents and lesions in fatal feedlot cases. Academy of Veterinary Consultants; 2003. Available at: http://avc-beef.org/proceedings/2003-3/Respiratory%20Disease%20in%20Cattle%20-%20Fulton.pdf#search=%22Fulton%22.
7. Agnes JT, Zekarias B, Shao M, et al. Bovine Respiratory Synctial Virus and *Histophilus somni* interaction at the alveolar barrier. Infect Immun 2013;81(7):2592–7. Available at: https://www.ncbi.nlm.nih.gov/pmc/articles/PMC3697614/.
8. Zekarias B, Matoo S, Worby C, et al. *Histophilus somni* IbpA DR2/Fic in virulence and immunoprotection at the natural host alveolar epithelial barrier. Infect Immun 2010;78(5):1850–8. Available at: https://www.ncbi.nlm.nih.gov/pmc/articles/PMC2863524/.
9. Gershwin LJ, Berghaus LJ, Arnold K, et al. Immune mechanisms of pathogenetic synergy in concurrent bovine pulmonary infection with *Haemophilus somnus* and bovine respiratory syncytial virus. Vet Immunol Immunopathol 2005;107:119–30.
10. Confer AW. Update on bacterial pathogenesis in BRD. Anim Health Res 2009;10:145–8. Available at: https://www.ncbi.nlm.nih.gov/pubmed/20003651.

11. Panciera RJ, Dahlgren RR. Rinker HB observations on septicemia of cattle caused by a Haemophilus-like organism. Pathol Vet 1968;5:212–26. Available at: https://journals.sagepub.com/doi/pdf/10.1177/030098586800500303.

12. O'Toole D, Sonderoth KS. Histophilosis as a natural disease. Curr Top Microbiol Immunol 2016;396:15–48. Available at: https://www.ncbi.nlm.nih.gov/pubmed/26847357.

13. Hunsaker B. *Histophilus somni*: impacts on high risk cattle sourced from the southeastern U.S. Academy of Veterinary Consultants Proceedings. 2013. Available at: http://avc-beef.org/proceedings/2013-3/Hunsaker.pdf#search=%22Histophilus%22. Accessed December 6, 2013.

14. Kennedy PC, Biberstein EL, Howarth JA, et al. Infectious meningo-encephalitis in cattle, caused by a *haemophilus*-like organism. Am J Vet Res 1960;21:403–9. Available at: https://www.ncbi.nlm.nih.gov/pubmed/13853365.

15. Radostits OM, Gay CC, Blood DC, et al. *Haemophilus somnus* In: veterinary medicine: a textbook of the diseases of cattle, sheep, pigs, goats and horses. 9th edition. New York: WB Saunders; 2004. p. 832, 895-901.

16. Firehammer BD. Bovine abortion due to *Haemophilus* species. J Am Vet Med Assoc 1959;135:421–2. Available at: http://europepmc.org/abstract/MED/13823032.

17. Songer JG, Post KW. The genera haemophilus, histophilus, and taylorella. In: Songer JG, Post KW, editors. Veterinary microbiology: bacterial and fungal agents of animal disease. St Louis (MO): Elsevier- Saunders; 2005. p. 195-6.

18. Angen O, Ahrens P, Kuhnert P, et al. Proposal of *Histophilus somni* gen. nov., sp. Nov. for the three species *incertae sedis* "Haemophilus somnus", "Haemophilus agni" and "Histopilus ovis". Int J Syst Evol Microbiol 2003;53:1449–56. Available at: https://www.microbiologyresearch.org/content/journal/ijsem/10.1099/ijs.0.02637-0.

19. Sandal I, Inzanza T. A genomic window into the virulence of *Histophilus somni*. Trends Microbiol 2009;18(2):90–9. Available at: https://www.sciencedirect.com/science/article/pii/S0966842X0900256X.

20. Lederer JA, Brown JF, Czuprynski CJ. *Haemophilus somnus*, a facultative intracellular pathogen of bovine mononuclear phagocytes. Infect Immun 1987;55: 381–7. Available at: https://www.ncbi.nlm.nih.gov/pmc/articles/PMC260338/.

21. Corbeil LB. Host immune response to *Histophilus somni*. In: Inzana TW, editor. *Histophilus somni* part of current topics in microbiology and immunology series, vol. 366. Switzerland: Springer International Publishing; 2016. p. 109–29. Available at: https://link.springer.com/chapter/10.1007%2F82_2015_5012.

22. Corbeil LB, Arthur JE, Widders PR, et al. Antigenic specificity of convalescent serum from cattle with *Haemophilus somnus* induced experimental abortion. Infect Immun 1987;55:1381–6. Available at: https://www.ncbi.nlm.nih.gov/pmc/articles/PMC260524/.

23. Gogolewski RP, Kania SA, Inzana TJ, et al. Protective ability and specificity of convalescent serum from calves with *Haemophilus somnus* pneumonia. Infect Immun 1987;55(6):1403–11. Available at: https://www.ncbi.nlm.nih.gov/pubmed/3570472.

24. Gogolewski RP, Kania SA, Liggitt HD, et al. Protective ability of antibodies against 78- and 40- kilodalton outer membrane antigens of *Haemophilus somnus*. Infect Immun 1988;56(9):2307–16. Available at: https://www.ncbi.nlm.nih.gov/pmc/articles/PMC259565/.

25. Corbeil LB, Gogolewski RP, Stephens LR, et al. *Haemophilus somnus:* antigen analysis and immune responses. In: Donachie W, Lainson FA, Hodgson JC, editors. *Haemophilus, actinobacillus*, and *pasteurella*. New York: Plenum Press;

1995. p. 63–73. Available at: https://link.springer.com/chapter/10.1007%2F978-1-4899-0978-7_6.

26. Corbeil LB, Blau K, Prieur DJ, et al. Serum susceptibility of *Haemophilus somnus* from bovine clinical cases and carriers. J Clin Microbiol 1985;22:192–8. Available at: https://www.ncbi.nlm.nih.gov/pmc/articles/PMC268357/.

27. Sethi S, Murphy TF. Bacterial infection in chronic obstructive pulmonary disease in 2000: a state of the art review. Clin Microbiol Rev 2001;14:336–63. Available at: https://www.ncbi.nlm.nih.gov/pmc/articles/PMC88978/.

28. Sanders JD, Bastida-Corcuera FD, Arnold KF, et al. Genetic manipulation of immunoglobulin binding proteins of *Haemophilus somnus*. Microb Pathog 2003;34:131–9. Available at: https://www.sciencedirect.com/science/article/pii/S0882401002001882.

29. Tagawa Y, Haritani M, Ishikawa H, et al. Characterization of a heat-modifiable outer membrane protein of *Haemophilus somnus*. Infect Immun 1993;61:1750–5. Available at: https://www.ncbi.nlm.nih.gov/pmc/articles/PMC280761/.

30. Inzana TJ, Gogolewski RP. Corbeil LB phenotypic phase variation in *Haemophilus somnus* lipooligosaccharide during bovine pneumonia and after in vitro passage. Infect Immun 1992;60:2943–51. Available at: https://www.ncbi.nlm.nih.gov/pmc/articles/PMC257258/.

31. Ellis JA, Jong C. Systemic adverse reactions in young Simmental calves following administration of a combined vaccine. Can Vet J 1997;38:45–7. Available at: https://www.researchgate.net/publication/14214062_Systemic_adverse_reactions_in_young_Simmental_calves_following_administration_of_a_combination_vaccine.

32. Perez DS, Perez FA, Bretschneider G. Pathogenicity of *Histophilus somni*. An Vet (Murcia) 2010;26:5–21. Available at: https://digitum.um.es/digitum/bitstream/10201/20617/1/Histophilus%20somni%20actualizacion%20de%20la%20patogenicidad%20en%20vacuno.pdf.

33. Siddaramppa D, Inzana TJ. – *Haemophilus somnus* virulence factors and resistance to host immunity. Anim Health Res Rev 2004;5(1):79–93. Available at: https://www.researchgate.net/profile/Thomas_Inzana/publication/8254131_IHaemophilus_somnus_virulence_factors_and_resistance_to_host_immunity/links/0fcfd5119014d85275000000/IHaemophilus-somnus-virulence-factors-and-resistance-to-host-immunity.pdf?origin=publication_detail.

34. Donlan RM, Costerton JW. Biofilms: survival mechanisms of clinically relevant microorganisms. Clin Microbiol 2002;15:167–93. Available at: https://www.ncbi.nlm.nih.gov/pubmed/11932229.

35. Madampage CA, Rawlyk N, Crockford G, et al. Single nucleotide polymorphisms in the bovine *Histophilus somni* genome; a comparison of new and old isolates. Can J Vet Res 2015;79(3):190–200. Available at: https://www.ncbi.nlm.nih.gov/pmc/articles/PMC4445511/.

36. Sandal I, Shao JQ, Annadata S, et al. *Histophilus somni* biofilm formation in cardiopulmonary tissues of the bovine host following respiratory challenge. Microbes Infect 2009;11(2):254–63. Available at: https://www.sciencedirect.com/science/article/pii/S1286457908003389.

37. Elswaifi SF, Scarratt WK, Inzana TJ. The role of lipooligosaccharide phosphorylcholine in colonization and pathogenesis of *Histophilus somni* in cattle. Vet Res 2012;43(1):49. Available at: https://www.ncbi.nlm.nih.gov/pmc/articles/PMC3406970/.

38. Corbeil LB, Bastida-Corcuera FD. Beveridge TJ Haemophilus somnus immunoglobulin binding proteins and surface fibrils. Infect Immun 1997;65:4250–7. Available at: https://www.ncbi.nlm.nih.gov/pmc/articles/PMC175610/pdf/654250.pdf.

39. Yarnall M, Widders PR, Corbeil LB. Isolation and characterization of Fc receptors from *Haemophilus somnus*. J Immunol 1988;28:1129–37. Available at: https://onlinelibrary.wiley.com/doi/abs/10.1111/j.1365-3083.1988.tb02424.x.
40. Deal C. Characterization of multidrug resistant *Histophilus somni* associated with bovine respiratory disease. University of Nebraska Undergraduate Honors Thesis; 2019. Available at: https://digitalcommons.unl.edu/honorsembargoed/68/.
41. Corbeil LB, Arnold KF, Kimball R, et al. Specificity of IgG and IgE antibody responses to *Haemophilus somnus* infection of calves. Vet Immunol Immunopathol 2006;113:191–9. Available at: https://www.sciencedirect.com/science/article/pii/S0165242706001395.
42. Howard MD, Cox AD, Weiser JN, et al. Antigenic diversity of *Haemophilus somus* lipooligosaccharide: phase variable accessibility of the phosphorylcholine epitope. J Clin Microbiol 2000;38:4412–9. Available at: https://www.ncbi.nlm.nih.gov/pmc/articles/PMC87614/.
43. Widders PR, Dorrance LA, Yarnall M, et al. Immunoglobulin-binding activity among pathogenic and carrier isolates of *Haemophilus somnus*. Infect Immun 1989;57:639–42. Available at: https://www.ncbi.nlm.nih.gov/pmc/articles/PMC313146/.
44. Yarnall M, Carbeil LB. Antibody response to *Haemophilus somnus* Fc receptor. J Clin Microbiol 1989;27:111–7. Available at: https://www.ncbi.nlm.nih.gov/pmc/articles/PMC267244/.
45. Corbeil LB, Gogolewski RP, Kacskovics I, et al. Bovine IgG2a antibodies to *Haemophilus somnus* and allotype expression. Can J Vet Res 1997;61:207–13. Available at: https://www.ncbi.nlm.nih.gov/pmc/articles/PMC1189405/pdf/cjvetres00019-0049.pdf.
46. Berghaus LJ, Corbeil LB, Berghaus RD, et al. Effects of dual vaccination for bovine respiratory syncytial virus and Haemophilus somnus on immune responses. Vaccine 2006;24(33–34):6018–27.
47. Garcia-Delgado GA, Little PB, Barnum DA. A comparision of various *Haemophilus somnus* strains. Can J Comp Med 1977;41:380–8. Available at: https://www.ncbi.nlm.nih.gov/pubmed/922555.
48. Appuhamy S, Parton R, Coote JG, et al. Genomic fingerprinting of *Haemophilus somnus* by a combination of PCR methods. J Clin Microbiol 1997;35(1):288–91. Available at: https://www.ncbi.nlm.nih.gov/pmc/articles/PMC229560/.
49. Fussing V, Wegner HC. Characterization of bovine *Haemophilus somnus* by biotyping, plasmid profiling, REA-patterns and ribotyping. Zentralbl Bakteriol 1993;279:60–74. Available at: https://www.sciencedirect.com/science/article/abs/pii/S0934884011804925.
50. Wiener B, Lawrence P. Genomic comparision of *Histophilus somni* strains show genetic drift. AABP Research Summaries Poster Presentation. 2018. Available at: http://aabp.org/members/publications/2018/proceedings/49%20Posters.pdf. Accessed September 13, 2018.
51. Ruby K. Histophilus vaccine research. Academy of Veterinary Consultants Proceedings. 2019. Available at: http://avc-beef.org/proceedings/2019-2/Ruby.pdf. Accessed August 8, 2019.

Respiratory Bacterial Microbiota in Cattle

From Development to Modulation to Enhance Respiratory Health

Edouard Timsit, DVM, PhD[a],*, Chris McMullen, BSc[b,1],
Samat Amat, MSc, PhD[b,c,d,2], Trevor W. Alexander, PhD[c,3]

KEYWORDS

- Microbiome • Bovine respiratory disease • 16S rRNA sequencing • Metagenome
- Alternative to antimicrobials

KEY POINTS

- The respiratory bacterial microbiota is dynamic, changing significantly during periods of increased risk for bovine respiratory disease.
- The respiratory microbiota is inhabited predominantly by 5 bacterial phyla: Proteobacteria, Firmicutes, Tenericutes, Actinobacteria, and Bacteroidetes; the relative abundance of each differs by animal age and production system.
- Upper respiratory tract and lower respiratory tract microbiotas differ in diversity and composition. The nasopharyngeal microbiota contributes the most to the lower respiratory microbiota and thus should be the primary target for sampling or modulation strategies.
- Composition of the respiratory microbiota is associated with respiratory health; increased abundances of respiratory *Lactobacillus* and/or *Lactococcus* are associated with good respiratory health.
- Intranasal application of selected *Lactobacillus* strains modifies the composition of the nasopharyngeal microbiotas in cattle and can provide colonization resistance against opportunistic bacterial pathogens such as *Mannheimia haemolytica*.

[a] Ceva Santé Animale, 10 Avenue de la Ballastière, Libourne 33500, France; [b] Faculty of Veterinary Medicine, University of Calgary, Calgary, Alberta, Canada; [c] Lethbridge Research and Development Center, Agriculture and Agri-Food Canada, Lethbridge, Alberta, Canada; [d] Department of Agricultural, Food and Nutritional Science, University of Alberta, Edmonton, Alberta, Canada
[1] Present address: 3280 Hospital Drive Northwest, Calgary, Alberta T2N 4Z6, Canada.
[2] Present address: Room 3-60D1 Ag/For Center Edmonton, Alberta T6G 2P5, Canada.
[3] Present address: 5403 1st Avenue South, Lethbridge, Alberta T1J 4B1, Canada.
* Corresponding author.
E-mail address: Edouard.timsit@ceva.com

INTRODUCTION

Over the past decade it has become clear that mammals live in symbiosis with their abundant resident microbes.[1] Advances in culture-independent techniques (eg, 16S ribosomal RNA [rRNA] sequencing) have enabled detection and quantification of bacterial species that are difficult or impossible to detect by culture-based methods (**Box 1**).[2] These advances in the field of molecular techniques, in particular metagenomics, have led to the definition of the animal microbiota, a term that refers to the complex microbial ecosystems in and on bodies of animals.[1]

Like other body sites, the respiratory tract of cattle is colonized by a variety of different bacterial microbiotas directly after birth.[3] Composition and diversity of these microbiotas have been recently associated with respiratory health in cattle.[4,5] More specifically, airway microbiotas enriched with known beneficial bacteria, such as *Lactobacillus*, have been associated with good respiratory health,[6,7] whereas microbiotas enriched with known bacterial pathogens, such as *Mycoplasma bovis, Mannheimia haemolytica*, or *Pasteurella multocida*, have been associated with bovine respiratory disease (BRD).[4,6]

Investigating the role of the respiratory microbiota in health and disease is a relatively new, rapidly developing field of research that provides new opportunities for the prevention and treatment of BRD.[8] This review summarizes current knowledge regarding composition of the respiratory bacterial microbiota in dairy cattle and beef cattle and its relationship with the development of BRD. Approaches to modulate the respiratory bacterial microbiota to promote enhanced heath (eg, probiotics, bacteriophages, and prebiotics) also are discussed.

Box 1
16S rRNA sequencing

Typically, short segments of the 16S rRNA that include hypervariable regions are sequenced for bacterial classification in microbiota studies (**Fig. 1**). Therefore, composition of the respiratory microbiota often is reported at the phylum, family, or genus level but not at the species level because only a small proportion (30%–50%) of these short 16S rRNA sequences can be classified as OTUs beyond the genus level.

COMPOSITION OF THE BACTERIAL RESPIRATORY MICROBIOTA IN HEALTHY CATTLE

The diversity of bacteria on earth is vast, comprising 55 phyla.[9] The cattle respiratory tract is inhabited predominantly by 5 of these phyla (Proteobacteria, Firmicutes, Tenericutes, Actinobacteria, and Bacteroidetes [**Table 1**]), which underlines its suitability for the growth of only a limited number of bacteria. This diversity is largely due to the biophysical properties of respiratory mucosal surfaces, that is, temperature, moisture, and pH.[10]

The composition of the airway microbiotas evolves over time due to a variety of selection pressures, which further influence the colonization process of the respiratory tract, including (**Fig. 2**) (1) endogenous forces, such as mucus, IgA, and innate/adaptative immune recognition,[10] and (2) exogenous forces, such as the maternal vaginal microbiota,[3] environmental biodiversity,[11] diet,[12] infection,[4,6] stressful events (weaning, transportation, and commingling)[13-15] and parenteral antibiotics.[16,17] Unfortunately, to date, no study has described the composition of the developing airway microbiotas across the life span of either dairy cattle or beef cattle.

A systematic review of the literature (performed in PubMed on December 12, 2019; key words [respiratory] AND [cattle] AND [microbiota OR microbiome]) revealed that

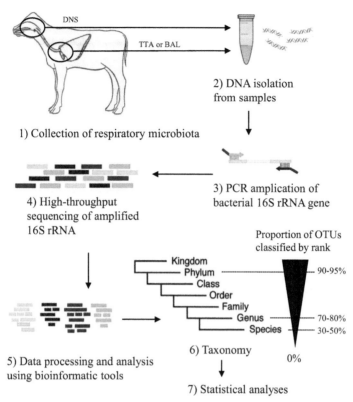

1) Collection of respiratory microbiota

2) DNA isolation from samples

3) PCR amplification of bacterial 16S rRNA gene

4) High-throughput sequencing of amplified 16S rRNA

5) Data processing and analysis using bioinformatic tools

6) Taxonomy

7) Statistical analyses

Proportion of OTUs classified by rank

Kingdom
Phylum — 90-95%
Class
Order
Family
Genus — 70-80%
Species — 30-50%

0%

Fig. 1. Schematic illustration of basic workflow for respiratory microbiota research (16S rRNA sequencing). Only a small proportion of the OTUs are classified at the species level (30%–50%). BAL, bronchoalveolar lavage; DNS, deep nasal swab; TTA, transtracheal aspiration. (*Adapted from* Jo JH, Kennedy EA, Kong H. Research techniques made simple: bacterial 16s ribosomal RNA gene sequencing in cutaneous research. *J Invest Dermatol.* 2016; 136, e23ee27; with permission).

most published studies have focused on the respiratory microbiota of postweaned beef cattle (n = 16), with only a limited number of studies describing the composition of the nasopharyngeal microbiota in preweaned dairy calves (n = 3)[3,4,18] or beef calves (n = 2).[19,20] Furthermore, these studies focused on the upper respiratory tract (URT), with only 6 studies reporting the composition of the lower respiratory tract (LRT) microbiota (sampled by transtracheal aspiration[6,11,13,21] or bronchoalveolar lavage [McMullen C, Alexander TW, Leguillette R, et al. Topography of the respiratory tract bacterial microbiota in feedlot beef calves, submitted for publication][22]).

The Nasopharyngeal Microbiota from Birth to 1 Month of Age in Dairy Calves

Colonization of the airways in dairy calves begins immediately after birth and evolves quickly during the first weeks of life.[3] Abundance of bacteria in the nasopharynx (measured by the number of 16S rRNA gene copies) increases significantly from birth to 14 days of age and then either decreases slightly until day 35[4] or remains the same until day 42.[23] The interval from birth to day 14, therefore, is highly critical for microbial establishment[23] and can predispose calves to a healthy state or pneumonia/otitis during the first weeks of age (discussed later).

The nasopharyngeal microbiota of preweaned dairy calves is dominated by Proteobacteria, especially at 3 days and 14 days of age, when this phylum can represent up to 70% of total bacterial diversity[3,4,18] (see **Table 1**). After day 14, however, the diversity (combined richness and evenness) of the nasopharynx increases, with other phyla becoming more abundant (including Tenericutes, Firmicutes, Actinobacteria, and Bacteroidetes).[3,4,18] The most abundant bacterial genera in the nasopharynx of dairy calves are *Mannheimia, Moraxella, Mycoplasma, Psychrobacter,* and *Pseudomonas.* Relative abundances of these genera change over time, with the relative abundance of *Moraxella* decreasing between day 14 and day 35 and the relative abundances of *Mannheimia* and *Mycoplasma* concurrently increasing substantially.[3,4]

In dairy calves, composition of the nasopharyngeal microbiota is highly influenced by the maternal vaginal microbiota.[3] In 81 dairy cow-calf pairs, 73%, 76%, and 87% of the bacteria detected by next-generation sequencing (ie, operational taxonomic units [OTUs]) were shared between the maternal vaginal microbiota and the calf nasopharyngeal microbiota at 3 days, 14 days, and 35 days of age, respectively.[3] The most abundant shared bacterial genera in the dam vaginal and calf nasopharyngeal samples across all sampling days were *Mannheimia, Moraxella, Bacteroides, Streptococcus,* and *Pseudomonas.*[3] The significant overlap between the 2 microbiotas was attributed to the transfer of maternal microbes to the neonate at birth via the vaginal canal. *Mannheimia* was found to be relatively more abundant in the vaginal microbiota of dams whose calves did not develop pneumonia and/or otitis compared with the microbiota of dams whose calves did develop disease.[3] Therefore, it appears that the prepartum higher abundance of *Mannheimia* in the vagina of dairy cows may confer a protective effect on the health of the respiratory tract and middle ear of their progeny.

The Nasopharyngeal Microbiota from Initial Vaccination to Preconditioning or Weaning in Beef Cattle (ie, Preweaned Beef Cattle)

The nasopharyngeal microbiota changes significantly between initial vaccination (approximately 40 days of age) and preconditioning (approximately 130 days of age) or weaning (approximately 150 days of age) in beef calves.[19,20] At initial vaccination, the diversity of the nasopharyngeal microbiota is low, with a high abundance of bacteria from the phylum Actinobacteria (more specifically, from the *Promicromonosporaceae* and *Microbacteriaceae* families).[19,20] Nasopharyngeal diversity then increases, with higher proportions of Tenericutes, Proteobacteria, and Firmicutes at the time of preconditioning or weaning.[19,20] At the genera level, relative abundances of *Mycoplasma,*[19,20] *Moraxella,*[19,20] and *Psychrobacter*[20] were higher at weaning than at initial vaccination. Although some commonalities of evolution among calves exist, groups of preweaned calves that were raised on different farms evolved differently (even when managed similarly),[19,20] implying that factors other than age (eg, environment and contact with older animals) have important roles in development of the nasopharyngeal microbiota.

The Nasopharyngeal Microbiota from Weaning to the First Weeks on Feed in Beef Cattle (ie, Postweaned Beef Cattle)

The structure of the nasopharyngeal microbiota evolves significantly from weaning at the ranch to 40 days to 60 days after entrance to a feedlot.[13–16] The largest shift occurs between departure from the ranch of origin and the first 7 days on feed, with a sharp increase in diversity of the nasopharyngeal microbiota during this short interval.[13–16] For example, the number of bacterial taxons (ie, OTUs) almost doubled (100 OTUs

Table 1
Composition of the nasopharyngeal microbiota in preweaned and postweaned beef calves and preweaned dairy calves

Type	Study Design	Phylum Level	Genus Level	Reference[a]
Postweaned feedlot beef calves	Cross-sectional; 2 populations (BRD, n = 82; healthy, n = 82)	Proteobacteria (69.3%), Tenericutes (22.5%), Firmicutes (3.3%), Actinobacteria (2.3%), Bacteroidetes (2.3%)	Mycoplasma (22.2%), Moraxella (19.5%), Histophilus (19.0%), Psychrobacter (9.8%), Mannheimia (6.3%), Pasteurella (4.4%), Pseudomonas (1.8%)	McMullen et al,[39] 2019
	Longitudinal; 4 populations (BRD at entry, n = 22; BRD at diagnosis; n = 22, healthy at entry, n = 44; healthy at diagnosis, n = 10)	Proteobacteria (34.8%), Firmicutes (18.6%), Actinobacteria (17.2%), Bacteroidetes (12.1%), Tenericutes (11.2%), Fusobacteria (1.2%)	Moraxella (10.9%), Mycoplasma (10.7%), Acinetobacter (9.7%), Rathayibacter (5.0%), Promicromonospora (4.4%), Mannheimia (4.1%), Solibacillus (3.5%), Clostridium (3.3%), Corynebacterium (3.8%), Pasteurella (1.9%)	Zeineldin et al,[31] 2017
	Longitudinal; 2 populations of 30 calves sampled at the ranch (d 0), at feedlot entry (d 2), and on d 7 and d 28 after entry	Tenericutes (41.1%), Proteobacteria (31.8%), Firmicutes (4.6%)	Mycoplasma (40.8%), Moraxella (18.7%), Pasteurella (6.8%), Mannheimia (3.8%)	Stroebel et al,[13] 2018
	Longitudinal; 1 population of 4 calves	Proteobacteria (68.9%), Firmicutes (19.2%)	At entry: Pseudomonas (23.7%), Shewanella (23.5%), Acinetobacter	Holman et al,[2] 2015

(continued on next page)

Table 1
(continued)

Type	Study Design	Phylum Level	Genus Level	Reference[a]
	sampled at feedlot entry and on d 60 after entry		(17.5%), *Carnobacterium* (12.2%). At d 60: *Staphylococcus* (20.8%), *Mycoplasma* (14.9%), *Mannheimia* (10.4%), *Moraxella* (9.4%)	Timsit et al,[14] 2016
	Longitudinal; 1 population of 30 calves sampled at the ranch (d 0), at feedlot entry (d 2), and on d 40 after entry	Tenericutes (53.2%), Proteobacteria (34.7%), Firmicutes (4.2%), Bacteroidetes (3.7%), Actinobacteria (3.4%)	NR	
	Longitudinal; 2 populations (treated with NORS [n = 10] or tilmicosin [n = 10] at entry) sampled at entry, and on d 1, d 5, and d 10 after entry	Tenericutes (92.8%), Proteobacteria (5.9%), Firmicutes (0.6%), Actinobacteria (0.6%), Bacteroidetes (0.1%)	NR	Timsit et al,[25] 2017
	Cross-sectional; 3 populations (controls, n = 5; medium selenium, n = 6; high selenium, n = 5)	Proteobacteria (31.7%), Bacteroidetes (27.5%), Firmicutes (24.3%), Actinobacteria (7.1%), Tenericutes (4.4%)	NR	Hall et al,[12] 2017
	Longitudinal; 1 population of 13 calves sampled at the ranch (d 0), at feedlot entry (d 2) and on d 5 and d 12 after entry	Proteobacteria (36.1%), Firmicutes (20.1%), Tenericutes (19.3%), Actinobacteria (12.7%), Bacteroidetes (8.6%)	NR	Amat et al,[24] 2019

Preweaned and postweaned beef calves	Longitudinal; 3 populations of 40 calves sampled at initial vaccination, weaning and on d 40 after entry at feedlots	Proteobacteria (27.5%), Actinobacteria (25.9%), Tenericutes (24.3%), Firmicutes (13.5%)	Mycoplasma (24.1%), Lactococcus (10.7%), Moraxella (7.4%), Histophilus (6.78%), Pasteurella (6.0%)	McMullen et al,[19] 2018
Preweaned dairy calves	Longitudinal; 1 population of 81 calves sampled at 3 d, 14 d, and 35 d of age	Proteobacteria (52.1%), Firmicutes (23.0%), Bacteroidetes (11.4%), Tenericutes (3.4%)	NR	Lima et al,[3] 2019

Abbreviation: NR, data not reported; NORS, nitric oxide releasing solution.
a Only studies reporting the general composition of the nasopharyngeal microbiota are presented.
Data from Refs.[2,3,12–14,19,24,25,31,39]

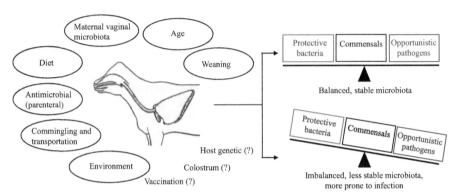

Fig. 2. Factors influencing the composition of the respiratory microbiota in cattle. The microbiota can develop toward a balanced, stable microbiota, which is more resistant against pathogens colonization and/or proliferation. Conversely, the microbiota also can develop toward a community that is imbalanced, less stable, and more prone to infection. (*Adapted from* van den Broek MFL, De Boeck I, Kiekens F, Boudewyns A, Vanderveken OM, Lebeer S. Translating recent microbiome insights in otitis media into probiotic strategies. *Clin Microbiol Rev.* 2019; 3, 32; with permission).

vs 200 OTUs) in the nasopharynx of 13 beef steer calves during the 48-hour interval from leaving ranch of origin to on-arrival processing at a feedlot.[24]

The nasopharyngeal microbiota stabilizes after the first week on feed, with diversity either remaining the same or slightly decreasing until 40 days to 60 days on feed.[14,15,17] The nasopharyngeal microbiota also becomes more homogeneous among cattle during this interval.[15,25] For example, at day 0 prior to transport, 76 OTUs were shared in the nasopharyngeal microbiota of 14 Angus-Herford cross heifers, whereas at 5 days and 12 days after arrival at a research feedlot, there were 373 and 274 OTUs, respectively, that were shared among these cattle.[15]

Numerous factors can explain significant shifts in the structure of the nasopharyngeal microbiota around cattle marketing (**Fig. 2**). First, transportation and adaptation to a feedlot environment have a major effect on the nasopharyngeal bacterial community.[13–16] By sampling the nasopharynx of preconditioned calves that were transported directly to a research feedlot, Holman and colleagues[15] (2017) determined that presence and relative abundance of numerous bacteria changed significantly before (day 0) and after (day 2) transportation, with a higher abundance of *Acinetobacter* and *Streptococcus* and a lower abundance of *Pasteurella* and *Bacillus* after transportation. This shift in the nasopharyngeal microbiota occurred even in the absence of commingling or change in diet, because cattle were fed the same diet at both locations and were kept separate from other cattle housed at the feedlot.

Adaptation to new diets and mixing cattle from multiple origins also alter the structure of the nasopharyngeal microbiota in cattle.[12,13] For example, recently weaned beef calves fed selenium-biofortified alfalfa hay had a higher bacterial diversity in their nasal cavities compared with healthy controls.[12] Concerning the impact of mixing cattle on the nasopharyngeal microbiota, a minimum duration and frequency of contact among cattle is needed for horizontal transmission of commensal and pathogenic bacteria to occur. Commingling cattle for 24 hours at an auction market did not significantly affect the diversity or the composition of the nasopharyngeal bacteria in 2 groups of 15 recently weaned beef calves.[13] This suggests that being held for 24 hours at an auction market was not enough time to allow bacterial transfer or that the environment of the auction market was not conducive to interanimal bacterial transfer.

Finally, parenteral antibiotics given at or soon after arrival to control BRD (ie, meta-phylaxis) modifies diversity and composition of the nasopharyngeal microbiota.[13,16,17] A single parenteral injection of either oxytetracycline or tulathromycin at feedlot place-ment altered the nasopharyngeal microbiota in comparison with cattle receiving only in-feed antibiotics for up to 60 days postadministration; oxytetracycline significantly reduced relative abundance of *Mannheimia* from feedlot entry to 60 days postarrival and cattle given either oxytetracycline or tulathromycin had a significantly lower rela-tive abundance of *Mycoplasma* at day 60 compared with those given only an in-feed antibiotics.[17] Effects of parenteral oxytetracycline and tulathromycin on the naspha-ryngeal microbiota were most important at days 2 and 5 post-treatment.[16] At that time, both oxytetracycline and tulathromycin appeared to confer some protection against *Pasteurella* spp colonization in the nasopharynx.

The nasopharyngeal microbiota of postweaned beef cattle often is dominated largely by Proteobacteria and Tenericutes, with lower proportions of Firmicutes, Acti-nobacteria, and Bacteroidetes (see **Table 1**). Of the dominant genera, *Mycoplasma*, *Moraxella, Acinetobacter, Psychrobacter, Mannheimia, Pasteurella*, and *Corynebacte-rium* are identified most frequently. There is considerable variability, however, in composition of the nasopharyngeal microbiota among groups of cattle and even among individual cattle within a group.[13,19] Furthermore, as discussed previously, the nasopharyngeal microbiota evolves significantly from entrance to the first weeks on feed. Therefore, it is difficult to identify a so-called normal microbiota in feedlot cattle.

In summary, the nasopharyngeal microbiota of beef cattle changes significantly be-tween weaning and the first weeks on feed. This evolution may explain why beef cattle are more susceptible to BRD during the first 40 days to 60 days on feed,[26] because an unstable microbiota is less resistant to colonization by pathogens.[27]

Composition of the Lower Respiratory Tract Microbiota

The LRT, previously thought to be sterile, is now known to harbor a unique microbiota (**Fig. 3**).[6,11,13,21,22] Characterization of the tracheal[6,11,13] and bronchial[22] microbiotas in cattle revealed that these bacterial communities are distinct from nasal and naso-pharyngeal microbiotas. Bacterial communities in the LRT are less rich and less diverse than the URT microbiotas,[6,11] consistent with URT being directly exposed to ambient airborne microbial communities. Furthermore, some bacteria, such as *My-coplasma*[6,11,13] and *Pasteurella*,[11,22] typically are enriched in the LRT compared with the URT.

Despite differences between URT and LRT microbiotas, most bacterial genera iden-tified in the LRT also are present in the URT (McMullen C, Alexander TW, Leguillette R, et al. Topography of the respiratory tract bacterial microbiota in feedlot beef calves, submitted for publication).[11,22] This is explained by the fact that, in healthy animals, bacterial composition of the LRT is determined more by a constant flow (immigration and elimination) of transient bacteria originating from the URT than replication of resi-dent bacteria.[28] In humans, the bacteria reaching the lung primarily originate from the oropharynx and the mouth.[28] In cattle, however, the nasopharynx seems to be the pri-mary source of bacteria for the LRT. In a recent study by the authors' team (McMullen C, Alexander TW, Leguillette R, et al. Topography of the respiratory tract bacterial microbiota in feedlot beef calves, submitted for publication), which compared bacte-rial communities of 17 locations across the respiratory tract, the lung microbiota was more compositionally similar to the nasopharynx than any other URT microbiota, including the mouth, oropharynx, palatine tonsils, or nostrils. Consequently, the naso-pharyngeal microbiota should be the primary target for sampling strategies and the

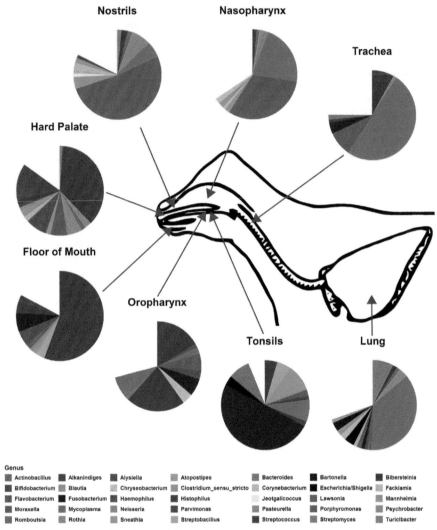

Fig. 3. Mean relative abundance of bacteria present at greater than or equal to 1% abundance at the genus level of different URT and LRT sampling locations in 15 healthy beef steer calves. URT, upper respiratory tract; LRT, lower respiratory tract. (*From* McMullen C, Alexander TW, Leguillette R, et al. Topography of the respiratory tract bacterial microbiota in feedlot beef calves. submitted for publication; with permission).

principal niche in the URT to modulate in order to promote good respiratory health (ie, prebiotics, probiotics, and bacteriophages).

INFLUENCE OF THE BACTERIAL MICROBIOTA ON RESPIRATORY HEALTH

Composition, diversity, and stability of the respiratory microbiota can play a role in either predisposing cattle to BRD or providing protection against colonization and/ or proliferation of bacterial pathogens in the respiratory tract (also known as colonization resistance) (see **Fig. 2**).[5]

Role of the Composition of the Microbiota on Respiratory Health

Primary bacteria involved in BRD are *M haemolytica*, *P multocida*, *H somni*, and *Mycoplasma bovis* (**Table 2**). Although these bacteria are opportunistic in nature, cattle with them in their respiratory tract are at higher risk of developing BRD.[29] For example, recently weaned beef cattle positive for *M haemolytica* on deep nasopharyngeal swabs at feedlot entry were more likely (odds ratio 1.7; 95% CI, 1.1–2.4) to be affected with BRD within 10 days after arrival than cattle negative for this bacterium.[30] Furthermore, in 174 dairy calves, relative abundance of *Mannheimia* and *Mycoplasma* was higher at days 14 and/or 28 in the nasopharynx of calves that subsequently developed BRD versus those that remained healthy.[4] Therefore, limiting colonization of opportunistic bacterial pathogens in the respiratory tract can reduce the prevalence of BRD in cattle.

Based on recent 16S rRNA sequencing, presence of bacteria other than *Pasteurellaceae* or *Mycoplasma bovis* in the respiratory tract also may predispose cattle to BRD (see **Table 2**). For example, *Moraxella* was enriched in the nasopharynx of calves that developed BRD.[4,31,32] Furthermore, a bacterium from the Leptotrichiaceae family was more abundant among postmortem lung tissue samples from dairy calves that died from BRD compared with lesion-free lung tissue of clinically healthy calves.[33] These findings indicate that there may be other bacterial species with the potential to be secondary BRD pathogens that the veterinary community is unaware of. Before implementing mitigation strategies against them, however, further research is needed to confirm a causal relation between their presence in the respiratory microbiota and BRD.

Comparison of the respiratory tract microbiota of healthy calves with those that developed BRD revealed the presence of specific commensal bacteria in the respiratory tract that can confer protection against the disease (see **Table 2**). For example, cattle having a higher relative abundance of *Lactobacillaceae* and *Bacillaceae* in their nasopharynx at feedlot entry were less likely to develop BRD during the first 60 days on feed.[7] Furthermore, in a comparison of the nasopharyngeal and tracheal microbiotas of 60 feedlot cattle with BRD to 60 healthy pen-mates, tracheal microbiota of healthy cattle was enriched with *Mycoplasma dispar*, *Lactococcus lactis*, and *Lactobacillus casei*.[6]

Commensal bacteria can confer resistance against colonization and proliferation of opportunistic bacterial pathogens through several mechanisms. First, resistance can be provided through occupation of an otherwise vacant respiratory niche. As a result, invading pathogens have to compete for adhesion receptors and nutrients. For example, numerous lactic acid bacteria (LAB) had greater adhesion to bovine bronchial epithelial cells than *M haemolytica*.[34] Commensals in the nasopharynx also can directly inhibit growth of bacterial pathogens by modifying their environment (ie, production of lactic or acetic acid) or producing antimicrobial molecules (eg, bacteriocins and hydrogen peroxide).[35] Finally, commensals can enhance colonization resistance against pathogens via immune stimulation of the host and modulation of mucosal inflammation. For example, *Streptococcus salivarius* inhibited inflammatory responses in human bronchial epithelial cells (ie, down-regulation of the nuclear factor κB pathway) and promoted host microbe homeostasis.[36]

New knowledge that commensal bacteria are not mere bystanders but have a role in maintaining respiratory health in cattle has led to advent of respiratory probiotics (discussed later).

Role of the Overall Diversity and Stability of the Microbiota on Respiratory Health

Because biodiversity correlates to efficiency of nutrient utilization by a community,[37] a more diverse bacterial community is, in theory, more likely to resist colonization by

Table 2
Changes in the upper and lower respiratory tract microbiota associated with bovine respiratory disease

Type	Study Design	Sample Type	Main Findings	Reference
Postweaned feedlot beef calves	Cross-sectional: 2 populations (dead calves with lung lesions at necropsy, n = 15; non-BRD related mortality, n = 3)	BAL collected at necropsy	M haemolytica, Mycoplasma bovis, and H somni were relatively abundant (>5%) in most but not all BRD samples. Other relatively abundant genera (>1%) included Acinetobacter, Bacillus, Bacteroides, Clostridium, Enterococcus, and Pseudomonas. Mycoplasma bovis was not detected in non-BRD lung samples.	Klima et al,[58] 2019
	Cross-sectional: 2 populations (BRD, n = 82; healthy pen-matched, n = 82)	DNS	Bacterial communities differed between BRD and CTRL groups. Relative abundance of H somni, M haemolytica, Mycoplasma bovis, or P multocida did not differ between BRD and CTRL groups. The proportion of samples that contained Mycoplasma bovis was higher, however, in the BRD group (43.90%) compared with the CTRL group (18.29%). Richness was lower in cattle with BRD.	McMullen et al,[39] 2019
	Cross-sectional over 5 wk after feedlot entry: 4 populations (calves sampled in 2015: BRD, n = 25 [5 pooled samples]; healthy, n = 30 [6 pooled samples]) and calves sampled in 2016: BRD, n = 8 [16 pooled samples]; healthy, n = 38 [10 pooled samples])	NS and DNS	Bacterial communities differed between BRD and CTRL groups only in 2016 (not in 2015). In 2016, Psychrobacter was more abundant in calves with BRD compared with CTRL in weeks 4 and 5 after feedlot entry, whereas Moraxella was greater in calves with BRD compared with CTRL throughout all 5 wk after feedlot entry.	McDaneld et al,[32] 2018

Cross-sectional: 2 populations (BRD, n = 60; healthy pen-matched, n = 60)	DNS and TTA	Bacterial communities present within the airways clustered into 4 distinct metacommunities that were associated with sampling locations and health status. Metacommunity 1, enriched with *Mycoplasma bovis*, *M haemolytica*, and *P multocida*, was dominant in the nasopharynx and trachea of cattle with BRD. In contrast, metacommunity 3, enriched with *Mycoplasma dispar*, *Lactococcus lactis*, and *Lactobacillus casei*, was present mostly in the trachea of CTRL cattle. Metacommunity 4, enriched with *Corynebacterium*, *Jeotgalicoccus*, *Psychrobacter*, and *Planomicrobium*, was present in the nasopharynx only. Metacommunity 2, enriched with *H somni*, *Moraxella*, and *L lactis*, was present in both BRD and CTRL cattle. Richness and diversity were lower in the trachea and nasopharynx of cattle with BRD.	Timsit et al,[6] 2018
Longitudinal; 4 populations (BRD at entry, n = 22; BRD at diagnosis; n = 22; healthy at entry, n = 44; healthy at diagnosis, n = 10)	DNS	Bacterial communities differed between BRD and CTRL groups. At the phylum level, *Proteobacteria* was higher in BRD calves vs CTRL (32.12% vs 16.32%). Actinobacteria (38.20% vs 16.58%) and Fusobacteria (3.86% vs 0.03%) were higher in CTRL. At the genus level, *Acinetobacter* (12.54% vs 2.16%), *Solibacillus* (3.71% vs 0.02%), and *Pasteurella* (2.38% vs 0.03%) were higher in BRD. *Mycoplasma* and *Moraxella* were numerically higher in BRD (but *P* > .05). *Rathayibacter* (20.09% vs 3.96%) was higher in CTRL. No difference in bacterial diversity and	Zeineldin et al,[31] 2017

(continued on next page)

Table 2
(continued)

Type	Study Design	Sample Type	Main Findings	Reference
	Longitudinal: 2 populations of calves sampled at feedlot entry and on 60 d after entry (BRD, n = 5; healthy, n = 5)	DNS	richness was observed between BRD and CTRL. Bacterial communities differed between BRD-CTRL groups at 0 and 60. At the phylum level, abundance of Actinobacteria was lower in BRD cattle. At the family level, there was a greater relative abundance of Micrococcaceae (d 0), Lachnospiraceae (d 60), Lactobacillaceae (d 0), and Bacillaceae (d 0) in CTRL. Richness and diversity were lower in the nasopharynx of cattle with BRD at d 0 and 60.	Holman et al,[7] 2015
Post-weaned beef calves (not feedlot)	Cross-sectional: 2 populations (BRD, n = 8; healthy, n = 11)	DNS and TTA	No difference in bacterial communities between BRD and CTRL groups.	Nicola et al,[11] 2017
Preweaned and post-weaned dairy calves	Cross-sectional: 3 populations (clinical BRD with lung lesions at necropsy, n = 6; clinically healthy with lung lesions at necropsy, n = 12; clinically healthy without lung lesions at necropsy, n = 8)	Lung tissue (cranial lung lobes) and lymph nodes	*Leptotrichiaceae, Fusobacterium, Mycoplasma, Trueperella,* and *Bacteroides* had greater relative abundances in lung samples collected from fatal BRD cases, compared with clinically healthy calves without lung lesions. *Leptotrichiaceae, Mycoplasma* and *Pasteurellaceae* had higher relative abundances in lymph nodes collected from fatal BRD cases, compared with clinically healthy calves without lung lesions.	Johnston et al,[33] 2017
Preweaned dairy calves	Longitudinal: 1 population sampled at 14 d and 28 d of life. During the study period, calves had BRD (n = 6) or remained healthy (n = 10).	DNS	The relative abundance of *Pseudomonas fluorescens* was higher in BRD calves at d 14 compared with CTRL. *M haemolytica* S1 and non-S1 were numerically higher at d 14 in calves with BRD compared with CTRL.	Gaeta et al,[18] 2017

Population	Study design	Sample	Findings	Reference
	Longitudinal: 1 population sampled at 3 d, 14 d, 28 d, and 35 d of life. During the study period, calves had BRD (n = 37), otitis media (n = 62), or BRD and otitis media (n = 11) or remained healthy (n = 64).	DNS	At d 3, heathy calves had significantly lower total bacterial loads in their nasopharynx than calves with BRD. The relative abundances of Mannheimia and Moraxella were higher in BRD calves at d 14. The relative abundance of Mannheimia and Mycoplasma were higher in BRD calves at d 28. Richness and diversity did not differ among groups.	Lima et al,[4] 2016
Preweaned dairy calves and their dams	Longitudinal; 1 population of calves sampled at 3 d, 14 d, and 35 d of age. During the study period, calves had BRD (n = 16), otitis media (n = 28), or BRD and otitis media (n = 5) or remained healthy (n = 32). Their dams were sampled just before calving.	DNS and vaginal swabs (for the dams)	The relative abundance of Mannheimia was significantly higher at d 14 in animals that eventually developed BRD than in calves that remained healthy. The genera Porphyromonas and Campylobacter were relatively more abundant in the vaginal microbiota of dams whose progeny developed disease, and Mannheimia and Caloramator were relatively more abundant in the vaginal microbiota of dams whose progeny remained healthy.	Lima et al,[3] 2019

Abbreviations: BAL, bronchoalveolar lavage; CTRL, control; DNS, deep nasal swab (≥20 cm long); NS, nasal swab (<20 cm long); S1, serotype 1; TTA, transtracheal aspiration.

Data from Refs.[3,4,6,7,11,18,31–33,39,58]

pathogens. For example, in children, colonization of the URT by acute otitis media pathogens (*Streptococcus pneumoniae*, *Haemophilus influenzae*, and *Moraxella catarrhalis*) was associated with lower levels of diversity in the URT microbiota.[38] In cattle, diversity of the URT and LRT was lower in cattle with BRD than in their healthy pen-mates.[6,7,39] Because overgrowth of pathogens in the respiratory tract could lead to a loss of diversity, however, it is difficult to determine whether reduced diversity predisposes cattle to BRD or is merely a consequence of proliferation of bacterial pathogens preceding clinical BRD. Therefore, additional longitudinal studies investigating the role of the microbiota diversity in respiratory health are needed.

A lack of stability in the URT microbiota during the first year of life has been associated with an increased risk of URT disease (such as otitis media) in human infants.[40] Perhaps disturbances in the bovine nasopharyngeal microbiota observed around the first month of age in dairy calves and during weaning/marketing in beef cattle predispose to colonization and/or proliferation of bacterial pathogens in the respiratory tract. Impact of microbiota stability on respiratory health in cattle, however, has not been reported.

MODULATION OF THE BACTERIAL RESPIRATORY MICROBIOTA TO PROMOTE HEALTH

Currently, modulation of the respiratory microbiota to promote health is based primarily on the use of parenteral antimicrobials in cattle.[41] This therapeutic strategy is effective in reducing URT colonization by *M haemolytica* or *P multocida*[16,42] and thus typically decreases incidence of BRD for 2 weeks to 3 weeks after administration.[41] Parenteral antimicrobials, however, also significantly disrupt microbial interactions among bacterial communities of the respiratory tract (Amat S, Timsit E, Workentine M, et al. Intranasal administration of bacterial therapeutics induces longitudinal modulation of the nasopharyngeal microbiota in post-weaned beef calves, submitted for publication). These communities then can become potentially more permissive to colonization by exogenous bacteria or proliferation of endogenous ones (Amat S, Timsit E, Workentine M, et al. Intranasal administration of bacterial therapeutics induces longitudinal modulation of the nasopharyngeal microbiota in post-weaned beef calves, submitted for publication). For example, on-arrival mass medication with tulathromycin was followed by rapid horizontal spread of a tulathromycin-resistant strain of *M haemolytica*.[43] Furthermore, parenteral administration of antimicrobials such as tulathromycin or oxytetracycline increased abundance of resistant genes, such as *erm*(X), *sul*2, *tet*(M), *msr*(E), and *tet*(H), in the nasopharyngeal microbiota.[16,17]

Fortunately, other approaches to modulate the respiratory microbiota and promote health (eg, probiotics, prebiotics, and bacteriophages) have potential as viable alternatives to parenteral antimicrobials.

Definition, Mechanisms of Action, and Possible Application Route of Probiotics

Probiotics are defined as "live microorganisms that when administered in adequate amounts, confer a health benefit to the host."[44] It is noteworthy that a higher abundance in heathy animals compared with sick animals is not enough for a strain to be designated as probiotic. A causative relationship with health promoting effects also should be demonstrated.

New probiotic postulates (based on Koch's postulates) have been recently suggested in development of next-generation probiotics.[45] They are defined as follows:

1. The microorganism is present in high abundance in healthy animals and decreased abundance in those suffering from a disease.
3. The microorganism can be isolated from healthy animals and grown in pure culture.
3. The cultured organism should promote health when introduced into a diseased animal.
4. Because probiotics are, by definition, administered as live organisms, it should be possible to reisolate these microorganisms from the healthy experimental host and confirm that they are identical to the original specific causative agents.

Based on these postulates, numerous LAB are potential candidates for next-generation probiotics.[34]

Probiotics promote respiratory health through 3 main mechanisms (**Fig. 4**).[45] First, they can have a direct antimicrobial action against bacterial respiratory pathogens by producing antimicrobial molecules, for example, lactic and acetic acid, bacteriocins, and hydrogen peroxide, in their microenvironment.[35] Second, probiotics can enhance the epithelial barrier by, for example, stimulating production of mucin or antimicrobial peptides (ie, defensins, lysozymes, and cathelicidins).[46,47] Finally, administration of probiotics also can modulate host immune responses (both innate and adaptive immunity) by interacting with host pattern recognition receptors of the mucosa.[48] For example, probiotic bacteria can modulate maturation of dendritic cells toward an anti-inflammatory interleukin (IL)-10 profile or stimulate regulatory T-cell activity to control overt inflammatory conditions.[48] In addition, they can modulate cytokine production and stimulate B-cell and antibody production (IgA and IgG).[48] Numerous other immunomodulatory effects of probiotics have been described, but a complete review of these mechanisms is outside the scope of this article (consult reviews by Lebeer and colleagues[48] [2010] and van den Broek and colleagues[45] [2019] for additional information). Most reports on effects of probiotics on host immunity are from humans or mice and not cattle.

Traditionally, probiotics have been administered by an oral route. Orally applied probiotics could benefit the URT via systemic immune effects.[49] They do not, however, have a direct antimicrobial action against bacterial respiratory pathogens, and they do not affect the URT's local immune response. Conversely, nasal application of probiotics has the advantage of promoting more direct contact of the applied organisms with the respiratory tract mucosa and microbiota.[45] Furthermore, by using the nasal route, probiotics do not have to survive transit through the gastrointestinal tract (especially the rumen). Therefore, the next logical step is to design probiotics that can be applied intranasally.

Intranasal Administration of Probiotics in Cattle

To investigate whether nasal application of probiotics can modulate the respiratory microbiota to promote health in cattle, the authors' team first selected in vitro probiotic strains originating from the nasopharynx of healthy cattle with properties that are important for URT probiotics (discussed later).[35] Then, these probiotics strains were administered to dairy calves[21] and beef calves (Amat S, Timsit E, Workentine M, et al. Intranasal administration of bacterial therapeutics induces longitudinal modulation of the nasopharyngeal microbiota in post-weaned beef calves, submitted for publication) to investigate their health-promoting effects.

For selection of probiotic strains, the authors used a stepwise approach.[35] Bacteria isolated from the nasopharynx of healthy cattle for their ability to inhibit *M haemolytica* (178 isolates from 12 genera). Subsequently, abilities of selected isolates were evaluated to adhere to bovine turbinate (BT) cells (n = 47), compete against *M haemolytica*

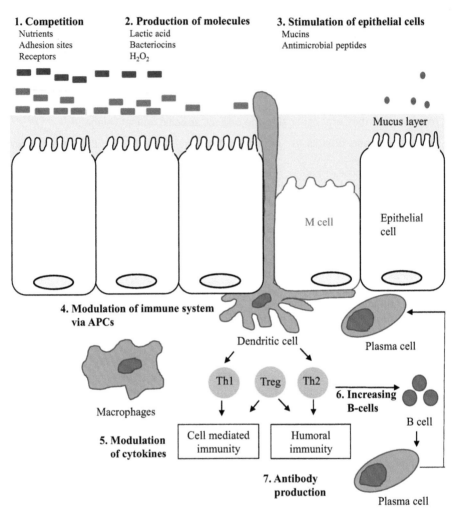

Fig. 4. Postulated beneficial modes of action of respiratory probiotics: (1) competition with pathogens for nutrients, adhesion sites, and receptors; (2) production of antimicrobial molecules, such as lactic acid, bacteriocins, and hydrogen peroxide (H_2O_2); (3) stimulation of epithelial cells to modulate mucin and antimicrobial peptide production; (4) modulation of the immune system via antigen-presenting cells (APCs); (5) modulation of cytokine production; (6) stimulation of increased B-cell production; and (7) stimulation of antibody production (IgA and IgG). Th1/2, T helper 1/2 cells; Treg, regulatory T cells. (*Adapted from* van den Broek MFL, De Boeck I, Kiekens F, Boudewyns A, Vanderveken OM, Lebeer S. Translating recent microbiome insights in otitis media into probiotic strategies. *Clin Microbiol Rev.* 2019; 3, 32; with permission.)

for BT cell adherence (n = 15), and modulate gene expression in BT cells (n = 10). *Lactobacillus* strains had the strongest inhibition against *M haemolytica*, with 88% of isolates having inhibition zones ranging from 17 mm to 23 mm. All isolates tested in competition assays reduced *M haemolytica* adherence to BT cells (32% to 78%). Among the 84 bovine genes evaluated, selected isolates slightly upregulated expression of IL-8 and IL-6. After ranking isolates for greatest inhibition, adhesion, competition, and immunomodulation properties, 6 *Lactobacillus* strains from 4 different species were selected as the best URT probiotic candidates: *L amylovorous*, *L buchneri* (2 strains), *L curvatus*, and *L paracasei* (2 strains). The authors primarily focused on LAB because these bacteria have a long history of safe use (eg, generally recognized as safe). Other bacteria, however, such as *Mycoplasma dispar*, also could have some probiotic properties, because they were present in higher abundance in healthy animals versus sick animals.[6]

Health-promoting effects of the 6 selected *Lactobacillus* strains were first evaluated in dairy calves.[21] For this evaluation, 1-week-old to 3-week-old dairy calves received either an intranasal cocktail of the 6 probiotic strains (3×10^9 colony-forming units [CFUs] per strain; n = 12) 24 hours prior to an intranasal *M haemolytica* challenge (3×10^8 CFUs), or only phosphate buffered saline (PBS) prior to challenge (control group; n = 12). Nasal swabs were collected over the course of 16 days after probiotic inoculation. Probiotic strains were reisolated up to 13 days after inoculation, with variation existing among strains and calves. Their administration significantly reduced nasal colonization by *M haemolytica*. It also modified composition and reduced the diversity of the nasal microbiota and altered interbacterial relationships among the 10 most abundant genera. This study demonstrated, for the first time, that intranasal probiotics developed from bovine nasopharyngeal *Lactobacillus* could reduce nasal colonization by *M haemolytica* in dairy calves.

In a second study, the authors investigated the health promoting effects of the same probiotic cocktail in beef cattle (Amat S, Timsit E, Workentine M, et al. Intranasal administration of bacterial therapeutics induces longitudinal modulation of the nasopharyngeal microbiota in post-weaned beef calves, submitted for publication). In that study, on arrival at the feedlot, newly received beef steers either received (1) an intranasal cocktail of the 6 strains (3×10^9 CFUs per strain; n = 20); (2) intranasal PBS (negative control; n = 20); or (3) parenteral tulathromycin (Draxxin [Zoetis (Kirkland, Ontario, Canada)]) (positive control; 2.5 mg/kg; n = 20). Nasopharyngeal swabs were collected for up to 42 days post-treatment. Nasopharyngeal colonization by probiotics was most apparent at day 2 postinoculation; however, administration of probiotics modified composition and reduced the diversity of the nasopharyngeal microbiota for up to 42 days. Compared with PBS and probiotics, parenteral tulathromycin decreased bacterial load in the nasopharynx and increased abundance of the antibiotic-resistant gene *msr*(E). There were no significant effects among treatments on relative abundance of *M haemolytica*, *P multocida*, or *H somni*. This second study demonstrated that a unique intranasal inoculation of probiotics could modify the nasopharyngeal microbiota for up to 42 days in postweaned beef cattle. Unfortunately, it did not provide useful information on potential health promoting effects of the probiotic cocktail, because the disease challenge was very low, with only 5 of the 60 calves diagnosed with BRD during the study period (3 in the PBS group and 2 in the probiotic group).

In summary, a single intranasal administration of 6 selected *Lactobacillus* strains modified the nasopharyngeal microbiota of dairy cattle and beef cattle and provided colonization resistance against *M haemolytica*. Additional research is needed to define the optimal dose and duration of application of this probiotic cocktail to maximize health benefits as well as to further confirm its health promoting effect (ie, can it reduce incidence of BRD after administration, which is the outcome of interest for the cattle industry). Perhaps a single inoculation is not enough to prevent BRD. In human studies, intranasal probiotics to prevent otitis media in infants typically are given multiples times over a few days or weeks; for example, 10 days per month over 2 consecutive months or twice daily for 10 days.[45] Furthermore, it is noteworthy that probiotics have different abilities to colonize and influence a particular individual. For example, it has been reported that transient colonization by probiotic strains is highly variable in the lower gastrointestinal tract of humans, with some humans being more permissive to colonization and others being resistant.[50] It, therefore, is possible that the composition of the probiotic cocktail should be adapted to animal age and production system, that is, preweaned dairy calves, preweaned or postweaned beef cattle, and veal calves.

Other Strategies: Bacteriophages and Prebiotics

Bacteriophage therapy is another way to modulate the bacterial structure of the respiratory microbiota.[51] Bacteriophages are viruses that infect bacteria. They either can be stably integrated into bacterial genomes (lysogenic phase) or can replicate and lyse bacteria, releasing virus particles (lytic phase).[52] Bacteriophages are highly specific and typically infect only 1 bacterial species, serotype, or strain. Their inoculation in the nasopharynx of cattle, therefore, can remove bacterial respiratory pathogens without having an impact on the commensal flora.[51] Furthermore, bacteriophages can amplify exponentially after administration and thus do not always need multiple administrations. Bacteriophages with lytic properties against *M haemolytica* have been isolated and characterized.[53] Unfortunately, to the authors' best knowledge, there are no published data on their use to remove *M haemolytica* from the nasopharynx of cattle. The increasing prevalence of antibiotic resistance in *M haemolytica* and *P multocida* isolated in the United States,[43,54] Canada,[29] and Europe[55] nevertheless is creating an impetus to further investigate bacteriophage therapies in cattle.

Prebiotics are nonviable substrates that serve as nutrients for beneficial microorganisms harbored by the host, including administered probiotic strains and indigenous (resident) microorganisms.[56] Commonly studied prebiotics include fructooligosaccharides, galacto-oligosaccharides, inulin, and resistant starch.[57] Administration of prebiotics alone or in combination with probiotics in the URTs of cattle could promote the selective growth of bacteria considered beneficial, for example, *Lactobacilli*. Unfortunately, to date, prebiotics have been used solely to selectively enhance the growth of beneficial bacteria in the digestive tract, and further research is needed before recommending their use for modulating the respiratory tract microbiota of cattle.

SUMMARY

The respiratory tract of cattle is colonized by complex bacterial ecosystems also known as bacterial microbiotas. These microbiotas evolve over time and are shaped by numerous factors, including maternal vaginal microbiota, environment, age, diet, parenteral antimicrobials, and stressful events (eg, transportation and commingling). The resulting microbiota can be diverse and enriched with known beneficial bacteria (ie, *Lactobacillus* and *Lactococcus*) that can provide colonization resistance against opportunistic bacterial pathogens or, on the contrary, with bacterial pathogens, such as *M haemolytica*, *P multocida*, *H somni*, or *Mycoplasma bovis*, predisposing cattle to respiratory disease. Beneficial bacteria promote health through 3 main mechanisms: (1) direct antimicrobial action against bacterial pathogens, (2) enhancement of the epithelial barrier, and (3) modulation of the host immune response. Among beneficial bacteria, *Lactobacillus* are of particular interest because they generally are regarded as safe. Intranasal inoculation of a cocktail of 6 *Lactobacillus* strain modified the structure of the nasopharyngeal microbiota over a few weeks in beef calves and dairy calves and provided colonization resistance against *M haemolytica*. That the respiratory microbiota can be modulated by nonantimicrobial approaches to promote health creates new potential strategies for prevention and treatment of BRD.

ACKNOWLEDGMENTS

The authors gratefully acknowledge Dr. John Kastelic for editing the article.

DISCLOSURE

Dr E. Timsit is an Innovation Scientist at Ceva Animal Health and is responsible for early phases of drug discovery and development. None of the authors of this article has a financial or personal relationship with other people or organizations that could inappropriately influence or bias the content of the article. This article reflects the views of the authors and should not be construed as representing the views of Ceva Animal Health.

REFERENCES

1. Turnbaugh PJ, Ley RE, Hamady M, et al. The human microbiome project. Nature 2007;449:804–10.
2. Holman DB, Timsit E, Alexander TW. The nasopharyngeal microbiota of feedlot cattle. Sci Rep 2015;5:15557.
3. Lima SF, Bicalho MLS, Bicalho RC. The *Bos taurus* maternal microbiome: Role in determining the progeny early-life upper respiratory tract microbiome and health. PLoS One 2019;14:e0208014.
4. Lima SF, Teixeira AG, Higgins CH, et al. The upper respiratory tract microbiome and its potential role in bovine respiratory disease and otitis media. Sci Rep 2016; 6:29050.
5. Timsit E, Holman DB, Hallewell J, et al. The nasopharyngeal microbiota in feedlot cattle and its role in respiratory health. Anim Front 2016;6:44–50.
6. Timsit E, Workentine M, van der Meer F, et al. Distinct bacterial metacommunities inhabit the upper and lower respiratory tracts of healthy feedlot cattle and those diagnosed with bronchopneumonia. Vet Microbiol 2018;221:105–13.
7. Holman DB, McAllister TA, Topp E, et al. The nasopharyngeal microbiota of feedlot cattle that develop bovine respiratory disease. Vet Microbiol 2015; 180:90–5.
8. Koppen IJN, Bosch A, Sanders EAM, et al. The respiratory microbiota during health and disease: a paediatric perspective. Pneumonia 2015;6:90–100.
9. Ley RE, Peterson DA, Gordon JI. Ecological and evolutionary forces shaping microbial diversity in the human intestine. Cell 2006;124:837–48.
10. Wypych TP, Wickramasinghe LC, Marsland BJ. The influence of the microbiome on respiratory health. Nat Immunol 2019;20:1279–90.
11. Nicola I, Cerutti F, Grego E, et al. Characterization of the upper and lower respiratory tract microbiota in Piedmontese calves. Microbiome 2017;5:152.
12. Hall JA, Isaiah A, Estill CT, et al. Weaned beef calves fed selenium-biofortified alfalfa hay have an enriched nasal microbiota compared with healthy controls. PLoS One 2017;12:e0179215.
13. Stroebel C, Alexander T, Workentine ML, et al. Effects of transportation to and comingling at an auction market on nasopharyngeal and tracheal bacterial communities of recently weaned beef cattle. Vet Microbiol 2018;223:126–33.

14. Timsit E, Workentine M, Schryvers AB, et al. Evolution of the nasopharyngeal microbiota of beef cattle from weaning to 40 days after arrival at a feedlot. Vet Microbiol 2016;187:75–81.

15. Holman DB, Timsit E, Amat S, et al. The nasopharyngeal microbiota of beef cattle before and after transport to a feedlot. BMC Microbiol 2017;17:70.

16. Holman DB, Yang W, Alexander TW. Antibiotic treatment in feedlot cattle: a longitudinal study of the effect of oxytetracycline and tulathromycin on the fecal and nasopharyngeal microbiota. Microbiome 2019;7:86.

17. Holman DB, Timsit E, Booker CW, et al. Injectable antimicrobials in commercial feedlot cattle and their effect on the nasopharyngeal microbiota and antimicrobial resistance. Vet Microbiol 2018;214:140–7.

18. Gaeta NC, Lima SF, Teixeira AG, et al. Deciphering upper respiratory tract microbiota complexity in healthy calves and calves that develop respiratory disease using shotgun metagenomics. J Dairy Sci 2017;100:1445–58.

19. McMullen C, Orsel K, Alexander TW, et al. Evolution of the nasopharyngeal bacterial microbiota of beef calves from spring processing to 40 days after feedlot arrival. Vet Microbiol 2018;225:139–48.

20. McDaneld TG, Kuehn LA, Keele JW. Microbiome of the upper nasal cavity of beef calves prior to weaning. J Anim Sci 2019;97:2368–75.

21. Amat S, Alexander TW, Holman DB, et al. Intranasal bacterial therapeutics reduce colonization by the respiratory pathogen *Mannheimia haemolytica* in dairy calves. mSystems 2020;5(2) [pii:e00629-19].

22. Zeineldin MM, Lowe JF, Grimmer ED, et al. Relationship between nasopharyngeal and bronchoalveolar microbial communities in clinically healthy feedlot cattle. BMC Microbiol 2017;17:138.

23. Osman R, Malmuthuge N, Gonzalez-Cano P, et al. Development and function of the mucosal immune system in the upper respiratory tract of neonatal calves. Annu Rev Anim Biosci 2018;6:141–55.

24. Amat S, Holman DB, Timsit E, et al. Evaluation of the nasopharyngeal microbiota in beef cattle transported to a feedlot, with a focus on lactic acid-producing bacteria. Front Microbiol 2019;10:1988.

25. Timsit E, Workentine M, Crepieux T, et al. Effects of nasal instillation of a nitric oxide-releasing solution or parenteral administration of tilmicosin on the nasopharyngeal microbiota of beef feedlot cattle at high-risk of developing respiratory tract disease. Res Vet Sci 2017;115:117–224.

26. Babcock AH, Renter DG, White BJ, et al. Temporal distributions of respiratory disease events within cohorts of feedlot cattle and associations with cattle health and performance indices. Prev Vet Med 2010;97:198–219.

27. Ducarmon QR, Zwittink RD, Hornung BVH, et al. Gut microbiota and colonization resistance against bacterial enteric infection. Microbiol Mol Biol Rev 2019;83: e00007–19.

28. Dickson RP, Erb-Downward JR, Freeman CM, et al. Bacterial topography of the healthy human lower respiratory tract. mBio 2017;8:e02287-16.

29. Timsit E, Hallewell J, Booker C, et al. Prevalence and antimicrobial susceptibility of *Mannheimia haemolytica, Pasteurella multocida,* and *Histophilus somni* isolated from the lower respiratory tract of healthy feedlot cattle and those diagnosed with bovine respiratory disease. Vet Microbiol 2017;208:118–25.

30. Noyes NR, Benedict KM, Gow SP, et al. *Mannheimia haemolytica* in feedlot cattle: prevalence of recovery and associations with antimicrobial use, resistance, and health outcomes. J Vet Intern Med 2015;29:705–13.

31. Zeineldin M, Lowe J, de Godoy M, et al. Disparity in the nasopharyngeal microbiota between healthy cattle on feed, at entry processing and with respiratory disease. Vet Microbiol 2017;208:30–7.

32. McDaneld TG, Kuehn LA, Keele JW. Evaluating the microbiome of two sampling locations in the nasal cavity of cattle with bovine respiratory disease complex (BRDC). J Anim Sci 2018. https://doi.org/10.1093/jas/sky032.

33. Johnston D, Earley B, Cormican P, et al. Illumina MiSeq 16S amplicon sequence analysis of bovine respiratory disease associated bacteria in lung and mediastinal lymph node tissue. BMC Vet Res 2017;13:118.

34. Amat S, Subramanian S, Timsit E, et al. Probiotic bacteria inhibit the bovine respiratory pathogen *Mannheimia haemolytica* serotype 1 in vitro. Lett Appl Microbiol 2017;64:343–9.

35. Amat S, Timsit E, Baines D, et al. Development of bacterial therapeutics against the bovine respiratory pathogen *Mannheimia haemolytica*. Appl Environ Microbiol 2019;85 [pii:e01359-19].

36. Cosseau C, Devine DA, Dullaghan E, et al. The commensal Streptococcus salivarius K12 downregulates the innate immune responses of human epithelial cells and promotes host-microbe homeostasis. Infect Immun 2008;76:4163–75.

37. Cardinale BJ, Duffy JE, Gonzalez A, et al. Biodiversity loss and its impact on humanity. Nature 2012;486:59–67.

38. Pettigrew MM, Laufer AS, Gent JF, et al. Upper respiratory tract microbial communities, acute otitis media pathogens, and antibiotic use in healthy and sick children. Appl Environ Microbiol 2012;78:6262–70.

39. McMullen C, Orsel K, Alexander TW, et al. Comparison of the nasopharyngeal bacterial microbiota of beef calves raised without the use of antimicrobials between healthy calves and those diagnosed with bovine respiratory disease. Vet Microbiol 2019;231:56–62.

40. Bosch A, de Steenhuijsen Piters WAA, van Houten MA, et al. Maturation of the infant respiratory microbiota, environmental drivers, and health consequences. a prospective cohort study. Am J Respir Crit Care Med 2017;196:1582–90.

41. Nickell JS, White BJ. Metaphylactic antimicrobial therapy for bovine respiratory disease in stocker and feedlot cattle. Vet Clin North Am Food Anim Pract 2010; 26:285–301.

42. Frank GH, Briggs RE, Loan RW, et al. Effects of tilmicosin treatment on *Pasteurella haemolytica* organisms in nasal secretion specimens of calves with respiratory tract disease. Am J Vet Res 2000;61:525–9.

43. Snyder E, Credille B, Berghaus R, et al. Prevalence of multi drug antimicrobial resistance in isolated from high-risk stocker cattle at arrival and two weeks after processing. J Anim Sci 2017;95:1124–31.

44. Hill C, Guarner F, Reid G, et al. Expert consensus document. The International Scientific Association for Probiotics and Prebiotics consensus statement on the scope and appropriate use of the term probiotic. Nat Rev Gastroenterol Hepatol 2014;11:506–14.

45. van den Broek MFL, De Boeck I, Kiekens F, et al. Translating recent microbiome insights in otitis media into probiotic strategies. Clin Microbiol Rev 2019;32 [pii: e00010-18].

46. Madsen K, Cornish A, Soper P, et al. Probiotic bacteria enhance murine and human intestinal epithelial barrier function. Gastroenterology 2001;121:580–91.

47. Bron PA, Kleerebezem M, Brummer RJ, et al. Can probiotics modulate human disease by impacting intestinal barrier function? Br J Nutr 2017;117:93–107.

48. Lebeer S, Vanderleyden J, De Keersmaecker SC. Host interactions of probiotic bacterial surface molecules: comparison with commensals and pathogens. Nat Rev Microbiol 2010;8:171–84.
49. Budden KF, Gellatly SL, Wood DL, et al. Emerging pathogenic links between microbiota and the gut-lung axis. Nat Rev Microbiol 2017;15:55–63.
50. Zmora N, Zilberman-Schapira G, Suez J, et al. Personalized gut mucosal colonization resistance to empiric probiotics is associated with unique host and microbiome features. Cell 2018;174:1388–405.e21.
51. Wienhold SM, Lienau J, Witzenrath M. Towards inhaled phage therapy in Western Europe. Viruses 2019;11:E295.
52. Kutateladze M, Adamia R. Bacteriophages as potential new therapeutics to replace or supplement antibiotics. Trends Biotechnol 2010;28:591–5.
53. Urban-Chmiel R, Wernicki A, Stegierska D, et al. Isolation and characterization of lytic properties of bacteriophages specific for *M. haemolytica* strains. PLoS One 2015;10:e0140140.
54. Woolums AR, Karisch BB, Frye JG, et al. Multidrug resistant *Mannheimia haemolytica* isolated from high-risk beef stocker cattle after antimicrobial metaphylaxis and treatment for bovine respiratory disease. Vet Microbiol 2018;221:143–52.
55. Schonecker L, Schnyder P, Overesch G, et al. Associations between antimicrobial treatment modalities and antimicrobial susceptibility in *Pasteurellaceae* and *E. coli* isolated from veal calves under field conditions. Vet Microbiol 2019;236: 108363.
56. Gibson GR, Hutkins R, Sanders ME, et al. Expert consensus document: The International Scientific Association for Probiotics and Prebiotics (ISAPP) consensus statement on the definition and scope of prebiotics. Nat Rev Gastroenterol Hepatol 2017;14:491–502.
57. Vitetta L, Vitetta G, Hall S. Immunological tolerance and function: associations between intestinal bacteria, probiotics, prebiotics, and phages. Front Immunol 2018;9:2240.
58. Klima CL, Holman DB, Ralston BJ, et al. Lower respiratory tract microbiome and resistome of bovine respiratory disease mortalities. Microb Ecol 2019;78:446–56.

Viruses in Bovine Respiratory Disease in North America

Knowledge Advances Using Genomic Testing

Robert W. Fulton, DVM, PhD*

KEYWORDS

- Genetic sequencing • Bioinformatics • Cattle • Influenza D virus
- Bovine coronaviruses • Bovine viral diarrhea viruses • Bovine herpesvirus 1

KEY POINTS

- In recent years, new bovine respiratory disease (BRD) viruses have been identified in bovine respiratory tract materials by viral sequencing and bioinformatics.
- Advances in viral identification have mirrored the use of viral sequencing, leading to identification of influenza D virus, bovine coronaviruses, and others.
- Diagnostic laboratories have moved to the use of viral sequencing and expanded the use of polymerase chain reaction for virus detection.
- New viruses sometimes are found in healthy cattle as well as in cattle with BRD, and more research is needed to confirm the importance of such viruses.
- Clinicians and diagnostic laboratories must work to confirm the role of new viruses in BRD and to determine whether vaccines have a place in their control.

INTRODUCTION

During the past several years, there have been conferences/symposiums for bovine respiratory disease (BRD) and research with several presentations on various aspects of BRD, including clinical disease, diagnosis, etiology, epidemiology, government and commercial diagnostic laboratories, treatment, prevention, economics of disease and prevention, and immunity. Participants included clinicians in private practice; university and government researchers; diagnostic laboratories; animal health firms; cattle owners including feedlots, beef cow calf operations, dairies for milk production, and dairy calf ranches for heifer replacements and dairy calves entering feedlots. A review published in 2009 summarized BRD research from 1983 (the initial BRD symposium) to

Department of Veterinary Pathobiology, College of Veterinary Medicine, Oklahoma State University, Stillwater, OK, USA
* 7405 East Oak Ridge Street, Broken Arrow, OK 74014.
E-mail address: robert.fulton@okstate.edu

Vet Clin Food Anim 36 (2020) 321–332
https://doi.org/10.1016/j.cvfa.2020.02.004
0749-0720/20/© 2020 Elsevier Inc. All rights reserved.

2009.[1] This review covered infectious agents, including viruses, bacteria, and myco-plasmas. Coverage of viruses included the 4 most commonly discussed respiratory tract viruses in BRD: bovine herpes virus 1 (BoHV1), bovine parainfluenza type 3 virus (PI3V), bovine viral diarrhea viruses (BVDVs), and bovine respiratory syncytial virus (BRSV). There are commercial vaccines containing immunogens to these viruses. These 4 viruses were investigated extensively prior to 2009 in research studies and were described in published reports from state and federal diagnostic laboratories. These viruses were identified by the virologic methods in place at that time.[2] These included isolation in cell culture based on cytopathology and confirmed by fluorescent antibody test using virus monospecific antisera. Other confirmatory tests included neutralization of infectivity using monospecific antisera. Numerous serosurveys permitted detection of viral exposure in selected populations. In the years prior to 2009, selected viruses such as BVDV were sequenced, resulting in the knowledge of genomic regions that could be used to identify these viruses. Eventually, technology produced many automated sequencing procedures and the field of bioinformatics facilitated alignment of newly identified sequences with reference sequences, permit-ting the identification of the entire or near full length of viral genomes. Terms, such as metagenomics, whole-genome sequencing, and next-generation sequencing, have become commonplace for both research and diagnostic laboratories. These new genomic tests permitted expansion of knowledge of the big 4 viruses: BoHV1, BVDV, PI3V, and BRSV.

EXAMPLES OF EXPANDED KNOWLEDGE OF BOVINE RESPIRATORY DISEASE VIRUSES: GENOMICS OF BOVINE HERPES VIRUS 1, BOVINE VIRAL DIARRHEA VIRUS, AND BOVINE PARAINFLUENZA TYPE 3 VIRUS

The BoHV1 represents one of the original viruses in BRD that was isolated and char-acterized in the 1950s with the advent of cell cultures. BoHV1 is a common component of bovine viral vaccines, including both modified live virus (MLV) vaccine and killed/inactivated viral vaccine. The MLV vaccine origin strains of BoHV1 have been identi-fied in clinical cases postvaccination and in aborted fetuses. Thus, it became neces-sary to differentiate field strains from the MLV strains, but this posed significant challenges. Using whole-genome sequencing and analysis of the resulting nucleic segments, the viral genomes of BoHV1 reference strains, BoHV1.1 reference strains Cooper and Los Angeles, were sequenced.[3,4] The resulting information on the BoHV1.1 genome was investigated further using the reference strain, Cooper, and multiple BoHV1.1 strains in the MLV vaccines available in North America.[5] This genetic analysis found single-nucleotide polymorphisms (SNPs) among the viruses, which permitted the viruses to be classified into groups. The SNPs for various regions permitted the selection of multiple primers to be used and the polymerase chain reac-tion (PCR) products sequenced. These SNPs patterns then permitted the ability to separate the viruses into groups and each strain to have a specific identity. This infor-mation permitted isolates from clinic cases to be categorized as field/wild-type or MLV strain. Use of the SNPs and the sequencing of the PCR products of the primers were applied in multiple studies identifying wild-type strains of BoHV1.1 as vaccine or wild-type strains.[5-10] In addition to the separation of vaccine from field strains, these genomic sequencing procedures identified a recombinant BoHV1.1 strain (including components of both a wild-type and a vaccine strain) from an aborted bovine fetus.[10] Using this genetic sequencing, the BoHV1.2b reference strain K22 and multiple wild-type genital and respiratory BoHV1.2b strains were sequenced.[11]

The BVDV strains are referred to as biotypes based on cytopathology in cell culture: cytopathic and noncytopathic, with 2 species, BVDV1 and BVDV2, based on genomics.[12,13] Application of genetic testing of BVDV strains initially had focused on the sequencing of PCR products from multiple regions of the BVDV genome. Initial studies of the presence of BVDV subtypes in surveys of US and other North American cattle populations, diagnostic accession of bovine samples, or reports of respiratory disease outbreaks with viral identification led to detection of subgenotypes, BVDV1a, BVDV1b, and BVDV2a. Studies of the distribution of these 3 subtypes from diagnostic laboratory accessions indicated BVDV1b as the predominant BVDV subtype,[14] and BVDV1b was the predominant subtype in multiple studies of beef calves with BRD, based on recovery of virus from acute cases of BRD and necropsy tissues.[15] Investigation of the source of BVDV exposure identified the persistently infected calf as the most important source of virus exposure, with persistently infected calves resulting from infection of susceptible heifers/cows during a critical stage of pregnancy.[12]

A study to evaluate diagnostic tests used to detect persistently infected calves was performed, with the additional objective of determining prevalence of BVDV1a, BVDV1b, and BVDV2a subtypes in persistently infected calves entering a southwest Kansas feedlot.[16] In a 2004 study, there were 86/21,743 (0.4%) persistently infected calves with the distribution of subtypes: BVDV1b (77.9%), BVDV1a (11.6%), and BVDV2a (10.5%). To determine if the distribution of the subtypes was consistent in succeeding years, samples from this same feedlot were tested over the following years and are summarized in **Table 1**. The distribution of the subtypes seems consistent for each collection from 2004 to 2008.

Another study, using complete genome sequences from samples from this same feedlot in August 2013 to April 2014, determined the distribution of subgenotypes among 119 samples.[17] There were 82% BVDV1b, 9% BVDV1a, and 8% BVDV2. It was reported that the BVDV2 belong to at least 3 distinct genetic groups. This study indicated 2 points:

1. BVDV1b remained the predominant persistently infected subgenotype from 2004 to 2014.
2. BVDV2 may belong to at least 3 distinct genetic groups.

These studies demonstrated prevalence of the subgenotypes in beef cattle, yet information regarding the distribution in dairy cattle is limited. A study of samples from

Table 1
Bovine viral diarrhea virus subtypes in persistently infected cattle entering a feedlot for beef cattle

Study	Number of Calves	Bovine Viral Diarrhea Virus 1a	Bovine Viral Diarrhea Virus 1b	Bovine Viral Diarrhea Virus 2a
2004–2005	86	(10) 11.6%	(67) 77.9%	(9) 10.5%
2005–2006	302	(33) 10.9%	(229) 75.8%	(40) 13.3%
2007 Spring	201	(28) 13.9%	(161) 80.1%	(12) 6.0%
2007 Summer	184	(13) 7.1%	(152) 82.6%	(19) 10.3%
2007 Fall	163	(24) 14.7%	(124) 76.1%	(15) 9.2%
2008 Spring	180	(28) 15.6%	(135) 75.0%	(17) 9.4%
2008 Fall	147	(14) 9.5%	(122) 83.0%	(11) 7.5%
Total: 2004–2008	1263	(150) 11.9%	(990) 78.4%	(123) 9.7%

39 persistently infected calves in a dairy calf ranch showed the distribution of BVDV subgenotypes: BVDV1a (2.6%), BVDV2a (12.8%), and BVDV1b (84.6%) (R. Fulton, unpublished data, 2020).

To identify BVDV persistently infected calves in beef cow herds, 4530 calves from 30 ranches in south central Oklahoma and north central Texas were tested for BVDV PI status.[18] There were 25/4530 (0.55%) persistently infected calves and 5/30 (16.7%) of the herds contained persistently infected calves. All of the PI BVDV strains were BVDV1b. In a summary of diagnostic laboratory samples over a 20-year period, the BVDV1b subtype predominated.[19] In a 2019 study using clinical samples from diagnostic laboratories and the US Department of Agriculture National Animal Disease Center, BVDV Laboratory, BVDV2b and BVDV2c were identified.[20] Thus, it appears with new genomics testing there may additional BVDV subtypes identified. A recent report on the global distribution of BVDV subgenotypes cited at least 21 subgenotypes for BVDV1 and 4 subgenotypes for BVDV2.[21]

The application of genomics, PCR testing, and antigenic comparison has been applied to another of the BRD viruses, PI3V. There are 3 PI3V genotypes in the United States: PI3Va, PI3Vb, and PI3Vc.[22,23] In addition to the genetic differences, there also are antigenic differences. These antigenic differences may have an impact on vaccine responses because the current PI3V vaccines contain PI3Va strains.

ADVANCES IN GENOMICS PERMITS IDENTIFICATION OF ADDITIONAL VIRUSES IN NORTH AMERICA: BOVINE CORONAVIRUS, INFLUENZA D VIRUS, AND OTHERS
Bovine Coronavirus

The bovine coronavirus (BoCV) has received considerable attention in recent years as another viral pathogen in respiratory disease. Although initially studied as a pathogen causing neonatal diarrhea/enteritis in young calves, growing evidence has suggested involvement in BRD, especially because of the recovery of BoCV from clinically ill cattle with BRD and necropsy cases of fatal pneumonias. The use of viral serology and more extensive use of PCR testing on respiratory tract swabs from BRD cases and necropsy cases by diagnostic laboratories have provided further evidence that BoCV plays a role in BRD. Interpretation of these diagnostic reports, however, often is difficult, especially because there is no US Department of Agriculture licensed BoCV vaccine for BRD prevention and control. A recent article by Ellis[24] gives an excellent review of the history of BoCV in respiratory cases, both in field cases and in experimental studies. The purpose of the review was to seek evidence that BoCV is a biologically significant respiratory pathogen in cattle.

A study using nasal swabs from calves treated for BRD and BRD necropsy cases from multiple feedlots identified viruses with PCR testing and virus isolation.[9] Of the 121 cases, the positives include: 14.9% (BoHV1), 15.7% (BVDV), 62.8% (BoCV), 9.1% (BRSV), and 8.3% (PI3V). In contrast to prior studies, the virus positives were tested by sequencing to differentiate vaccine strains from field strains. Often surveys collect samples from cattle recently vaccinated with MLV vaccines containing BoHV1, BVDV, PI3V, and BRSV. In a study of virus recovery from fatal cases in Ontario, Canada, feedlots, BoCV was recovered from 2/99 (2.0%) cases.[25] A subsequent report in 2009 dealt with a year-long study of pathology and identification of infectious agents in fatal feedlot pneumonias.[26] In that study, which used PCR testing of fresh lung samples, 21/194 (10.8%) were positive for BoCV. The BoCV has been isolated from both healthy calves and sick calves.[27–30] Using a virus neutralization serotest, however, individual calf serums collected at feedlot entry in a retained ownership study (fresh from the ranch and no mixed-source auction calves) were tested for neutralizing antibodies, and those calves with low antibody levels to BoCV (16 or less) were more likely to be treated for BRD during the feeding phase compared with calves with higher titers.[27] In other research, BoCV from nasal swabs and bronchoalveolar washing fluids were evaluated for genetic and antigenic differences.[28] A region of the viral spike protein in the envelope was the target of genomic sequencing, and virus neutralization tests in cell culture were used to compare antigenic relatedness. Testing demonstrated genetic differences that allowed classification of 2 clades, BoCV1 and BoCV2, which also demonstrated antigenic differences. The current reference BoCV is of enteric origin and is classified as BoCV1. This strain is included in most licensed BoCV vaccines for enteric disease in the United States. Another study of 15 isolates from 3 herds, using sequencing of the spike hypervariable gene region, indicated that there were 4 polymorphisms in the 15 isolates.[30]

A critical question posed for BoCV as a respiratory pathogen has been whether BoCV infection with isolates of respiratory tract origin (as opposed to the reference enteric strain or other enteric strains) in susceptible cattle results in measurable gross and microscopic lesions on the respiratory tract. Such challenge studies are required in order to have a model to measure efficacy of BoCV vaccines in the respiratory tract protection. A series of studies was performed with multiple isolates from the respiratory tract of calves and the reference enteric strain to study dynamics of the BoCV infection.[31] BVDV exposure was used in dual infections (BVDV and BoCV) as well as BVDV alone, BoCV alone, and controls.[31] Respiratory disease was observed in calves inoculated with BoCV 6 days or 9 days after BVDV. Lung lesions were present in calves in dual infection groups; however, lesions were more pronounced in calves inoculated with BVDV followed by BoCV inoculation 6 days later. Immunohistochemistry (IHC) confirmed the presence of BoCV antigen in the respiratory tract. Gross lung lesions of the dual infected calves were multifocal and randomly distributed throughout the lungs in most cases. Histologically, lung lesions consisted of interstitial to bronchointerstitial pneumonia (BIP), with inflammatory changes ranging from mononuclear infiltrates to fibrin and neutrophils in more severely affected lungs. Similarly, less severe changes could be seen in several of the BVDV or BoCV inoculated calves. In this study, BoCV antigen was found via IHC in bronchial and tracheal epithelium, alveolar interstitium, and macrophages, whereas BVDV antigen was not detected by IHC. This study confirms the potential for BoCV isolates from the respiratory tract to cause clinical disease detected by gross and microscopic lesions, in particular, with a sequential dual infection with BVDV. In addition, IHC detected the present of BoCV antigen in multiple respiratory tract sites. This study indicates that sequential dual infections may have potential as models for vaccine and therapy development and efficacy studies.

Additional information on BoCV will follow in the section on various surveys using metagenomics and PCR testing as well as serotesting in samples from North America.

Influenza D Virus

The influenza D virus (IDV) has gained considerable attention in the etiology of BRD. Use of genomic testing, including sequencing of the viral genome and use of PCR testing, along with antibody testing has resulted in numerous studies indicating the widespread presence of IDV in North America. The virus ultimately identified as IDV initially was isolated from swine, and designated C/swine/Oklahoma/1223/2011 (C/OK); this virus was found to have homology to human influenza C viruses.[32] Respiratory tract samples from cattle were submitted to a commercial laboratory for testing for BRD diagnosis using PCR testing, which included testing with primers derived from this swine influenza C virus. Viruses from these PCR positives were isolated from cell cultures and confirmed to be influenza virus by hemagglutination and PCR. The viral genomes were sequenced and found different from the influenza C viruses. Using serotesting, these bovine isolates also were found antigenically different from the influenza C viruses. The swine strain C/OK, and these new bovine influenza viruses are now classified as D influenza viruses referred to as IDVs (influenza D viruses).

With this new information, multiple studies have reported the presence of IDV in several regions of North America using respiratory tract samples for detection of the viral genome, PCR positives, and/or serology.[32–41] These reports are summarized later, not only for presence of IDV but also for other viruses. As with other viruses detected in BRD cases, the question of whether the virus causes disease (acts as a pathogen) or is a resident in healthy cattle without disease potential has been raised. Another question posed for IDV in cattle is whether a vaccine might provide protection in vaccinated and challenged cattle. A subsequent report found that an inactivated IDV vaccine using an isolate from cattle provided partial protection in vaccinated calves compared with controls, and the challenge virus caused inflammation in the nasal turbinates and trachea but not appreciably in the lungs.[42] These results give evidence for the role of IDV of cattle in BRD and that partial protection may result from an inactivated vaccine.

STUDIES OF ADDITIONAL VIRUSES BEYOND BOVINE HERPES VIRUS 1, BOVINE VIRAL DIARRHEA VIRUS, BOVINE PARAINFLUENZA TYPE 3 VIRUS, AND BOVINE *Respiratory Syncytial Virus*

Use of testing for influenza viruses in cattle in the United States first was published in 2014.[32] Nasal swabs or lung samples were submitted for testing for BRD diagnosis and consisted of 45 samples. These samples were from 6 different states and were tested using a real-time/reverse transcriptase (RT)-PCR assay, which included primers for the influenza C viruses. There were 8 samples (18%) positive for the influenza C virus, representing samples from Minnesota and Oklahoma. Five of the positives were isolated in cell culture and were tested further by PCR and hemagglutination assays. Four positives were from 1 herd in Minnesota and 2 were chosen for further study, C/bovine/Minnesota/628/2013 and C/bovine/Minnesota/729/2013, and 1 remaining isolate was from a case in Oklahoma, C/bovine/Oklahoma/660/2013. Eventually these viruses were placed into a new group based on genomic and antigenic differences from influenza C virus group, leading to designation of a new genus (D) in the viral family *Orthomyxoviridae*. Seroprevalence of IDV in bovine populations was examined with hemagglutination inhibition (HI) with the C/swine/Oklahoma/1334/2011 (C/OK) virus and C/bovine/660/2013 (C/660) as antigen and bovine sera from 8 herds in 5 different states tested individually. With the exception of 1 herd, all herds had high geometric mean titers of greater than 40, and antibodies against the bovine C/OK virus and C/660 virus were cross-reactive in the HI assay. These results indicated that cattle are a reservoir for these viruses.

The epidemiology of IDV was reported further in 2015 using samples from cattle in Mississippi.[33] Sera, nasal swabs, and nasopharyngeal swabs were collected from calves at a cattle buying facility in Mississippi. Respiratory swabs testing positive by RT-PCR revealed that 16/55 (29.1%) of the sick calves and 2/84 (2.4%) of the healthy calves were positive for IDV, and the virus was isolated in cell culture from 15 of these 18 RT-PCR positive samples. The genome of D/bovine/Mississippi/C00046/2014 was fully sequenced. Phylogenetic analysis of the HE gene aligned the IDV isolates from Mississippi into 2 clades. Using serology with the HI test on serum samples from neonatal samples indicated transfer of IDV antibodies to the calf from the dam. Also, testing of sera archived from 2004, 2005, and 2006 found the seroprevalance by year of 18.3% (n = 241), 14.8% (n = 223), and 13.5% (n = 141), respectively, indicating presence of IDV in Mississippi since at least 2004.

Distinct genetic and antigenic lineages of IDV in cattle were reported.[34] Samples from BRD cases submitted to the Kansas State University Veterinary Diagnostic Laboratory were screened by BRD PCR panel, which detects BoHV1, BVDV, PI3V, BRSV, and BoCV. The samples were later tested for IDV by an RT-PCR assay. These 208 samples represented nasal and pharyngeal swabs and lung tissues from 12 Midwestern states. There were 10 (4.8%) positive for IDV along with other positives: 36% (BoCV), 7% (BoHV1), 5% (BVDV), 3% (BRSV), and less than 1% (PI3V). The 10 IDV positives were from Kansas, Texas, and Nebraska. Of the 10 PCR IDV positives, 6 were positive via cell culture inoculation. Full-genome sequencing was performed on all 6 cell culture IDV positives. The phylogenetic analysis showed 2 distinct lineages of the IDV from cattle. Using polyclonal antiserum against 2 IDV, D/OK (D/swine/Oklahoma/1334/2011 and the D/660 (D/bovine/Oklahoma/660/2013 in the HI serotest, antigenic differences were noted based on varied HI results.

Metagenomics and PCR testing were used to detect viruses in a study of BRD in California dairy calves.[35] Dairy calves between the ages of 27 days and 60 days were enrolled as either BRD cases or controls. Nasopharyngeal and pharyngeal recess swabs were collected. Using metagenomics and subsequent PCR testing, numerous viruses were identified. Viruses were detected in 68% of the BRD cases and 16% of the healthy controls. Multiple viruses were found in 38% of the sick animals versus 8% of the controls. Based on the viral hits of the genome sequences, the following viruses were detected in descending order: bovine rhinitis A virus, which was greater than bovine adenovirus 3, which was greater than bovine adeno-associated virus, which was greater than bovine rhinitis B virus, which was greater than astrovirus, which was greater than bovine IDV, which was greater than picobirnavirus, which was greater than bovine parvovirus 2, which was greater than bovine herpesvirus 6. Those viruses significantly associated with BRD compared with matched controls included bovine adenovirus 3 ($P<.0001$), bovine rhinitis A virus ($P = .009$), and bovine IDV ($P = .012$).

A metagenomics study investigated viral genomes in nasal swabs from 103 cattle from Mexico (63) and the United States (40), representing 6 Mexican feedlots and 4 Kansas feedlots in 2015.[36] Cattle with acute BRD and asymptomatic pen mates were included. There were 21 viruses detected, with bovine rhinitis A (52.7%), bovine rhinitis B (23.7%), and BoCV (24.7%) the most commonly reported. Comparing the recovery of viruses from cattle with BRD versus asymptomatic controls, bovine IDV tended to be significantly associated with BRD ($P = .134$; odds ratio 2.94). The other viruses historically associated with BRD, including BoHV1, BVDV, PI3V, and BRSV, were detected less frequently.

A Canadian survey of beef cattle utilized metagenomics to detect viruses in western Canadian feedlot cattle with or without BRD.[37] There were 116 cattle sampled with deep nasal swabs and transtracheal washes collected and included samples from animals with or without BRD. The cattle on arrival received an MLV vaccine containing BoHV1, BVDV1. BVDV2, PI3V, and BRSV. There were 21 viruses identified via metagenomics. Viruses associated with BRD based on statistical comparison included bovine IDV ($P<.015$), bovine rhinitis B virus ($P<.02$), BRSV ($P<.022$), and BoCV ($P<.021$). This report represents the first report of bovine IDV in western Canada. The BoHV1 was not identified in any sample, and BVDV1 and PI3V were found only in 1 sample and 2 samples, respectively. Perhaps the efficacy of the MLV resulted in reduced or absence of recovery of BVDV, PI3V, and BoHV1. The BRSV was found in 17% of BRD cases and 2% of the controls. There was weak agreement in the identification of viruses in the nasal swabs and transtracheal swabs, suggesting that sample location affects the recovery of viruses.

A study was performed to determine prevalence of BRD viruses and *Mycoplasma bovis* in US cattle.[38] Samples were from different production classes, including cow calf, stocker, feedlot, and dairy, and from varied seasons of the year. There were 3205 samples collected between May 2015 and July 2016 and from 80 different premises. The intent was to test healthy animals; however, disease status and other clinical data were not collected. These nasopharyngeal swabs were assayed using RT-PCR assay using primers for BoHV1, BVDV, BoCV, IDV, BRSV, and *Mycoplasma bovis*. The overall percent positive rates for each agent were 3.81% for BRSV, 1.59% for BoHV1, 3.56% for BVDV, 8.3% for IDV, 43.81% for BoCV, 20.12% for *M bovis*, and 17.32% for multiple-agent positives. The high percentage of IDV and BoCV positives suggested that more emphasis should be placed on these viruses in BRD. The BoCV was significantly more associated with stocker production class and the fall season. This study did not differentiate vaccine viruses from field strains.

A metagenomics study was performed using cases submitted to a western Canadian diagnostic laboratory BRD diagnosis.[39] The samples from pneumonia cases (130) were submitted between September 2017 and December 2018. There were 90.8% of the samples from beef cattle and 9.2% from dairy cattle. Formalin-fixed tissues were processed for histologic examination and fresh tissues frozen until further testing. Cases were classified as suppurative bronchopneumonia (SBP), fibrinous bronchopneumonia (BP), interstitial pneumonia, BP + BIP, and bronchiolitis. The metagenomics identification was performed on fresh lung tissues. From 34 samples with metagenomics sequencing results, an RT-PCR test with primers for BVDV, PI3V, BRSV, BoHV1, and BoCV was used in all cases of these viruses detected. In 4 cases, however, a virus was detected by RT-PCR that was not detected by metagenomics sequencing. The recovery of viruses was low, with only 36.9% (48/130) positive. There were 16 viruses identified. The bovine parvovirus 2 was the most prevalent virus, 11.5%, followed by ungulate tetraparvovirus 1 and BRSV, both 8.3%. The BRD viruses—BRSV, 8.5%, and BVDV1 and BVDV2, 2.3%, and 3.8%, respectively—and PI3V, 2.3%, were found infrequently. None of these viruses was associated with a particular pneumonia. Animal viruses were identified in only 1 animal each: bovine rhinitis B, IDV, fowl aviadenovirus, avian adenovirus–associated virus, and bovine polyomavirus. The most prevalent virus in each type of pneumonia was bovine parvovirus 2, at 5.9% in FDP; bovine astrovirus, at 3.1% in SBP; BRSV, at 1.5% in interstitial pneumonia; and ungulate tetraparvovirus 1 in BP and BIP, at 1.5%. However, for every type of pneumonia, samples in which no virus was detected, this was the most common result compared to the percentage virus recovery in each pneumonia category. None of these viruses detected were significantly associated with any type of pulmonary pathology. This virus detection in lung tissue provides low analytic sensitivity relative to ante mortem sampling of the upper respiratory tract for virus surveillance.[39] In this study, however, the bacterial agents *Histophilus somni, Mannheimia haemolytica*, and *Pasteurella multocida* were found to have strong associations with SBP, fibrinous BP, and BP and BIP, respectively.[39] These results were in contrast to a prior western Canadian study using swabs from the upper respiratory tract (nasal and tracheal) of beef cattle where IDV, bovine rhinitis B, BRSV, and BoCV were significantly associated with BRD.[37] A potential explanation for these divergent findings is that the lungs of the fatal cases may have cleared the viruses and the bacterial pathogens remained predominant.

Serologic surveys often are used to determine presence and prevalence of viruses in various populations of cattle, based on production class and/or geographic regions. Such surveys preferably should rely on samples from animals that have lost their maternal antibodies; thus, antibodies identified result from active infections. Using HI testing, the seropositive rate for IDV ranged from 13.5% to 80.2% in 2 studies.[33,40] In the latter study, sera from animals 2 years of age or older from beef cattle herds in Nebraska were tested for IDV antibodies via the HI assay. These were from samples collected from September 2003 to May 2004. The HI assay used 2 IDV from Mississippi, representing 2 reported IDV clusters that were antigenically distinct. There were 240 (81.9%) samples seropositive to 1 or both of the 2 IDVs. There were log_2 differences in titers in some samples, suggesting there were 2 antigenic clusters circulating in these Nebraska herds. The cattle from all the 40 farms had evidence of exposure and were from farms across Nebraska.

A subsequent serosurvey was performed using samples from throughout the United States as part of the US brucellosis surveillance program.[41] Both male and female cattle 2 years of age or older representing 42 US states were randomly sampled in 5 slaughter plants. The cattle represented 6 US regions: Pacific West, Mountain West, Upper Midwest, South Central, Northeast, and Southeast. The antigen in the HI test was selected as D/bovine/Kansas/14-22/12. Of the 1992 samples, 1545 (77.5%) were positive for IDV antibodies. Positives were found in samples from 41 of 42 states, with a seropositive rate by state ranging from 25% to 93.8%. Sample size by state or titer level may have caused bias. The range among geographic regions for seropositivity was 47.7% to 84.6%. The Mountain West region had the highest, 84.6%, and the Northeast the lowest, 47.7%.

SUMMARY

Advances in viral detection in BRD mirrors advances in viral sequencing using respiratory tract samples. Additional viruses beyond BoHV1, BVDV, PI3V, and BRSV include, as examples, IDV, BoCV, bovine rhinitis A, bovine rhinitis B, adenoviruses, astrovirus, bovine parvovirus, and others. Diagnostic laboratories are now using PCR testing based on primers learned from sequencing. In selected instances, such as IDV and BoCV, serosurveys have demonstrated the widespread presence of these viruses in North American cattle. In limited studies, these viruses, such as IDV and BoCV, have caused disease in animal studies. In various studies, some of these viruses, but not all, have been found in BRD cases more frequently than in healthy cattle. It is important that reagents be developed by diagnostic laboratories to use in diagnostic testing for the new viruses. The pathogenicity of these new viruses should be determined in controlled challenge studies. Vaccine development and evaluation in controlled studies for these viruses should be considered to determine if vaccinations have a role in their control.

DISCLOSURE

The author has nothing to disclose.

REFERENCES

1. Fulton RW. Bovine respiratory disease research: 1983 to 2009. Anim Health Res Rev 2019;10:131–9.
2. Fulton RW, Confer AW. Laboratory test descriptions for bovine respiratory disease diagnosis and their strengths and weaknesses: Gold standards for diagnosis, do they exist? Can Vet J 2012;53:754–61.

3. d'Offay JM, Fulton RW, Eberle R. Complete genome sequence of the NVSL BoHV-1.1 Cooper reference strain. Arch Virol 2013;158:1109–13.

4. d'Offay JM, Fulton RW, Eberle R, et al. Complete genome sequence of bovine herpesvirus type 1.1 (BoHV-1.1) Los Angeles (LA) and its genotypic relationship to BoHV-1.1 Cooper and more recently isolated wild-type field strains. Arch Virol 2018;164:2843–8.

5. Fulton RW, d'Offay JM, Eberle R. Bovine herpesvirus-1: Comparison and differentiation of vaccine and field strains based on genomic sequence variation. Vaccine 2013;31:1471–9.

6. Chase CCL, Fulton RW, O'Toole D, et al. Bovine herpesvirus 1 modified live virus vaccines for cattle reproduction: balancing protection with undesired effects. Vet Microbiol 2017;69:69–77.

7. Fulton RW, d'Offay JM, Eberle R, et al. Bovine herpesvirus-1: evaluation of genetic diversity of subtypes derived from field strains of varied clinical syndromes and their relationship to vaccine strains. Vaccine 2015;21:549–58.

8. Fulton RW, d'Offay JM, Dubovi EJ, et al. Bovine herpesvirus-1: genetic diversity of field strains from cattle with respiratory disease, genital, fetal disease and systemic neonatal disease and their relationship to vaccine strains. Virus Res 2016;223:115–21.

9. Fulton RW, d'Offay JM, Landis C, et al. Detection and characterization of viruses as field and vaccine strains in feedlot cattle with bovine respiratory disease. Vaccine 2016;34:3478–92.

10. d'Offay JM, Fulton RW, Fishbein M, et al. Isolation of a naturally occurring vaccine/wild-type recombinant herpesvirus type 1 (BoHV-1) from an aborted fetus. Vaccine 2019;37:3518–4524.

11. d'Offay JM, Eberle R, Fulton RW, et al. Complete genomic sequence and comparative analysis of four genital and respiratory isolates of bovine herpesvirus subtype 1.2b (BoHV1.2b) including prototype virus strain K22. Arch Virol 2016;161:2369–3274.

12. Ridpath JF, Fulton RW. Knowledge gaps impacting the development of bovine viral diarrhea virus control programs in the United States. J Am Vet Med Assoc 2009;235:1171–9.

13. Ridpath JF, Fulton RW, Kirkland PD, et al. Prevalence and antigenic differences observed between bovine viral diarrhea virus subgenotypes isolated from cattle in Australia and feedlots in the southwestern United States. J Vet Diagn Invest 2010;22:184–91.

14. Fulton RW, Ridpath JF, Ore S, et al. Bovine viral diarrhea virus (BVDV) subgenotypes in diagnostic laboratory accessions: distribution of BVDV1a, BVDV1b, and BVDV2a subgenotypes. Vet Microbiol 2005;111:35–40.

15. Fulton RW, Ridpath JF, Saliki JT, et al. Bovine viral diarrhea virus (BVDV1b): predominant BVDV subtype in calves with respiratory disease. Can J Vet Res 2002;66:181–90.

16. Fulton RW, Hessman B, Johnson BJ, et al. Evaluation of diagnostic tests used for detection of bovine viral diarrhea virus and prevalence of BVDV subtypes 1a, 1b, and 2a in persistently infected cattle entering a feedlot. J Am Vet Med Assoc 2006;228:578–84.

17. Workman AM, Heaton MP, Harhay GP, et al. Resolving bovine viral diarrhea virus subtypes from persistently infected U.S. beef calves with complete genome sequence. J Vet Diagn Invest 2016;28:519–28.

18. Fulton RW, Whitley EM, Johnson BJ, et al. Prevalence of bovine viral diarrhea virus (BVDV) in persistently infected cattle and BVDV subtypes in affected cattle in beef herds in South Central United States. Can J Vet Res 2009;73:283–91.

19. Ridpath JF, Lovell G, Neill JD, et al. Change in predominance of bovine viral diarrhea virus subgenotypes among samples submitted to a diagnostic laboratory over a 20-year time span. J Vet Diagn Invest 2011;23:185–93.

20. Neill JD, Workman AM, Hesse R, et al. Identification of BVDV2b and 2c subgenotypes in the United States: genetic and antigenic characterization. Virology 2019; 528:19–29.

21. Yesilbag K, Alpay G, Becher P. Variability and global distribution of subgenotypes of bovine viral diarrhea virus. Viruses 2017;9:1–19.

22. Neill JD, Ridpath JF, Valayudhan BT. Identification and genome characterization of genotype B and genotype C bovine parainfluenza type 3 viruses isolated in the United States. BMC Vet Res 2015;11:1–6.

23. Fulton RW, Neill JD, Saliki JT, et al. Genomic and antigenic characterization of bovine parainfluenza-3 viruses in the United States including modified live virus vaccine (MLV) strains and field strains from cattle. Virus Res 2017;235:77–81.

24. Ellis J. What is the evidence that bovine coronavirus is a biologically significant respiratory pathogen in cattle? Can Vet J 2019;60:147–52.

25. Gagea M, Bateman KG, vanDreumel T, et al. Diseases and pathogens associated with mortality in Ontario feedlots. J Vet Diagn Invest 2006;18:18–28.

26. Fulton RW, Blood KS, Panciera RJ, et al. Lung pathology and infectious agents in fatal feedlot pneumonias and relationship with mortality, disease onset, and treatments. J Vet Diagn Invest 2009;21:462–77.

27. Fulton RW, Step DL, Wahrmund J, et al. Bovine coronavirus infections in transported commingled beef cattle and sole source ranch calves. Can J Vet Res 2011;75:191–9.

28. Fulton RW, Ridpath JF, Burge LJ. Bovine coronaviruses from the respiratory tract: antigenic and genetic diversity. Vaccine 2013;31:886–92.

29. Workman AM, Kuehn LA, McDaneld TG, et al. Evaluation of the effect of serum antibody abundance against bovine coronavirus on bovine coronavirus shedding and risk of respiratory tract disease in beef calves from birth through the first five weeks in a feedlot. Am J Vet Res 2017;78:1065–76.

30. Workman AM, Kuehn LA, McDaneld TG, et al. Longitudinal study of humoral immunity to bovine coronavirus, virus shedding, and treatment for bovine respiratory disease in pre-weaned calves. BMC Vet Res 2019;15:1–15.

31. Ridpath JM, Fulton RW, Bauermann FV, et al. Sequential exposure to bovine viral diarrhea virus and bovine coronavirus results in increased respiratory disease lesions, clinical, immunological, pathological, and immunohistochemical findings. J Vet Diagn Invest, in press.

32. Hause BM, Collin EA, Liu R, et al. Characterization of a novel influenza virus in cattle and swine: proposal for a new genus in the *Orthomyxoviridae* family. mBio 2014;6:1–14.

33. Ferguson L, Eckard L, Epperson WB, et al. Influenza D virus infection in Mississippi beef cattle. Virology 2015;486:28–34.

34. Collin EA, Sheng Z, Lang Y, et al. Cocirculation of two distinct genetic and antigenic lineages of proposed influenza D virus in cattle. J Virol 2015;89:1036–42.

35. Ng TFF, Kondov NO, Deng X, et al. A metagenomics study and case control study to identify viruses associated with bovine respiratory disease. J Virol 2015;89:5340–9.

36. Mitra N, Cernicchiaro N, Torres S, et al. Metagenomic characterization of the virome associated with bovine respiratory disease in feedlot cattle identified with novel viruses and suggests and etiologic role for influenza D virus. J Gen Virol 2016;97:1771–84.
37. Zhang M, Hill JE, Fernando C, et al. Respiratory viruses identified in western Canadian beef cattle by metagenomics sequencing and their association with bovine respiratory disease. Transbound Emerg Dis 2019;66:1379–86.
38. Lubbers BV, Renter DG, Hesse RA, et al. Prevalence of respiratory viruses and Mycoplasma bovis in U.S. cattle and variability among herds of origin, production systems and season of year. Bov Pract (Stillwater) 2017;51:159164.
39. Zhang M, Hill JE, Godson DL, et al. The pulmonary virome, bacteriological and histopathological findings in bovine respiratory disease from western Canada. Transbound Emerg Dis 2020;67:924–34.
40. Luo J, Ferguson L, Smith DR, et al. Serological evidence for high prevalence of influenza D viruses in cattle: Nebraska, United States, 2003-2004. Virology 2017;501:88–91.
41. Silveira S, Falkenberg SM, Kaplan BS, et al. Serosurvey for influenza D virus exposure in cattle, United States, 2014-2015. Emerg Infect Dis 2019;25:2074–80.
42. Hause BM, Huntimer L, Falkenberg S, et al. An inactivated influenza D virus vaccine partially protects cattle from respiratory disease caused by homologous challenge. Vet Microbiol 2017;199:47–53.

The Immunology of Bovine Respiratory Disease

Recent Advancements

Jodi L. McGill, MS, PhD[a],*, Randy E. Sacco, PhD[b]

KEYWORDS

- Bovine • Respiratory disease • Lung • Innate immunity • Adaptive immunity
- Immunomodulation

KEY POINTS

- Bovine respiratory disease (BRD) is a syndrome caused by multiple factors, including environmental and management-related stressors and multiple viral and bacterial pathogens.
- The innate immune system is the first line of defense against BRD. Epithelial cells and immune sentinel cells prevent infection through mucociliary action and secretion of antimicrobial molecules, and secretion of proinflammatory cytokines.
- Neutrophils are essential for eliminating bacterial infections but also play an important role in the pathogenesis of BRD by contributing to lung tissue destruction and inflammation.
- After infection, cattle mount antibody and antigen–specific T-cell responses; however, pathogens frequently evade these immune responses using multiple strategies.
- Immunomodulation and innate training are future alternatives to antibiotics for the prevention and control of BRD.

INTRODUCTION

Susceptibility to bovine respiratory disease (BRD) is multifactorial, influenced by a complex interaction between stress, multiple viral and bacterial pathogens, and the host immune response (**Table 1**). Despite the widespread availability of vaccines and antimicrobial compounds, BRD remains a leading cause of morbidity, mortality, and economic loss to the cattle industry. The continued high prevalence of the disease underlines a fundamental gap in understanding of the host immune response to respiratory infection. In recent years, several advancements have been made in the

[a] Department of Veterinary Microbiology and Preventative Medicine, Iowa State University, 1907 ISU C-Drive, VMRI Building 5, Ames, IA 50010, USA; [b] Ruminant Diseases and Immunology Research Unit, Agricultural Research Services, USDA, PO Box 70, 1920 Dayton Avenue, Ames, IA 50010, USA
* Corresponding author.
E-mail address: jlmcgill@iastate.edu

Vet Clin Food Anim 36 (2020) 333–348
https://doi.org/10.1016/j.cvfa.2020.03.002
0749-0720/20/© 2020 Elsevier Inc. All rights reserved.

Table 1		
The multiple factors with a role in bovine respiratory disease		
Stress Factors	Viral Agents	Bacterial Agents
Heat	PIV type 3	M haemolytica
Cold	BHV-1, BHV-4	P multocida
Dampness	BVDV	H somni
Dust	BRSV	Mycoplasma bovis
Injury	Adenovirus	Trueperella pyogenes
Fatigue	Coronavirus	
Dehydration	Enterovirus	
Nutritional	Reovirus	
Weaning	Influenza D virus	
Shipping		

understanding of the immune system's role in protecting—and potentially harming—the host and how multiple pathogens of the BRD complex interact to evade the host response. There have been comprehensive reviews on the immune response to BRD in previous issues of *Veterinary Clinics of North America: Food Animal Practice*[1,2]; this article focuses on the developments that have occurred over the past decade.

INNATE IMMUNOLOGY OF BOVINE RESPIRATORY DISEASE
Pattern Recognition Receptors

The innate immune system utilizes an array of soluble, surface-bound and intracellular receptors to detect the presence of invading pathogens. These receptors, termed *pattern recognition receptors (PRRs)*, recognize conserved molecular patterns, known as *pathogen-associated molecular patterns (PAMPs)*. Common PAMPs include peptidoglycan and lipotechoic acids from gram-positive bacteria, lipopolysaccharide (LPS) from gram-negative bacteria, CpG-rich DNA, and single-stranded and double-stranded RNA. Together, the cells that comprise the bovine respiratory tract express a full arsenal of surface-bound and intracellular PRRs, including Toll-like receptors (TLRs), NOD-like receptors, and RNA helicases, such as RIG-I and MDA-5. All pathogens of the BRD complex produce some type of PAMP that activate the innate immune system.

Infection induces up-regulation of many PRRs, preparing an animal to mount a robust response to the insult. In vitro infection of bovine bronchial epithelial cells by bovine herpesvirus (BHV)-1 or *Mannheimia haemolytica* results in up-regulation of TLR2,[3] a PRR generally involved in the recognition of gram-positive bacteria. In vivo infection with BHV-1 induces up-regulation of TLR3, TLR7, TLR8, and TLR9 in the nasal mucosa, tracheal epithelium, and lung.[4] A transcriptome analysis of the bronchial lymph nodes of calves singly infected with BRD pathogens revealed a global up-regulation of many PRR-associated genes, although there was some specificity in the response to particular pathogens.[5] Although *M haemolytica* infection induced selective up-regulation of TLR1 and TLR6, infection with BHV-1, bovine respiratory syncytial virus (BRSV) or bovine viral diarrhea virus (BVDV) induced more pronounced up-regulation of TLR2 and TLR4.[5] The biological significance of these differences is not immediately clear but warrants further investigation. In an in vitro coinfection model, exposure of alveolar type 2 epithelial cells to *Histophilus somni* induced activation of the type I interferon (IFN) response, which subsequently protected the cells from BRSV infection. Thus, global activation in innate immune sensors may be an important defense strategy. Other reports, however, have shown that this response may not always be beneficial. Acute stress, such as that caused by abrupt weaning and shipping, results in increased expression of TLR4, CD14, and the IFN-responsive gene 2,5-OAS by circulating peripheral blood mononuclear cells (PBMCs).[6] Although this increase resulted in an enhanced capacity by the cells to respond to LPS (also known as endotoxin) stimulation, a significant positive association was found between PRR expression and risk of mortality from a subsequent BHV and M haemolytica challenge.[6]

Airway and Lung Epithelia and Resistance to Bovine Respiratory Disease

Although not often included under the purview of the immune system, airway epithelial cells play a critical role in the first line of defense against infection. The mucociliary escalator is responsible for the removal of inhaled particles, including invading pathogens. One study of healthy animals showed that greater than 90% of aerosolized M haemolytica could be eliminated from the lung within 4 hours of administration, primarily due to ciliary action.[7] Viral pathogens, however, such as BRSV, BHV, and parainfluenza virus (PIV), cause ciliary dysfunction and necrosis,[1,8] which can lead to significant delays in the clearance of inhaled particles.[9] Thus, interference with normal ciliary function may be 1 explanation by which primary viral infections predispose cattle to secondary bacterial pneumonia.

Bovine airway epithelial cells express many PRRs, and are responsive to common TLR agonists, such as LPS, which signals through TLR4, and Pam3CSK4, which activates TLR2.[10,11] Epithelial cells of the respiratory tract produce several antimicrobial molecules, including lactoferrin, tracheal antimicrobial peptide (TAP), lingual antimicrobial peptide (LAP), and bovine myeloid antimicrobial peptide (BMAP-28), which accumulate in the mucus and periciliary layers of the air-surface interface. Stimulation with LPS or Pam3CSK induces secretion of LAP, TAP, and lactoferrin, preparing the tissues to ward off invading bacterial pathogens.[11,12] TAP has bactericidal activity against M haemolytica, H somni, and Pasteurella multocida,[13] whereas BMAP-28 can kill P multocida in vitro.[14] Viral infections can interfere with the production of antimicrobial peptides by epithelial cells. For example, prior infection with BVDV inhibits pathogen-induced expression of both LAP and lactoferrin by tracheal epithelial cells.[12]

Airway epithelial cells also can play a role in the antiviral immune response. In vivo infection with BHV-1 results in rapid activation of the type I IFN response in the trachea, including secretion of type I and type II IFNs and induction of the interferon-stimulated genes Mx1, OAS, and BST-2.[15] BHV, and many other viruses of the BRD complex, including BVDV, BRSV, and PIV, however, have mechanisms in place to actively suppress the host IFN response.[16–19] In 1 report, coinfection of bovine epithelial cells with BVDV inhibited type I IFN production, enabling significantly increased replication of BRSV in the same cell cultures,[19] suggesting a synergistic interaction between the 2 viruses.

Perhaps the most critical result of an insult to the airway epithelia is the engagement of the effector arm of the innate immune system. In vitro, invasion of bovine bronchial epithelial cells by M haemolytica, or infection with BHV-1, induces rapid secretion of the proinflammatory cytokines interleukin (IL)-6, tumor necrosis factor (TNF)-α, and IL-8, leading to the recruitment and activation of innate immune effector cells, such as neutrophils.[3,20] Coinfection of bronchial epithelial cells with both BHV-1 and M haemolytica has been shown to exacerbate proinflammatory responses by bovine epithelial cells, resulting in greater cytokine expression by dually infected cells compared with either single pathogen alone.[3,20] Similar results also have been shown after coinfection of bovine bronchial epithelial cells with BRSV and P multocida.[21] Proinflammatory cytokines, however, are not the only factors that can contribute to lung damage. In vitro infection of bovine alveolar type 2 cells with BRSV and *H somni* results in significant up-regulation of matrix metalloproteinases 1 and 3, enzymes that break down collagen, thus enhancing the invasion of *H somni* across the alveolar barrier.[22]

Airway epithelial cells also may play a role in regulating the inflammatory response in the respiratory tract. Annexin A1 and annexin A2 are anti-inflammatory proteins produced by airway epithelial cells that regulate neutrophil recruitment and activation, similar to glucocorticoids. Increased concentrations of annexin A1 and annexin A2 in the bronchoalveolar lavage (BAL) fluid prior to challenge have been shown to correlate with improved resistance to the later development of BRD.[23]

Effector Cells of the Innate Immune System

Neutrophils

Neutrophils are among the first cell type to be recruited to the site of infection, migrating from the blood in response to proinflammatory cytokines and chemotactic factors, such as IL-8. Neutrophils are highly phagocytic cells that play an important role in protecting the host against extracellular bacterial infections. It is clear, however, that neutrophils also play a major role in lung tissue destruction during BRD. Depletion of neutrophils,[24] or inhibition of neutrophil infiltration to the respiratory tract,[25] prior to *M haemolytica* infection results in a significant decrease in inflammatory cytokine and lung pathology.

Neutrophil extracellular traps (NETs) have emerged as 1 important factor contributing to BRD pathogenesis. Neutrophils have the capacity to undergo NETosis, a form of cell death in which neutrophils release their nuclear DNA and associated proteins into the extracellular environment. *M haemolytica*[26], *Mycoplasma bovis*,[27] and *H somni*[28] cause neutrophil NET formation in vitro, and evidence of NETS has been observed in the lungs of calves infected with both *M haemolytica*[26] and *H somni*.[28] There is some debate as to whether NETs are an active form of host defense or simply an artifact of neutrophil cell death. In vitro, NETs can kill *M haemolytica* and *H somni*, suggesting some active role in immunity, but the relevance of this antimicrobial activity is difficult to investigate in vivo in the morbid animal. *Mycoplasma bovis* is not susceptible to NET-mediated killing in vitro,[27] potentially due to its ability to release nucleases and degrade the extracellular DNA.[29] Citrullinated histone 3, an indicator of NETs, is increased in the BAL fluid of calves with severe BRSV infection,[30] and NETs have been observed microscopically in the lungs of calves with BRSV infection,[31] demonstrating that NETosis is not specific to bacterial invasion. In calves with BRSV, NETs form dense networks, entrapping mucin and cells, leading to airway occlusion.[31] Consistent with the idea the NETs play a pathogenic role, aerosol administration of dornase alfa, a synthetic form of DNAse I that can degrade NETS, considerably reduced airway obstruction and improved lung pathology in a small group of calves infected with BRSV.[32]

Antigen-presenting cells: monocytes, macrophages and dendritic cells

Antigen-presenting cells (APCs), including monocytes, macrophages, and dendritic cells, are critical in bridging the innate and adaptive immune systems. Dendritic cells in particular are essential to the induction of an effective T-cell and B-cell response. Monocytes and macrophages also fulfill the role of an APC but are similarly active in phagocytosis of dead and dying cells; killing of extracellular pathogens and inflammatory cytokine production.

BVDV infection is a major predisposing factor for BRD due to its known immunosuppressive effects on cells of both the innate and adaptive immune systems. In alveolar macrophages, noncytopathic BVDV infection suppresses proinflammatory cytokine secretion and reduces phagocytic activity. In vitro infection of monocyte-derived macrophages with both cytopathic and noncytopathic strains of BVDV suppresses responsiveness to ligands for TLR2, TLR3, and TLR4 but does not alter signaling through TLR7.[33] Similarly, in vivo BVDV infection also modulates the capacity of monocytes and macrophages to respond via TLR4.[34]

Like BVDV, several other viruses have an impact on APC activation and function. PIV infection suppresses macrophage phagocytosis and inhibits oxidative burst.[35,36] PIV-infected macrophages, however, are hyperresponsive to LPS stimulation, producing significantly increased quantities of TNF-α.[37] BRSV infection also inhibits alveolar macrophage phagocytosis but does not appear to impair the oxidative burst response.[38] In vitro BRSV infection of ovine alveolar macrophages induces only low-level proinflammatory cytokine expression.[39] In vivo infection of lambs also results in only limited activation of lung-resident dendritic cells, with no significant changes in major histocompatibility complex (MHC) class I or the costimulatory molecules CD80 or CD86. Instead, both lung dendritic cells and alveolar macrophages significantly upregulate gene expression of IL-4 and IL-10.[39] In vivo BHV-1 infection induces recruitment of interstitial and alveolar macrophages to the lungs, and induces production of proinflammatory cytokines, such as TNFα, IL-1α, and induced nitric oxide synthase (iNOS).[40] Calves coinfected with BVDV and BHV-1 show greater numbers of infiltrating macrophages than animals that are singly infected but reduced production of iNOS and the proinflammatory mediators TNF-α and IL-1α.[40]

ADAPTIVE IMMUNOLOGY OF BOVINE RESPIRATORY DISEASE

The development of an adaptive immune response is critical for control and clearance of respiratory pathogens. After infection, cattle mount antibody (Ab) and antigen-specific T-cell responses; however, pathogens frequently evade these immune responses by using multiple strategies. Many of these immune evasion strategies have been covered in reviews of the specific pathogens.[41–44]

B cells and antibody responses

B-cell surface immunoglobulins recognize pathogen epitopes. After antigen recognition and additional downstream signals, B cells terminally differentiate into antibody (Ab)-secreting plasma cells. The Ab secreted play important roles in defending the host from infection with respiratory pathogens. Those roles include neutralizing Ab (nAb), complement activation, Fc Receptor-mediated phagocytosis, and Ab-dependent cellular cytotoxicity. On the other hand, specific Ab against respiratory pathogens and the resultant immune complexes may contribute to BRD pathogenesis.

The protective antigens of Pasteurellaceae family members have not been fully elucidated. There are studies, however, that have shown that Ab that neutralize toxins or Ab against LPS, outer membrane proteins, or secreted antigens can be protective.[45] For example, Ab to *M haemolytica* serotype 1 outer membrane lipoprotein PlpE cross-protects against other serotypes and these Ab promote complement-mediated bacterial killing.[46] Antibodies against the surface exposed outer membrane lipoprotein Gs60 can be protective and have been suggested as especially important in protection against *M haemolytica* when nAb titers to the *M haemolytica* leukotoxin are low.[47] Other Pasteurellaceae, including *P multocida* and *H somni*, have Gs60 homologues,[47] and these also may be targets of protective Ab. In addition, vaccination of calves with sialoglycoprotease enhances protection against experimental disease due to *M haemolytica*.[48] Fewer studies have been conducted to identify antigens associated with protection from *P multocida* challenge. As was the case for *M haemolytica*, however, Ab generated against outer membrane proteins of *P multocida* have been shown to be an important component of host defense. Intranasal treatment with *P multocida* outer membrane protein H induced both serum IgG and secretory IgA levels that protected calves from experimental challenge with *P multocida*.[49] Although studies have yet to be conducted in cattle, a recombinant outer membrane lipoprotein B from *P multocida* serotype A strain was shown to induce serum Ab in mice with significant bacterial killing activity.[50] Regarding *H somni* immunity, antibodies to a 40-kDa outer membrane protein (OMP) have been found protective, whereas those to a 78-kDa OMP are not.[41] Furthermore, 40-kDa OMP IgG1 antibodies protected less effectively than IgG2. In calves vaccinated with a commercial *H somni* vaccine and then experimentally challenged, IgG2 levels were shown to inversely correlate with disease severity in response to experimental infection.[51]

Seroconversion is detectable 14 days to 28 days after experimental respiratory infection with *Mycoplasma bovis*.[52] The primary serum Ab detected in calves is IgG1,[53] which corresponds with a predominance of IgG1 plasma cells in the lungs of calves experimentally infected with *Mycoplasma bovis*.[43] In cattle, IgG1 is known to be a poorer opsonin for phagocytosis and killing than IgG2, and this may be 1 strategy which *Mycoplasma bovis* uses for immune evasion.[43] Moreover, new antigenically distinct variants of *Mycoplasma bovis* variable surface proteins[54] arise in response to Ab that target these immunodominant surface lipoproteins which further facilitates evasion of host defenses, until adaptive immunity can again respond.

nAb are critical in the response to bovine respiratory viral pathogens. Viral glycoproteins (g) are targets of these Ab against BHV-1, including gB, gC, gD, and gH. Among these, gD has been shown to elicit especially strong nAb titers compared with gC or tegument protein VP8 when delivered via DNA vaccination.[55] Thus, researchers have sought to identify epitopes on gD important for virus neutralization, several of which have been defined, including recently described highly conserved, neutralizing epitopes within the amino and carboxy termini of BHV-1 gD.[56,57] Experimental evidence indicates that BVDV envelope E2 is not only the major immunodominant glycoprotein but also the most variable for BVDV isolates. nAb induced against E2 after natural infection or after vaccination is considered protective against BVDV.[58] To provide information for future vaccines, investigators have mapped neutralizing epitopes and characterized neutralizing monoclonal Ab that bind to E2.[58] Protective Ab responses to BRSV predominately target the F, G, and NP proteins, although calves mount responses to several antigens. Specific Ab can be detected in nasal secretions by day 8 postinfection. Time to detection of BRSV-specific serum IgG1 and IgG2 differs, with IgG1 observed at approximately day 13, whereas IgG2 is not detected until 1 month to 3 months after infection.[59] In either case, the IgG subclass responses wane rapidly. Important in protection from BRSV are nAb against F and G. Neutralizing epitopes have been defined for the prefusion and postfusion F proteins, with the most potent targeting the prefusion protein.[60] In addition, the conserved central core domain of G is an important target of broadly nAb.

Gamma delta T cells

Gamma delta ($\gamma\delta$) T cells play an early role in the host immune response and have functions related to both innate and adaptive immunity. High levels of $\gamma\delta$ T cells are found in the peripheral blood of cattle, especially in young calves, where they can comprise up to 60% of lymphocyte pool.[61] These cells are found in large proportions at mucosal sites, including the respiratory tract, where they serve as part of a first line of defense against invading pathogens.

Relatively few studies have examined $\gamma\delta$ T cell responses to bovine respiratory bacterial pathogens, which is somewhat remarkable given their relative abundance in calves. The authors have shown that *M haemolytica* can exacerbate the expression of the inflammatory cytokine IL-17 induced by BRSV infection and that $\gamma\delta$ T cells are a primary producer of IL-17 using an in vitro model system.[62] No enhancement of IL-17 was seen, however, when PBMCs were cocultured with BRSV and *P multocida*. After challenge of previously immunized calves with *P multocida*, an increase in CD5, CD8, and MHC class II expression was found on activated $\gamma\delta$ T cells in BAL samples.[63] After *Mycoplasma bovis* lung infection in calves, $\gamma\delta$ T cells isolated from peripheral blood and restimulated with heat-inactivated *Mycoplasma bovis* antigen exhibited higher levels of the activation marker CD25.[53] Activated $\gamma\delta$ T cells could be 1 source of the intracellular IFN-γ that was measured from in vitro activated PBMCs in that study.

In response to BHV-1 modified live vaccination and subsequent challenge in calves, increased peripheral blood $\gamma\delta$ T cells with an activated phenotype were observed.[64] In response to intrabronchial challenge with BVDV1, expansion of $\gamma\delta$ T cells in BAL fluid of calves has been reported.[65] The authors' group has found expression of the surface molecule WC1.1 correlates with increased $\gamma\delta$ T cell chemokine elaboration during BRSV infection in calves, suggesting that these cells may contribute to recruitment of inflammatory cells.[66] Earlier work of others had shown that depletion of WC1.1-expressing cells did not have an impact on the clinical course of disease in BRSV-infected calves but rather resulted in significantly increased local IgM and IgA responses.[67]

Alpha/beta T cells

As discussed previously for $\gamma\delta$ T cells, there has been limited investigation of bovine alpha/beta ($\alpha\beta$) T cells after infection with members of the Pasteurellaceae family. Experimental infection of naïve calves with *P multocida* resulted in a significant increase in the percentage of activated CD8$^+$ T cells in BAL that express MHC II compared with control-naïve calves; however, no significant differences in these cells were seen between immunized control and immunized challenged groups of calves.[63] In addition, increased bronchus-associated lymphoid tissue was noted in lung tissue and an increase in the number of MHC class II–expressing CD4$^+$ T cells was observed in draining lymph nodes after challenge.

Cellular immune responses have been measured using PBMCs isolated from calves after experimental lung infection with *Mycoplasma bovis*.[53] Heat-killed *M bovis* activated CD4$^+$ and CD8$^+$ peripheral blood subpopulations in vitro as measured by flow cytometric analyses. Moreover, as equal percentages of simulated cells produced IFN-γ and IL-4 cytokine responses,[53] indicative of a mixed systemic cytokine response. Local immune responses in lung tissue were evaluated after challenge with *Mycoplasma bovis*; however, no statistical differences in numbers of CD4$^+$ or CD8$^+$ T-cell subsets were noted.[68]

Although nAb are critical in protection against bovine respiratory viruses, there is an important role for cellular immunity involving both CD4$^+$ and CD8$^+$ T cells. CD4$^+$ T cells are considered essential for clearance of BHV-1, with recognition of glycoproteins gB, gC, gD, and VP8 by these immune cells.[44] Defining antigenic regions within these major glycoproteins recognized by CD4$^+$ T cells is important for novel vaccines strategies for BHV-1, and, in this regard, CD4$^+$ T cells epitopes have been mapped on gB[69] and gD.[70] Similarly, gC and gD have been shown to be targets of cytotoxic CD8$^+$

T cells. Importantly, CD8[+] T cells may play a role in control of re-establishment of active infection from latency.[44] CD4[+] and CD8[+] $\alpha\beta$ T cells are critical in the response to BRSV. The F and G proteins are the major class II–restricted targets in cattle, with multiple antigenic regions described for the F protein of BRSV. CD8[+] T cells are critical for clearance of BRSV, with M2, F, N, and G targets described.[71] Increased CD8[+] T-cell infiltration in several tissues has been seen during BRSV infection, with cytotoxic CD8[+] T-cell activity peaking at 7 days to 10 days postinfection.[72] BVDV infections generate peripheral CD4 T cells that can recognize structural and nonstructural epitopes, including those on E2 and NS3 as dominant MHC class II epitopes.[73] Increased numbers of activated CD4 and CD8 T cells have been noted in BAL in response to primary and secondary cytopathic BVDV intrabronchial challenge.[65]

FACTORS THAT HAVE AN IMPACT ON IMMUNITY AND SUSCEPTIBILITY TO BOVINE RESPIRATORY DISEASE
Stress and Immunity

Multiple studies have postulated a link between stress and incidence and severity of respiratory infections. Stress often is a broadly used term to describe adverse circumstances or an alteration induced in an individual as a result of those circumstances. In cases of BRD, the stresses may be categorized generally as psychological, physiologic, and/or nutritional. Thus, stresses in calves can include those associated with weaning, veterinary procedures, transport, comingling, crowding, and dietary changes, among other factors. There is conflicting evidence in the literature on the impact of some of these factors in inducing altered serum stress markers (eg, cortisol levels) and how these may influence bacterial or viral infections or viral-bacterial coinfections associated with BRD.[74] There seems to be strong evidence, however, that weaning and transportation are stressors that contribute to severity of BRD.[75]

Genetics of Disease Resistance

Over the past decades, it has become clear that genetics play a significant role in determining resistance and susceptibility to a wide variety of disease conditions in humans and livestock. In cases of BRD, cattle of the same age and housed under the same conditions vary greatly in their tendency to develop disease, and the severity of the resultant clinical signs. This individual variability strongly suggests some degree of genetic control. Genetic regulation of disease susceptibility was reviewed in a recent edition of *Veterinary Clinics of North America: Food Animal Practice*.[76] This section provides only a brief summary of recent findings related to BRD and the genetic component of disease susceptibility.

Quantitative-trait locus mapping has revealed some regions linked to BRD susceptibility. Two single-nucleotide polymorphisms (SNPs) on BTA20, identified as the *ANKRA2* gene and the *CD180* gene, were shown to associate with susceptibility to BRD.[77] *ANKRA2* plays a role in transcription of the MHC class II genes, whereas *CD180* is a gene in the TLR family and is important for B-cell responsiveness to LPS. Polymorphisms have been identified in other innate bovine PRRs, including TLR, RIG-I, NOD2, and mannose-binding lectin.[78] Although there currently is little evidence to directly link these SNPs to BRD susceptibility, 1 study has suggested that polymorphisms in TLR4 and TLR8 contribute to increased responsiveness to BRSV vaccination.[78] In a recent study, gene set enrichment analysis identified glucose as the most important upstream regulator of BRD susceptibility in dairy cattle. In the same study, TNF was identified as the most significant upstream regulator in beef cattle, influencing 64 downstream genes that were associated with the immune response.[79] Comparisons between the beef and dairy populations in this studied identified 6 BRD-associated SNPs that were shared between the groups, located in the genes *ADIPOQ, HTR2A, MIF, PDE6G, PRDX3,* and *SNCA.*[79] All 6 genes are known to be involved in down-regulating TNF production and in the metabolism of reactive oxygen species.[79] It is expected that the next decade will bring continued advancements in understanding of the genetic components of this pervasive syndrome.

NOVEL INTERVENTION STRATEGIES FOR USE AGAINST BOVINE RESPIRATORY DISEASE

Vaccination and effective management strategies are the foundation of BRD prevention. Metaphylactic use of antibiotics generally is effective against BRD and is an essential tool for controlling outbreaks. There are ongoing concerns, however, regarding the development of antimicrobial resistance, and significant research efforts currently are aimed at designing new approaches for BRD prevention. Vaccines are the focus of another article in this edition. Therefore, this section is focused on a few promising alternative intervention strategies, which are being developed to reduce the impact of BRD in the dairy and feedlot.

Antimicrobial Peptides as Alternatives to Antibiotics for Bovine Respiratory Disease Control

The bovine innate immune system produces several antimicrobial peptides and several have been explored for their use as therapeutic alternatives to antibiotics. NK-lysin is an antimicrobial peptide that has been described in the granules of cytotoxic T cells and NK cells in humans, pigs, and cattle. Although humans and pigs have only a single NK-lysin gene, cattle have 4 functional NK-lysin genes, *NK1, NK2A, NK2B,* and *NK2C.*[80,81] NK-lysin gene expression is up-regulated in the lungs of animals infected with *Mycoplasma bovis, M haemolytica, P multocida,* BVDV, BRSV, and BHV-1.[80] In vitro, NK-lysin has antimicrobial activities against *M haemolytica, P multocida,* and *H somni,* although susceptibility to the 4 individual NK-lysin peptides differs between species.[80,82] *Mycoplasma bovis* is susceptible only to NK2A and NK2C peptides, and these are effective only at relatively high concentrations,[83] suggesting that NK-lysin may not be an ideal therapeutic candidate for this organism.

TAP is a β-defensin produced by airway epithelial cells. TAP gene expression is induced in bovine epithelial cells in response to TLR stimulation or IL-17A[10,11] and is up-regulated in the lungs of calves with *M haemolytica* pneumonia.[84] In vitro, TAP has potent bactericidal activity against *M haemolytica, P multocida,* and *H somni,* although *Mycoplasma bovis* is resistant to TAP treatment.[13] In a recent study, TAP was administered therapeutically, via aerosol or intranasal administration, to neonatal calves that had been challenged with *M haemolytica.*[85] Unfortunately, TAP treatment had little effect on *M haemolytica* disease. Further investigation revealed that physiologic concentrations of sodium chloride, such as the concentrations present in nasal secretions or serum, inhibited TAP-mediated bactericidal activity in vitro.[85]

Innate Immunomodulation as a Novel Strategy for Controlling Bovine Respiratory Disease

Although vaccine development continues to be an active area of research, the past decade has seen increasing interest in strategies to influence the innate immune system. Immunology dogma has long taught that the innate immune system is nonspecific and does not improve with repeated exposure. It has become apparent, however, that, in fact, the innate immune system can be primed, or trained, by exposure to certain organisms or molecules, that results in an enhanced state of responsiveness to secondary stimuli. This enhanced state of responsiveness, termed trained immunity, is induced primarily in myeloid cells (monocytes and macrophages) and NK cells[86] and results in superior cytokine expression and ultimately, enhanced capacity to prevent infection. Mechanistic studies have demonstrated that trained immunity is independent of adaptive immunity and is caused by epigenetic reprogramming and alterations in basal intracellular metabolic pathways, which result in changes in gene expression and cell physiology leading to increased innate immune cells' capacity to respond to stimulation.[86] The idea of enhancing an animal's innate state of disease resistance is appealing, particularly during well-defined periods of stress, such as during weaning and shipping. Several recent therapies have emerged with potential to train or enhance the innate immune system during times of stress. One such DNA-based immunostimulant, marketed as the commercial product Zelnate (Bayer Animal Health, Shawnee Mission, KS, USA), has been shown to reduce lung pathology scores in cattle experimentally challenged with M haemolytica[87] and significantly reduce mortality in high-risk cattle after feedlot placement.[88,89] Although the product's exact mechanisms of action is not well defined, it may be stimulating the immune system via the innate cytosolic DNA sensing cGAS-STING pathway.[90] Another immunomodulatory product, marketed as Amplimune (Novavive, Inc, located in Napanee, Ontario, Canada), is a mycobacterium cell wall fraction derived from the nonpathogenic Mycobacterium phlei. Amplimune nonspecifically activates the innate immune system and has been successfully applied for prevention of K99 Escherichia coli in preweaned calves. A promising study revealed, however, that Amiplimune had beneficial effects in reducing incidence and mortality associated with BRD in newly received, light-weight beef calves.[91]

SUMMARY

The innate and adaptive immune systems are well equipped to protect the lung from pathogen invasion. BRD is a complex syndrome, however, caused by multiple factors, including environmental and management-related stressors and viral and bacterial pathogens. In combination, these factors overwhelm and dysregulate host immunity and lead to disease. Although vaccination and antimicrobial therapy remain the primary methods for controlling BRD, several novel strategies currently are being investigated as alternatives, including innate immunomodulation and selection of genetically resistant stock.

DISCLOSURE

Research was supported by funds from the Agriculture and Food Research Initiative Competitive Grant No. 2018-06904 from the USDA National Institute of Food and Agriculture to JLM; and appropriated funds from the USDA Agricultural Research Service CRIS projects 5030-32000-116-00D and 5030-32000-117-00D to RES.

REFERENCES

1. Ackermann MR, Derscheid R, Roth JA. Innate immunology of bovine respiratory disease. Vet Clin North Am Food Anim Pract 2010;26:215–28.
2. Ellis JA. The immunology of the bovine respiratory disease complex. Vet Clin North Am Food Anim Pract 2001;17:535–50, vi-vii.

3. N'jai AU, Rivera J, Atapattu DN, et al. Gene expression profiling of bovine bronchial epithelial cells exposed in vitro to bovine herpesvirus 1 and Mannheimia haemolytica. Vet Immunol Immunopathol 2013;155:182–9.

4. Marin MS, Quintana S, Faverín C, et al. Toll-like receptor activation and expression in bovine alpha-herpesvirus infections. Res Vet Sci 2014;96:196–203.

5. Tizioto PC, Kim J, Seabury CM, et al. Immunological response to single pathogen challenge with agents of the bovine respiratory disease complex: an RNA-sequence analysis of the bronchial lymph node transcriptome. PLoS One 2015; 10:e0131459.

6. Hodgson PD, Aich P, Stookey J, et al. Stress significantly increases mortality following a secondary bacterial respiratory infection. Vet Res 2012;43:21.

7. Lopez A, Maxie MG, Savan M, et al. The pulmonary clearance of Pasteurella haemolytica in calves infected with bovine virus diarrhea or Mycoplasma bovis. Can J Comp Med 1982;46:302–6.

8. Caswell JL. Failure of respiratory defenses in the pathogenesis of bacterial pneumonia of cattle. Vet Pathol 2014;51:393–409.

9. Gershwin LJ, Gunther RA, Hornof WJ, et al. Effect of infection with bovine respiratory syncytial virus on pulmonary clearance of an inhaled antigen in calves. Am J Vet Res 2008;69:416–22.

10. Taha-Abdelaziz K, Wyer L, Berghuis L, et al. Regulation of tracheal antimicrobial peptide gene expression in airway epithelial cells of cattle. Vet Res 2016;47:44.

11. Berghuis L, Abdelaziz KT, Bierworth J, et al. Comparison of innate immune agonists for induction of tracheal antimicrobial peptide gene expression in tracheal epithelial cells of cattle. Vet Res 2014;45:105.

12. Al-Haddawi M, Mitchell GB, Clark ME, et al. Impairment of innate immune responses of airway epithelium by infection with bovine viral diarrhea virus. Vet Immunol Immunopathol 2007;116:153–62.

13. Taha-Abdelaziz K, Perez-Casal J, Schott C, et al. Bactericidal activity of tracheal antimicrobial peptide against respiratory pathogens of cattle. Vet Immunol Immunopathol 2013;152:289–94.

14. Brogden KA, Nordholm G, Ackermann M. Antimicrobial activity of cathelicidins BMAP28, SMAP28, SMAP29, and PMAP23 against Pasteurella multocida is more broad-spectrum than host species specific. Vet Microbiol 2007;119:76–81.

15. Osman R, Gonzalez-Cano P, Brownlie R, et al. Induction of interferon and interferon-induced antiviral effector genes following a primary bovine herpesvirus-1 (BHV-1) respiratory infection. J Gen Virol 2017;98:1831–42.

16. Bossert B, Marozin S, Conzelmann KK. Nonstructural proteins NS1 and NS2 of bovine respiratory syncytial virus block activation of interferon regulatory factor 3. J Virol 2003;77:8661–8.

17. Eberle KC, McGill JL, Reinhardt TA, et al. Parainfluenza virus 3 blocks antiviral mediators downstream of the interferon lambda receptor by modulating stat1 phosphorylation. J Virol 2015;90:2948–58.

18. Palomares RA, Walz HG, Brock KV. Expression of type I interferon-induced antiviral state and pro-apoptosis markers during experimental infection with low or high virulence bovine viral diarrhea virus in beef calves. Virus Res 2013;173: 260–9.

19. Alkheraif AA, Topliff CL, Reddy J, et al. Type 2 BVDV Npro suppresses IFN-1 pathway signaling in bovine cells and augments BRSV replication. Virology 2017;507:123–34.

20. Rivera-Rivas JJ, Kisiela D, Czuprynski CJ. Bovine herpesvirus type 1 infection of bovine bronchial epithelial cells increases neutrophil adhesion and activation. Vet Immunol Immunopathol 2009;131:167–76.

21. Sudaryatma PE, Nakamura K, Mekata H, et al. Bovine respiratory syncytial virus infection enhances Pasteurella multocida adherence on respiratory epithelial cells. Vet Microbiol 2018;220:33–8.

22. Agnes JT, Zekarias B, Shao M, et al. Bovine respiratory syncytial virus and Histophilus somni interaction at the alveolar barrier. Infect Immun 2013;81:2592–7.

23. Senthilkumaran C, Clark ME, Abdelaziz K, et al. Increased annexin A1 and A2 levels in bronchoalveolar lavage fluid are associated with resistance to respiratory disease in beef calves. Vet Res 2013;44:24.

24. Breider MA, Walker RD, Hopkins FM, et al. Pulmonary lesions induced by Pasteurella haemolytica in neutrophil sufficient and neutrophil deficient calves. Can J Vet Res 1988;52:205–9.

25. Radi ZA, Caverly JM, Dixon RA, et al. Effects of the synthetic selectin inhibitor TBC1269 on tissue damage during acute Mannheimia haemolytica-induced pneumonia in neonatal calves. Am J Vet Res 2001;62:17–22.

26. Aulik NA, Hellenbrand KM, Klos H, et al. Mannheimia haemolytica and its leukotoxin cause neutrophil extracellular trap formation by bovine neutrophils. Infect Immun 2010;78:4454–66.

27. Gondaira S, Higuchi H, Nishi K, et al. Mycoplasma bovis escapes bovine neutrophil extracellular traps. Vet Microbiol 2017;199:68–73.

28. Hellenbrand KM, Forsythe KM, Rivera-Rivas JJ, et al. Histophilus somni causes extracellular trap formation by bovine neutrophils and macrophages. Microb Pathog 2013;54:67–75.

29. Mitiku F, Hartley CA, Sansom FM, et al. The major membrane nuclease MnuA degrades neutrophil extracellular traps induced by Mycoplasma bovis. Vet Microbiol 2018;218:13–9.

30. Hagglund S, Blodorn K, Naslund K, et al. Proteome analysis of bronchoalveolar lavage from calves infected with bovine respiratory syncytial virus-Insights in pathogenesis and perspectives for new treatments. PLoS One 2017;12:e0186594.

31. Cortjens B, de Boer OJ, de Jong R, et al. Neutrophil extracellular traps cause airway obstruction during respiratory syncytial virus disease. J Pathol 2016;238:401–11.

32. Cortjens B, de Jong R, Bonsing JG, et al. Local dornase alfa treatment reduces NETs-induced airway obstruction during severe RSV infection. Thorax 2018;73:578–80.

33. Schaut RG, Ridpath JF, Sacco RE. Bovine viral diarrhea virus type 2 impairs macrophage responsiveness to toll-like receptor ligation with the exception of toll-like receptor 7. PLoS One 2016;11:e0159491.

34. Schaut RG, McGill JL, Neill JD, et al. Bovine viral diarrhea virus type 2 in vivo infection modulates TLR4 responsiveness in differentiated myeloid cells which is associated with decreased MyD88 expression. Virus Res 2015;208:44–55.

35. Liggitt D, Huston L, Silflow R, et al. Impaired function of bovine alveolar macrophages infected with parainfluenza-3 virus. Am J Vet Res 1985;46:1740–4.

36. Slauson DO, Lay JC, Castleman WL, et al. Alveolar macrophage phagocytic kinetics following pulmonary parainfluenza-3 virus infection. J Leukoc Biol 1987;41:412–20.

37. Bienhoff SE, Allen GK, Berg JN. Release of tumor necrosis factor-alpha from bovine alveolar macrophages stimulated with bovine respiratory viruses and bacterial endotoxins. Vet Immunol Immunopathol 1992;30:341–57.

38. Trigo E, Liggitt HD, Evermann JF, et al. Effect of in vitro inoculation of bovine respiratory syncytial virus on bovine pulmonary alveolar macrophage function. Am J Vet Res 1985;46:1098–103.

39. Fach SJ, Olivier A, Gallup JM, et al. Differential expression of cytokine transcripts in neonatal and adult ovine alveolar macrophages in response to respiratory syncytial virus or toll-like receptor ligation. Vet Immunol Immunopathol 2010;136: 55–64.

40. Risalde MA, Molina V, Sánchez-Cordón PJ, et al. Pathogenic mechanisms implicated in the intravascular coagulation in the lungs of BVDV-infected calves challenged with BHV-1. Vet Res 2013;44:20.

41. Corbeil LB. Host immune response to Histophilus somni. Curr Top Microbiol Immunol 2016;396:109–29.

42. Srikumaran S, Kelling CL, Ambagala A. Immune evasion by pathogens of bovine respiratory disease complex. Anim Health Res Rev 2007;8:215–29.

43. Maunsell FP, Chase C. Mycoplasma bovis: interactions with the immune system and failure to generate an effective immune response. Vet Clin North Am Food Anim Pract 2019;35:471–83.

44. Levings RL, Roth JA. Immunity to bovine herpesvirus 1: II. Adaptive immunity and vaccinology. Anim Health Res Rev 2013;14:103–23.

45. Confer AW, Ayalew S. Mannheimia haemolytica in bovine respiratory disease: immunogens, potential immunogens, and vaccines. Anim Health Res Rev 2018;19: 79–99.

46. Ayalew S, Blackwood ER, Confer AW. Sequence diversity of the immunogenic outer membrane lipoprotein PlpE from Mannheimia haemolytica serotypes 1, 2, and 6. Vet Microbiol 2006;114:260–8.

47. Orouji S, Hodgins DC, Lo RY, et al. Serum IgG response in calves to the putative pneumonic virulence factor Gs60 of Mannheimia haemolytica A1. Can J Vet Res 2012;76:292–300.

48. Shewen PE, Lee CW, Perets A, et al. Efficacy of recombinant sialoglycoprotease in protection of cattle against pneumonic challenge with Mannheimia (Pasteurella) haemolytica A1. Vaccine 2003;21:1901–6.

49. Muangthai K, Tankaew P, Varinrak T, et al. Intranasal immunization with a recombinant outer membrane protein H based Haemorrhagic septicemia vaccine in dairy calves. J Vet Med Sci 2018;80:68–76.

50. Wei X, Wang Y, Luo R, et al. Identification and characterization of a protective antigen, PlpB of bovine Pasteurella multocida strain LZ-PM. Dev Comp Immunol 2017;71:1–7.

51. Berghaus LJ, Corbeil LB, Berghaus RD, et al. Effects of dual vaccination for bovine respiratory syncytial virus and Haemophilus somnus on immune responses. Vaccine 2006;24:6018–27.

52. Grissett GP, White BJ, Larson RL. Structured literature review of responses of cattle to viral and bacterial pathogens causing bovine respiratory disease complex. J Vet Intern Med 2015;29:770–80.

53. Vanden Bush TJ, Rosenbusch RF. Characterization of the immune response to Mycoplasma bovis lung infection. Vet Immunol Immunopathol 2003;94:23–33.

54. Le Grand D, Solsona M, Rosengarten R, et al. Adaptive surface antigen variation in Mycoplasma bovis to the host immune response. FEMS Microbiol Lett 1996; 144:267–75.

55. Toussaint JF, Coen L, Letellier C, et al. Genetic immunisation of cattle against bovine herpesvirus 1: glycoprotein gD confers higher protection than glycoprotein gC or tegument protein VP8. Vet Res 2005;36:529–44.
56. Ni H, Jia XX, Wang J, et al. Mapping a highly conserved linear neutralizing epitope at the N-terminus of the gD glycoprotein of bovine herpesvirus type I using a monoclonal antibody. Microb Pathog 2019;138:103815.
57. Wang X, Bi Y, Ran X, et al. Mapping a highly conserved linear neutralizing epitope on gD glycoprotein of bovine herpesvirus type I using a monoclonal antibody. J Vet Med Sci 2019;81:780–6.
58. Kalaycioglu AT, Russell PH, Howard CR. The characterization of the neutralizing bovine viral diarrhea virus monoclonal antibodies and antigenic diversity of E2 glycoprotein. J Vet Med Sci 2012;74:1117–20.
59. Kimman TG, Westenbrink F, Schreuder BE, et al. Local and systemic antibody response to bovine respiratory syncytial virus infection and reinfection in calves with and without maternal antibodies. J Clin Microbiol 1987;25:1097–106.
60. Zhang B, Chen L, Silacci C, et al. Protection of calves by a prefusion-stabilized bovine RSV F vaccine. NPJ Vaccines 2017;2:7.
61. Jutila MA, Holderness J, Graff JC, et al. Antigen-independent priming: a transitional response of bovine gammadelta T-cells to infection. Anim Health Res Rev 2008;9:47–57.
62. McGill JL, Rusk RA, Guerra-Maupome M, et al. Bovine gamma delta T cells contribute to exacerbated IL-17 production in response to co-infection with bovine RSV and Mannheimia haemolytica. PLoS One 2016;11:e0151083.
63. Mathy NL, Mathy JP, Lee RP, et al. Pathological and immunological changes after challenge infection with Pasteurella multocida in naive and immunized calves. Vet Immunol Immunopathol 2002;85:179–88.
64. Endsley JJ, Quade MJ, Terhaar B, et al. BHV-1-Specific CD4+, CD8+, and gammadelta T cells in calves vaccinated with one dose of a modified live BHV-1 vaccine. Viral Immunol 2002;15:385–93.
65. Silflow RM, Degel PM, Harmsen AG. Bronchoalveolar immune defense in cattle exposed to primary and secondary challenge with bovine viral diarrhea virus. Vet Immunol Immunopathol 2005;103:129–39.
66. McGill JL, Nonnecke BJ, Lippolis JD, et al. Differential chemokine and cytokine production by neonatal bovine gammadelta T-cell subsets in response to viral toll-like receptor agonists and in vivo respiratory syncytial virus infection. Immunology 2013;139:227–44.
67. Taylor G, Thomas LH, Wyld SG, et al. Role of T-lymphocyte subsets in recovery from respiratory syncytial virus infection in calves. J Virol 1995;69:6658–64.
68. Hermeyer K, Buchenau I, Thomasmeyer A, et al. Chronic pneumonia in calves after experimental infection with Mycoplasma bovis strain 1067: characterization of lung pathology, persistence of variable surface protein antigens and local immune response. Acta Vet Scand 2012;54:9.
69. Gao Y, Wang C, Splitter GA. Mapping T and B lymphocyte epitopes of bovine herpesvirus-1 glycoprotein B. J Gen Virol 1999;80(Pt 10):2699–704.
70. Tikoo SK, Campos M, Popowych YI, et al. Lymphocyte proliferative responses to recombinant bovine herpes virus type 1 (BHV-1) glycoprotein gD (gIV) in immune cattle: identification of a T cell epitope. Viral Immunol 1995;8:19–25.
71. Gaddum RM, Cook RS, Furze JM, et al. Recognition of bovine respiratory syncytial virus proteins by bovine CD8+ T lymphocytes. Immunology 2003;108:220–9.
72. Woolums AR, Gunther RA, McArthur-Vaughan K, et al. Cytotoxic T lymphocyte activity and cytokine expression in calves vaccinated with formalin-inactivated

bovine respiratory syncytial virus prior to challenge. Comp Immunol Microbiol Infect Dis 2004;27:57–74.

73. Collen T, Carr V, Parsons K, et al. Analysis of the repertoire of cattle CD4(+) T cells reactive with bovine viral diarrhoea virus. Vet Immunol Immunopathol 2002;87:235–8.
74. Hodgson PD, Aich P, Manuja A, et al. Effect of stress on viral-bacterial synergy in bovine respiratory disease: novel mechanisms to regulate inflammation. Comp Funct Genomics 2005;6:244–50.
75. Griebel P, Hill K, Stookey J. How stress alters immune responses during respiratory infection. Anim Health Res Rev 2014;15:161–5.
76. Emam M, Livernois A, Paibomesai M, et al. Genetic and epigenetic regulation of immune response and resistance to infectious diseases in domestic ruminants. Vet Clin North Am Food Anim Pract 2019;35:405–29.
77. Casas E, Garcia MD, Wells JE, et al. Association of single nucleotide polymorphisms in the ANKRA2 and CD180 genes with bovine respiratory disease and presence of Mycobacterium avium subsp. paratuberculosis(1). Anim Genet 2011;42:571–7.
78. Glass EJ, Baxter R, Leach RJ, et al. Genes controlling vaccine responses and disease resistance to respiratory viral pathogens in cattle. Vet Immunol Immunopathol 2012;148:90–9.
79. Neupane M, Kiser JN, Neibergs HL, et al. Gene set enrichment analysis of SNP data in dairy and beef cattle with bovine respiratory disease. Anim Genet 2018;49:527–38.
80. Chen J, Yang C, Tizioto PC, et al. Expression of the bovine NK-lysin gene family and activity against respiratory pathogens. PLoS One 2016;11:e0158882.
81. Chen J, Huddleston J, Buckley RM, et al. Bovine NK-lysin: copy number variation and functional diversification. Proc Natl Acad Sci U S A 2015;112:E7223–9.
82. Dassanayake RP, Falkenberg SM, Briggs RE, et al. Antimicrobial activity of bovine NK-lysin-derived peptides on bovine respiratory pathogen Histophilus somni. PLoS One 2017;12:e0183610.
83. Dassanayake RP, Falkenberg SM, Register KB, et al. Antimicrobial activity of bovine NK-lysin-derived peptides on Mycoplasma bovis. PLoS One 2018;13:e0197677.
84. Caverly JM, Diamond G, Gallup JM, et al. Coordinated expression of tracheal antimicrobial peptide and inflammatory-response elements in the lungs of neonatal calves with acute bacterial pneumonia. Infect Immun 2003;71:2950–5.
85. Vulikh K, Bassel LL, Sergejewich L, et al. Effect of tracheal antimicrobial peptide on the development of Mannheimia haemolytica pneumonia in cattle. PLoS One 2019;14:e0225533.
86. Netea MG, Joosten LA, Latz E, et al. Trained immunity: a program of innate immune memory in health and disease. Science 2016;352:aaf1098.
87. Nickell JS, Keil DJ, Settje TL, et al. Efficacy and safety of a novel DNA immunostimulant in cattle. Bov Pract (Stillwater) 2016;50:9–20.
88. Rogers KC, Miles DG, Renter DG, et al. Effects of delayed respiratory viral vaccine and/or inclusion of an immunostimulant on feedlot health, performance, and carcass merits of auction-market derived feeder heifers. Bov Pract (Stillwater) 2016;50:154–62.
89. Woolums AR, Karisch BB, Parish JA, et al. Effect of a DNA-based immunostimulant on growth, performance, and expression of inflammatory and immune mediators in beef calves abruptly weaned and introduced to a complete ration. J Anim Sci 2019;97:111–21.

90. Ilg T. Investigations on the molecular mode of action of the novel immunostimulator ZelNate: activation of the cGAS-STING pathway in mammalian cells. Mol Immunol 2017;90:182–9.
91. Nosky B, Biwer J, Alkemade S, et al. Effect of a non-specific immune stimulant (Amplimune™) on the health and production of light feedlot calves. J Dairy Vet Anim Res 2017;6:00179.

Host Tolerance to Infection with the Bacteria that Cause Bovine Respiratory Disease

Laura L. Bassel, DVM, MSc, Saeid Tabatabaei, DVM, PhD,
Jeff L. Caswell, DVM, DVSc, PhD*

KEYWORDS

- Cattle • Respiratory • Bacteria • Pneumonia • Tolerance • Resilience
- Inflammation • Immunology

KEY POINTS

- Studies of natural disease and of experimental infections indicate considerable variation in how calves respond to infection of the lung with bacteria.
- Some calves develop only mild lung lesions and minimal clinical signs despite substantial numbers of pathogenic bacteria in the lung.
- This may represent "tolerance" to pulmonary infection because these calves are able to control their inflammatory responses or protect the lung from damage without eliminating infection.
- Bovine respiratory disease risk factors might cause a loss of tolerance that leads to a harmful inflammatory and tissue-damaging response to infection.

INTRODUCTION

Veterinarians focus mostly on animals that become ill, such as those with pneumonia. In this article, we look to the rest of the herd, to ask why most calves remain healthy despite sharing similar life experiences and pathogen exposures as those who become sick. There are several explanations for why calves might show no clinical signs despite having pathogenic bacteria in the lung. Some calves have prior immunity and resist bacterial infection. Others become infected but mount a timely and effective innate or acquired immune response, clear the pathogen, and do not show clinical signs. A failure to adequately observe the cattle could also be considered, so that clinical signs are present but overlooked. These reasons are of great importance for beef production, but this article focuses on other reasons including bacterial factors, development of minimal lesions despite infection of the lung, and lack of clinical signs despite substantial lung lesions.

Department of Pathobiology, Ontario Veterinary College, University of Guelph, 50 Stone Road East, Guelph, Ontario N1G 2W1, Canada
* Corresponding author.
E-mail address: jcaswell@uoguelph.ca

Vet Clin Food Anim 36 (2020) 349–359
https://doi.org/10.1016/j.cvfa.2020.03.003
0749-0720/20/© 2020 Elsevier Inc. All rights reserved.

BACTERIAL FACTORS

Different strains of some bacterial pathogens, such as *Mannheimia haemolytica*, vary in their ability to cause disease, whereas other pathogens show minimal variation among strains. For bacteria that have strains of differing virulence, an absence of clinical signs might simply reflect infection with a nonpathogenic strain. In this case, the pathogen's subtype or genotype must be taken into account when considering the response to infection, and this is now easily done for *M haemolytica*. Isolates can be routinely genotyped as type 1 or type 2 using MALDI-TOF (matrix-assisted laser desorption/ionization–time of flight) mass spectrometry.[1] Similarly, it is now possible for any diagnostic laboratory to differentiate serotypes 1, 2, and 6 by multiplex polymerase chain reaction,[2] whereas the availability of serotyping was previously more limited. *M haemolytica* serotype 1 and genotype 2 isolates are more frequently associated with pneumonia and indeed with stress or viral infection, whereas serotype 2 and genotype 1 isolates are more often isolated from healthy calves. This finding seems to correspond to a difference in virulence following experimental infection, at least for some isolates.[3] Some older studies reported that *M haemolytica* was isolated from apparently healthy calves without determining the genotype or serotype of isolates, and this has been a basis for considering *M haemolytica* as a "commensal." However, readily available tools are now available to distinguish whether healthy calves are unsurprisingly infected with serotype 2/genotype 1 or more unexpectedly infected with serotype 1/genotype 2.

Mycoplasma bovis strains differ to a limited degree in their ability to adhere to, invade, and cause apoptosis of epithelial cells in vitro,[4,5] and an *M bovis* strain that was repeatedly passaged in vitro had attenuated in vivo virulence compared with the parent strain.[6] However, there is no solid evidence that natural isolates differ in their in vivo virulence, whereas there is evidence that the same strain can cause severe disease or no disease depending on the circumstances. For example, *M bovis* was first detected in New Zealand in 2017 as an outbreak of mastitis and arthritis affecting 50% of a cohort of dry cows as well as dysmaturity and death of neonatal calves born to this cohort.[7] Despite this evidence of virulence, clinical disease has been minimal or absent in other infected herds despite solid evidence that all isolates arose from a single introduction.[8] In the same way, *M bovis* isolates from outbreaks in bison caused severe disease in experimentally challenged bison but not in cattle,[9] implying that host factors rather than the bacterial strain determine the outcome. Thus, current knowledge does not support differences in virulence among *M bovis* strains as an explanation for why some infected calves develop disease and others do not.

M haemolytica, *Pasteurella multocida*, *Histophilus somni*, and *M bovis* are reported to form biofilms in vitro, where they have reduced metabolic activity and are shielded from antibiotics and the host immune response.[10–12] If the biofilm-encased bacteria were able to survive without triggering an inflammatory response, as is suggested for models of *Streptococcus pneumoniae* infection,[13] this could be another reason that calves could have pulmonary infection without significant lesions. However, this phenomenon has not been studied in vivo for bovine respiratory pathogens.

MINIMAL CLINICAL SIGNS OR LESIONS IN EXPERIMENTALLY INFECTED CALVES

As a focus of this review, an absence of clinical signs in an infected calf might reflect tolerance of the calf to infection. All bacteria contain molecular components that are recognized by the host and induce an inflammatory response. These molecules are known as pathogen-associated molecular patterns and include lipopolysaccharide and lipoproteins in the bacterial membrane, lipoteichoic acids and peptidoglycan in the cell wall, flagellar proteins, and CpG oligodeoxynucleotides. Thus, it might be assumed that if a bacterium is capable of surviving within the lung, it should trigger an inflammatory response that would cause an observable lesion. However, evidence from experimental infections and natural disease of cattle indicates that this is not the case, because calves can have pulmonary infection with virulent bacteria yet develop minimal lesions and no clinical signs of illness.

Holstein bull calves were raised in a BSL-2 facility with[14] or without[3] colostrum in the first hours after birth. The calves were challenged by aerosol with *M haemolytica* serotype 1 at about 1 month of age. These calves were uniform in many respects: they were sourced from the same herd, were free of *Mannheimia* based on culture of nasal swabs, lacked serum antibody to *M haemolytica* leukotoxin, and were challenged by aerosol with the same bacterial isolate. Nonetheless, the calves showed considerable variation in the severity of clinical signs and gross lung lesions following *M haemolytica* challenge, despite a lack of prechallenge antileukotoxin antibody. In 1 study, 3 of 8 challenged calves developed severe clinical signs, whereas 3 calves showed no or minimal clinical signs after the first 24 hours.[3] In a second study, 3 of 12 calves developed severe clinical signs, whereas 1 calf did not show clinical signs at any time after challenge.[14] There were also differences in the severity of gross and histologic lesions in the lung (**Fig. 1**). In 1 study, 4 of 11 challenged calves had consolidation of less than 2% of the lung; 3 had 3% to 15% lung consolidation, and 4 had 21% to 55% lung consolidation.[3,15] In another study, 6 of 12 challenged calves had less than 1% of the lung affected, even though another 3 calves challenged by the same protocol had consolidation of 7% to 22% of the lung.[14]

Similarly, in work by others, 1 of 3 control calves challenged intratracheally with *M haemolytica* had no gross lung lesions despite a positive lung culture at postmortem.[16] Furthermore, in a reflection on 44 experiments conducted at the same institution over 15 years, including aerosol challenge of 183 control (nonvaccinated) beef calves with bovine herpesvirus-1 (BHV-1) followed by *M haemolytica*, gross lung lesions affected ≤10% of the lung in 48% of challenged calves, 11% to 30% of the lung in 20% of calves, and greater than 30% of the lung in 32% of calves.[17] These studies illustrate that calves differ considerably in their pathologic and clinical responses to *M haemolytica* challenge, even in controlled experimental settings. It should be mentioned that experiments using endobronchial or transthoracic inoculation of naïve calves with *M haemolytica* report more consistent induction of lesions, so the above findings may reflect the less abrupt and arguably more natural aerosol route of infection.

Furthermore, the aerosol challenge studies identified discordance between bacterial infection and lung lesions when analyzed on the basis of individual lung lobes. *M haemolytica* was isolated in large numbers from 9 of 60 lung lobes that had no or minimal gross lesions, and there was poor correlation between quantitative bacterial cultures and gross lesions ($P = 0.4$).[14] In another study, the nebulizer was shown to deliver aerosol to all lobes of the lung, and the bacteria used for challenge were recovered from all lung lobes, yet lesions were mainly present in the cranial and middle lobes. In fact, in 2 of 8 challenged calves, *M haemolytica* was isolated from the caudodorsal lung, but there were no gross or histologic lesions in these lobes.[3] Together, these studies indicate that the amount of *M haemolytica* in the lung does not necessarily correlate with the severity of lesions (see **Fig. 1**), and calves can develop no or minimal lesions despite having pulmonary infection with pathogenic bacteria.

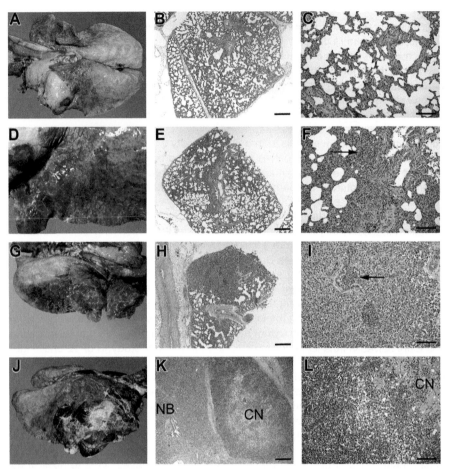

Fig. 1. (*A-L*) Individual-animal differences in the response to *Mannheimia haemolytica* challenge, and the disparity between lesions and bacterial load. Colostrum-deprived Holstein calves were raised in a BSL-2 facility, were free of *M haemolytica* and lacked serum antibody to leukotoxin, and were challenged by aerosol with *M haemolytica* serotype 1.[3,15] (*A-F*) One calf had minimal gross lesions (*A, D*), and the lung was histologically normal (*B, C, E*) except for one focus of neutrophil infiltration (arrow) in alveoli and bronchioles (*F*). The cranioventral lung (shown histologically in panels *B, C, E, F*) contained $10^{8.1}$ (*right*) and $10^{3.5}$ (*left*) CFU/100 mg of *M haemolytica*. (*G-I*) A second calf had mild gross and histologic lesions with patchy areas of neutrophil infiltration in bronchioles (arrow) and alveoli but no necrosis (*H, I*). The cranioventral lung (shown histologically in panels H and I) contained $10^{8.5}$ (right) and $10^{8.0}$ (left) CFU/100 mg of *M haemolytica*. (*J-L*) A third calf had severe gross lesions of consolidation with fibrinous pleuritis (J) and histologic lesions of neutrophil-rich bronchopneumonia (NB) with numerous foci of coagulation necrosis (CN) (*K, L*). Despite the severe lesions, the cranioventral lung (shown histologically in panels *K and L*) contained only $10^{6.6}$ (*right*) and $10^{6.5}$ (*left*) CFU/100 mg of *M haemolytica*. Hematoxylin and eosin. Scale bars: 400 μm (*B, E, H, K*); 100 μm (*C, F, I, L*).

MINIMAL CLINICAL SIGNS OR LESIONS IN NATURALLY INFECTED CALVES

Studies that apply the same diagnostic methods to calves with and without clinical disease also show that bacterial infection of the lung is not limited to calves with pneumonia. For example, bacterial culture of bronchoalveolar lavage fluid from healthy beef calves at the time of arrival to a feedlot yielded M haemolytica in 23%, P multocida in 12%, and H somni in 3%; at least 1 Pasteurellaceae or Mycoplasma species was isolated from 83% of these clinically healthy calves.[18] In the subsequent 2 weeks after arrival, bacterial pathogens were isolated from bronchoalveolar lavage fluid of healthy pen mates with comparable frequency to that of calves with clinical respiratory disease: 86% versus 64% for M bovis, 43% versus 23% for M haemolytica, 7% versus 5% for P multocida, and 7% versus 9% for H somni, respectively,[18] comparable to data reported by others.[19] Similarly, transtracheal aspirates from 56 healthy dairy calves and 34 calves with pneumonia yielded M haemolytica in 23% versus 29%, P multocida in 48% versus 82%, and H somni in 20% versus 41%, respectively.[20] Thus, many calves infected with pathogenic bacteria nonetheless show no or minimal clinical signs.

Furthermore, naturally infected calves can appear clinically healthy despite having substantial pulmonary lesions. For example, of dairy calves less than 12 weeks old with no or mild clinical signs, 16 of 24 had areas of lung consolidation detected by thoracic ultrasound or postmortem examination.[21] Similarly, of feedlot beef calves with postmortem lung lesions, only 27% showed clinical illness.[22]

Postmortem studies comparing animals with pneumonia to those dying of other causes also show that bacterial pathogens may be present in the lung in the absence of significant lesions. In a study of mortality in Ontario beef feedlots within 60 days of arrival, 13 calves had no gross or histologic lesions of pneumonia, yet M bovis was isolated from the lung of 6 of them and P multocida from 3, although neither M haemolytica nor H somni was isolated from these cases.[23,24] In a study of weaned beef and dairy calves in Ireland, 70 had no gross lung lesions, and of these, 10 had P multocida, 8 had M haemolytica, 7 had H somni, and 2 had M bovis identified in lung samples.[25] Comparable findings are reported in other studies.[26] In contrast, another study did not identify M bovis, M haemolytica, or H somni by immunohistochemistry in 9 feedlot calf mortalities that had no histologic lung lesions.[27]

Together, the above studies indicate that a high proportion of feedlot beef calves in the postarrival period have lung infection with substantial numbers of pathogenic bacteria despite appearing clinically healthy, and a considerable number of apparently healthy beef and dairy calves have bacterial pneumonia without showing clinical signs. What is to be learned from these observations? Why do some calves tolerate infection without showing clinical signs or reduced growth, whereas others develop clinical signs or succumb to the infection?

THE RELATIONSHIP BETWEEN INFECTION AND CLINICAL SIGNS

One way to approach this question is by considering how bacterial infection of the lung leads to clinical signs. In bovine respiratory disease (BRD), the bacteria themselves do not cause illness but do so by triggering a host response. Some aspects of the clinical picture result directly from changes in the lung itself. In the infected lung, the bronchiolar and alveolar airspaces fill with edema, neutrophils, and fibrin, impeding both ventilation and gas exchange. Inflammatory mediators cause vasodilation that disrupts ventilation-perfusion matching and can lead to shunting of nonoxygenated blood past nonventilated alveoli. Inflammatory mediators also cause bronchoconstriction, and edema and leukocyte infiltration within airway walls, all of which compromise ventilation of the lung. In an effort to repair damaged airways, cattle have a propensity to develop fibrous polyps within bronchioles (bronchiolitis obliterans) that are a permanent barrier to airflow. All of these changes lead to lung dysfunction, tachypnea, and respiratory distress. However, cattle can appear clinically healthy even when greater than 30% of the lung is rendered nonfunctional by chronic pneumonia. Thus, the duration of disease as well as individual variation in how calves regulate these disease-causing inflammatory and immune responses may affect which animals show clinical signs and which do not.

Other aspects of the clinical picture are not direct consequences of the lung lesion but instead result from sepsis, in which cytokines and other inflammatory mediators produced at the site of lung infection have body-wide effects, including induction of sickness behavior, fever, hypotension, hypercoagulability, acute phase protein production in the liver, release of leukocytes from the marrow, and cachexia. Sepsis may also cause damage to other organs, most notably the kidney, liver, and the lung itself, but also the intestine, heart, and brain. Sepsis is thought of mainly in the context of acute fulminant pneumonia, but the same processes can continue if infection persists and thus contribute to the fever, malaise, and cachexia of calves with chronic pneumonia. Experimental studies have shown that different calves have differing sepsis responses to intravenous injection of lipopolysaccharide.[28,29] Thus, it seems likely that different calves regulate their pulmonary and systemic inflammatory responses differently, and this is a possible explanation for individual variation in clinical signs.

TOLERANCE TO INFECTION

Infected calves that have minimal lesions or clinical signs might be considered to have "tolerance" to pulmonary infection because they do not mount an excessive inflammatory response. This tolerance probably depends on the microenvironment of the respiratory tract before infection, and how the respiratory tract responds in the first hours or days following infection. Compared with later time points, when clinical disease becomes apparent or when calves die of their disease, the responses to bacteria during the early postinfection period are less studied.

Transition beef calves (ie, those experiencing recent weaning, nutritional changes, transportation, comingling, adverse climatic conditions, castration, and dehorning) are traditionally considered to be immunosuppressed, and this immunosuppression is thought to allow bacteria to enter and colonize the lung, which in turn leads to disease.[30] However, the points raised above might suggest an alternative pathogenesis, that calves experiencing these risk factors mount an unusually harmful response to infection, and it may be this dysregulated response that leads to inflammation and disease. In this way, we might re-examine the observed changes in the respiratory and immune systems of transition beef calves through the lens of tolerance rather than (or in addition to) immunosuppression.

There is some evidence that inflammation in the respiratory tract of healthy calves increases the risk of later developing respiratory disease. First, prior treatment with dexamethasone was shown to protect against subsequent M haemolytica challenge in healthy calves, with lower clinical disease scores and extent of consolidated lung.[31] Second, administration of meloxicam significantly reduced the prevalence of respiratory disease after beef calves arrived to a feedlot and were castrated[32] (although it is not clear if this disease sparing resulted from an anti-inflammatory effect[33] or from pain reduction). It should be noted that these studies involve anti-inflammatory drug administration during the very early risk period before infection becomes established, not their therapeutic use in calves with established pneumonia. Finally, in beef calves that were healthy but at high risk of BRD, stimulating an inflammatory response in the airways resulted in increased rectal temperatures, treatment rate, and mortality.[15]

There is evidence that transition beef calves mount excessive inflammatory responses as a result of virus infection and perhaps of the stress response. Certainly, viruses induce inflammatory responses in the respiratory tract, and viral infections also influence how calves respond to other infectious agents. In vitro models show that viral infection enhances production of proinflammatory cytokines in response to stimulation with bacteria (or bacterial components), including infection of blood mononuclear cells with BHV-1 and subsequent stimulation with lipopolysaccharide,[34] infection of blood mononuclear cells with bovine respiratory syncytial virus (BRSV) and stimulation with M haemolytica,[35] or infection of bovine bronchial epithelial cells with BHV-1 and stimulation with M haemolytica.[36] Similarly, in vivo challenge of calves with either BHV-1 or BRSV induces secretion of tumor necrosis factor-α in the trachea and lung, respectively, as well as histologic evidence of inflammation[37–39], and infection with bovine viral diarrhea virus results in higher serum tumor necrosis factor-α levels after BHV-1 challenge.[40] Thus, infections with respiratory viruses induce inflammation directly and seem to enhance the response to other proinflammatory stimuli, suggesting that this dysregulated inflammatory response could be a mechanism by which viruses predispose to bacterial pneumonia.

In addition, although stress is normally alleged to be immunosuppressive, and this indeed seems true of chronic stress, acute stress can involve a proinflammatory state. For example, calves treated with glucocorticoid had greater lipopolysaccharide-induced neutrophil responses in their lung compared with untreated calves, consistent with enhanced neutrophil innate immune responses in stressed calves.[41] Similarly, acute stress is associated with increased numbers of blood neutrophils, increased neutrophil migration, and higher somatic cell counts in milk.[42,43] The lung lavage fluid of recently weaned and transported calves has reduced levels of the anti-inflammatory protein "odorant-binding protein."[44] Furthermore, lower levels of another anti-inflammatory protein "annexin A1" correlated with later development of disease.[45] Although more work is needed, these studies provide some support to the concept that viral infection and acute stress in healthy transition beef calves promote a proinflammatory environment that affects subsequent responses to bacterial infections.

The cellular and molecular mechanisms of how calves dampen the pulmonary and systemic inflammatory responses to bacteria have received little attention, yet an extensive variety of anti-inflammatory and proresolving molecules is known in other species.[46,47] The healthy lung microenvironment is known to promote tranquility: proteins in the lung fluids as well as cues from alveolar epithelial cells encourage resting pulmonary alveolar macrophages to not secrete inflammatory mediators during their daily business of ingesting inhaled particles,[47] and abundant proteins in the lung of cattle (including annexin A1, odorant-binding protein, and fatty acid–binding protein[44,48,49]) curtail neutrophil responses and scavenge any inflammatory mediators that are produced. Even when inflammation does occur, there is secretion not only of mediators that trigger an inflammatory response, but also of anti-inflammatory cytokines (including interleukin 10 and transforming growth factor-β1) and eicosanoid lipid mediators (including lipoxins and resolvins) that quell the harmful response once the stimulus is eliminated. Furthermore, the balance of cytokines within the lung microenvironment affects whether recruited monocytes develop into macrophages that tend to promote resolution of inflammatory responses and healing instead of those that promote inflammation. Finally, the process by which macrophages ingest dying (apoptotic) neutrophils is important in resolving inflammation: not only does this remove neutrophils before they further damage the inflamed tissue, but this process also sooths the macrophages to become proresolving rather than proinflammatory.[46,50] Understanding these mechanisms of how inflammation is prevented or resolved, and how BRD risk factors and other cattle management factors disrupt these anti-inflammatory mechanisms,[29,51] may explain why different calves respond in different ways to bacterial infection of the lung.[52]

An alternative mechanism of tolerance to pulmonary bacterial infection involves responses that reduce disease severity by protecting the lung from damage, without necessarily eliminating bacterial infection. Thus, the concept of disease tolerance contrasts with that of protective immunity, in which the focus is on elimination of the pathogen even at the expense of host tissue damage and disease. For example, consider that leukotoxin is an important *M haemolytica* virulence factor, and its harmful effect on bovine leukocytes is exacerbated by inflammation-induced upregulation of CD18, the leukotoxin receptor.[53] A military host defense strategy would be to mount an immune and inflammatory response that kills *Mannheimia*, even though the upregulation of CD18 associated with this response makes leukocytes more susceptible to leukotoxin. Alternatively, one might speculate that a tolerance strategy would dampen inflammatory responses, thus minimizing CD18 expression and leukotoxin-induced damage. Many acute phase proteins act to dampen inflammatory responses (eg, C-reactive protein and α2-macroglobulin) or prevent oxidative and proteolytic tissue damage (eg, haptoglobin and serine protease inhibitors). Studies in calves have shown that glucocorticoid[49] and stress[41] induce changes in the levels of these antioxidant proteins and protease inhibitors in lung fluids, and this may represent a mechanism to reduce disease severity without directly eliminating the pathogen. Consistent with this notion, the levels of the anti-inflammatory protein annexin A1 and the antioxidant proteins peroxiredoxin 1, calcyphosin, dihydrodiol dehydrogenase 3, and superoxide dismutase were higher in lung fluids of healthy transition beef calves that remained healthy compared with those that later developed respiratory disease.[45]

These findings support the hypothesis that when calves become infected with respiratory pathogens, those calves that can control their inflammatory responses and enhance tissue-protecting responses may be able to minimize lung lesions and remain clinically healthy. Whether these tolerance mechanisms are regulated by genetics, nutrition, calf-management factors, respiratory microbiome, coinfections, or concurrent diseases requires further study.

ACKNOWLEDGMENTS

The authors are supported by the Natural Sciences and Engineering Research Council of Canada (NSERC, RGPIN-2017-03872, RGPAS-2017-507803, CRDPJ 476331-14), Canadian Cattleman's Association (ANH.13.17), Beef Farmers of Ontario (17-02), Zoetis, and the Ontario Ministry of Agriculture, Food and Rural Affairs (27337).

DISCLOSURE

The authors have nothing to disclose.

REFERENCES

1. Loy JD, Clawson ML. Rapid typing of Mannheimia haemolytica major genotypes 1 and 2 using MALDI-TOF mass spectrometry. J Microbiol Methods 2017; 136:30–3.

2. Klima CL, Zaheer R, Briggs RE, et al. A multiplex PCR assay for molecular capsular serotyping of Mannheimia haemolytica serotypes 1, 2, and 6. J Microbiol Methods 2017;139:155–60.

3. Bassel LL, Kaufman EI, Alsop SNA, et al. Development of an aerosolized Mannheimia haemolytica experimental pneumonia model in clean-catch colostrum-deprived calves. Vet Microbiol 2019;234:34–43.

4. Josi C, Bürki S, Stojiljkovic A, et al. Bovine epithelial in vitro infection models for Mycoplasma bovis. Front Cell Infect Microbiol 2018;8:329.

5. Suleman M, Prysliak T, Clarke K, et al. Mycoplasma bovis isolates recovered from cattle and bison (Bison bison) show differential in vitro effects on PBMC proliferation, alveolar macrophage apoptosis and invasion of epithelial and immune cells. Vet Microbiol 2016;186:28–36.

6. Zhang R, Han X, Chen Y, et al. Attenuated Mycoplasma bovis strains provide protection against virulent infection in calves. Vaccine 2014;32(25):3107–14.

7. Hay M. Mycoplasma bovis infection on a South Canterbury dairy farm. In: Proceedings of the Society of Dairy Cattle Veterinarians of the NZVA Annual Conference. Oamaru, December 2017.

8. Hamill C. Clinical impact of Mycoplasma bovis in New Zealand 2019. Available at: https://www.biosecurity.govt.nz/dmsdocument/35661-clinical-impact-research. Accessed December 30, 2019.

9. Register KB, Olsen SC, Sacco RE, et al. Relative virulence in bison and cattle of bison-associated genotypes of Mycoplasma bovis. Vet Microbiol 2018;222: 55–63.

10. McAuliffe L, Ellis RJ, Miles K, et al. Biofilm formation by mycoplasma species and its role in environmental persistence and survival. Microbiology 2006;152(Pt 4): 913–22.

11. Pillai DK, Cha E, Mosier D. Role of the stress-associated chemicals norepinephrine, epinephrine and substance P in dispersal of Mannheimia haemolytica from biofilms. Vet Microbiol 2018;215:11–7.

12. Boukahil I, Czuprynski CJ. Mannheimia haemolytica biofilm formation on bovine respiratory epithelial cells. Vet Microbiol 2016;197:129–36.

13. Chao Y, Marks LR, Pettigrew MM, et al. Streptococcus pneumoniae biofilm formation and dispersion during colonization and disease. Front Cell Infect Microbiol 2014;4:194.

14. Vulikh K, Bassel LL, Sergejewich L, et al. Effect of tracheal antimicrobial peptide on the development of Mannheimia haemolytica pneumonia in cattle. PLoS One 2019;14(11):e0225533.

15. Bassel LL, Hewson J, Sharif S, et al. Effects of innate immune stimulation on naturally occurring respiratory disease in beef calves. In: American College of Veterinary Pathologists Annual Meeting. Vancouver, Canada, 5 November 2017.

16. Lhermie G, Ferran AA, Assié S, et al. Impact of timing and dosage of a fluoroquinolone treatment on the microbiological, pathological, and clinical outcomes of calves challenged with mannheimia haemolytica. Front Microbiol 2016;7:237.

17. Jericho KWF, Kozub GC. Experimental infectious respiratory disease in groups of calves: lobar distribution, variance, and sample-size requirements for vaccine evaluation. Can J Vet Res 2004;68(2):118–27.

18. Castillo-Alcala F, Bateman KG, Cai HY, et al. Prevalence and genotype of Mycoplasma bovis in beef cattle after arrival at a feedlot. Am J Vet Res 2012;73(12): 1932–43.

19. Allen JW, Viel L, Bateman KG, et al. Changes in the bacterial flora of the upper and lower respiratory tracts and bronchoalveolar lavage differential cell counts in feedlot calves treated for respiratory diseases. Can J Vet Res 1992;56(3): 177–83.

20. Angen O, Thomsen J, Larsen LE, et al. Respiratory disease in calves: microbiological investigations on trans-tracheally aspirated bronchoalveolar fluid and acute phase protein response. Vet Microbiol 2009;137(1–2):165–71.
21. Ollivett TL, Caswell JL, Nydam DV, et al. Thoracic ultrasonography and bronchoalveolar lavage fluid analysis in Holstein calves with subclinical lung lesions. J Vet Intern Med 2015;29(6):1728–34.
22. Timsit E, Dendukuri N, Schiller I, et al. Diagnostic accuracy of clinical illness for bovine respiratory disease (BRD) diagnosis in beef cattle placed in feedlots: a systematic literature review and hierarchical Bayesian latent-class meta-analysis. Prev Vet Med 2016;135:67–73.
23. Gagea MI, Bateman KG, Shanahan RA, et al. Naturally occurring Mycoplasma bovis-associated pneumonia and polyarthritis in feedlot beef calves. J Vet Diagn Invest 2006;18(1):29–40.
24. Gagea MI, Bateman KG, van Dreumel T, et al. Diseases and pathogens associated with mortality in Ontario beef feedlots. J Vet Diagn Invest 2006;18(1):18–28.
25. Murray GM, More SJ, Sammin D, et al. Pathogens, patterns of pneumonia, and epidemiologic risk factors associated with respiratory disease in recently weaned cattle in Ireland. J Vet Diagn Invest 2017;29(1):20–34.
26. Shoo MK, Wiseman A, Allan EM, et al. Distribution of Pasteurella haemolytica in the respiratory tracts of carrier calves and those subsequently infected experimentally with Dictyocaulus viviparus. Res Vet Sci 1990;48(3):383–5.
27. Booker CW, Abutarbush SM, Morley PS, et al. Microbiological and histopathological findings in cases of fatal bovine respiratory disease of feedlot cattle in Western Canada. Can Vet J 2008;49(5):473–81.
28. Plessers E, Wyns H, Watteyn A, et al. Characterization of an intravenous lipopolysaccharide inflammation model in calves with respect to the acute-phase response. Vet Immunol Immunopathol 2015;163(1–2):46–56.
29. Carroll JA, Arthington JD, Chase CC. Early weaning alters the acute-phase reaction to an endotoxin challenge in beef calves. J Anim Sci 2009;87(12):4167–72.
30. Caswell JL. Failure of respiratory defenses in the pathogenesis of bacterial pneumonia of cattle. Vet Pathol 2014;51(2):393–409.
31. Malazdrewich C, Thumbikat P, Maheswaran SK. Protective effect of dexamethasone in experimental bovine pneumonic mannheimiosis. Microb Pathog 2004; 36(4):227–36.
32. Coetzee JF, Edwards LN, Mosher RA, et al. Effect of oral meloxicam on health and performance of beef steers relative to bulls castrated on arrival at the feedlot. J Anim Sci 2012;90(3):1026–39.
33. Van Engen NK, Platt R, Roth JA, et al. Impact of oral meloxicam and long-distance transport on cell-mediated and humoral immune responses in feedlot steers receiving modified live BVDV booster vaccination on arrival. Vet Immunol Immunopathol 2016;175:42–50.
34. Sheridan MP, Regev-Shoshani G, Martins J, et al. Nitric oxide modulates the immunological response of bovine PBMCs in an in vitro BRDc infection model. Res Vet Sci 2016;109:21–8.
35. McGill JL, Rusk RA, Guerra-Maupome M, et al. Bovine gamma delta T cells contribute to exacerbated IL-17 production in response to co-infection with bovine RSV and mannheimia haemolytica. PLoS One 2016;11(3):e0151083.
36. N'jai AU, Rivera J, Atapattu DN, et al. Gene expression profiling of bovine bronchial epithelial cells exposed in vitro to bovine herpesvirus 1 and Mannheimia haemolytica. Vet Immunol Immunopathol 2013;155(3):182–9.

37. Røntved CM, Tjørnehøj K, Viuff B, et al. Increased pulmonary secretion of tumor necrosis factor-alpha in calves experimentally infected with bovine respiratory syncytial virus. Vet Immunol Immunopathol 2000;76(3–4):199–214.
38. Burucúa MM, Quintana S, Lendez P, et al. Modulation of cathelicidins, IFNβ and TNFα by bovine alpha-herpesviruses is dependent on the stage of the infectious cycle. Mol Immunol 2019;111:136–44.
39. Caswell JL, Williams KJ. Respiratory system. In: Maxie MG, editor. Jubb, Kennedy & Palmer's pathology of domestic animals. 6th edition. St. Louis, Missouri: Saunders; 2015. p. 465–591.
40. Risalde MA, Molina V, Sánchez-Cordón PJ, et al. Response of proinflammatory and anti-inflammatory cytokines in calves with subclinical bovine viral diarrhea challenged with bovine herpesvirus-1. Vet Immunol Immunopathol 2011; 144(1–2):135–43.
41. Mitchell GB, Clark ME, Siwicky M, et al. Stress alters the cellular and proteomic compartments of bovine bronchoalveolar lavage fluid. Vet Immunol Immunopathol 2008;125(1–2):111–25.
42. Yagi Y, Shiono H, Chikayama Y, et al. Transport stress increases somatic cell counts in milk, and enhances the migration capacity of peripheral blood neutrophils of dairy cows. J Vet Med Sci 2004;66(4):381–7.
43. O'Loughlin A, McGee M, Waters SM, et al. Examination of the bovine leukocyte environment using immunogenetic biomarkers to assess immunocompetence following exposure to weaning stress. BMC Vet Res 2011;7:45.
44. Mitchell GB, Clark ME, Lu R, et al. Localization and functional characterization of pulmonary bovine odorant-binding protein. Vet Pathol 2011;48(6):1054–60.
45. Senthilkumaran C, Clark ME, Abdelaziz K, et al. Increased annexin A1 and A2 levels in bronchoalveolar lavage fluid are associated with resistance to respiratory disease in beef calves. Vet Res 2013;44:24.
46. Sugimoto MA, Vago JP, Perretti M, et al. Mediators of the resolution of the inflammatory response. Trends Immunol 2019;40(3):212–27.
47. Iwasaki A, Foxman EF, Molony RD. Early local immune defences in the respiratory tract. Nat Rev Immunol 2017;17(1):7–20.
48. Senthilkumaran C, Hewson J, Ollivett TL, et al. Localization of annexins A1 and A2 in the respiratory tract of healthy calves and those experimentally infected with Mannheimia haemolytica. Vet Res 2015;46:6.
49. Mitchell GB, Clark ME, Caswell JL. Alterations in the bovine bronchoalveolar lavage proteome induced by dexamethasone. Vet Immunol Immunopathol 2007;118(3–4):283–93.
50. Fischer CD, Beatty JK, Zvaigzne CG, et al. Anti-inflammatory benefits of antibiotic-induced neutrophil apoptosis: tulathromycin induces caspase-3-dependent neutrophil programmed cell death and inhibits NF-kappaB signaling and CXCL8 transcription. Antimicrob Agents Chemother 2011;55(1):338–48.
51. Sharon KP, Liang Y, Sanchez NCB, et al. Pre-weaning plane of nutrition and Mannheimia haemolytica dose influence inflammatory responses to a bovine herpesvirus-1 and Mannheimia haemolytica challenge in post-weaning Holstein calves. J Dairy Sci 2019;102(10):9082–96.
52. Mulder WJM, Ochando J, Joosten LAB, et al. Therapeutic targeting of trained immunity. Nat Rev Drug Discov 2019;18(7):553–66.
53. Czuprynski CJ, Leite F, Sylte M, et al. Complexities of the pathogenesis of Mannheimia haemolytica and Haemophilus somnus infections: challenges and potential opportunities for prevention? Anim Health Res Rev 2004;5(2):277–82.

Bovine Respiratory Disease Influences on Nutrition and Nutrient Metabolism

Clinton R. Krehbiel, PhD, PAS

KEYWORDS

- Acute phase response • Feedlot cattle • Inflammation • Nutrient requirements
- Stress

KEY POINTS

- Inflammation caused by bovine respiratory disease (BRD) continues to be one of the greatest challenges facing beef cattle producers and feedlot managers.
- BRD results in decreased intake, daily gain, and feed efficiency in feedlot calves, decreasing growth rate and increasing required days on feed.
- Morbidity caused by BRD has been associated with decreased hot carcass weight and poor carcass characteristics.
- Acute phase protein production in the liver, initiated by proinflammatory cytokines, may shift the priority for amino acid and energy use by the host animal during periods of sickness.
- Nutrient requirements for stressed calves seem to be the same as for nonstressed calves; however, nutrients should be concentrated early in the receiving period to account for low dry matter intake.

INTRODUCTION

The bovine respiratory disease (BRD) complex is the major cause of morbidity and mortality in growing and finishing cattle. BRD is a multifaceted disease generally caused by a combination of stress and viral and bacterial infections. The primary stressors encountered by calves during the marketing process include removal from dam, feed and water deprivation, exposure to new animals and pathogens, and castration/dehorning.[1] These stressors can weaken the immune system and allow infection to occur. The major viruses normally involved in BRD are infectious bovine rhinotracheitis virus, bovine viral diarrhea viruses (BVDVs), parainfluenza type-3 virus, and/or bovine respiratory syncytial virus (BRSV). Viruses can weaken the immune defenses and allow secondary infection by bacteria to occur in the lungs of the compromised calf. Bacteria most commonly isolated from lungs of calves infected with BRD

Department of Animal Science, University of Nebraska-Lincoln, C203 Animal Science Complex, 3940 Fair Street PO Box 830908, Lincoln, NE 68583-0908, USA
E-mail address: ckrehbiel2@unl.edu

Vet Clin Food Anim 36 (2020) 361–373
https://doi.org/10.1016/j.cvfa.2020.03.010
0749-0720/20/© 2020 Elsevier Inc. All rights reserved.

vetfood.theclinics.com

are *Mannheimia haemolytica, Pasteurella multocida, Histophilus somni,* and *Mycoplasma bovis.* Bovine viral diarrhea virus has been isolated alone or in combination with other viral and bacterial pathogens in animals diagnosed with BRD. Cattle persistently infected with BVDV have been reported as the main source of disease transmission in feedlot settings,[2] and the presence of an animal persistently infected with BVDV in a feedlot pen has been reported to increase the risk of antimicrobial treatment of BRD by 43% compared with nonexposed cattle.[3]

The impact of BRD on nutrient requirements has been studied and debated for many years. Because nutrition and stress are interrelated, it is important to consider how both can be managed to minimize the potential impact of BRD on animal health and performance. Stress can produce or aggravate nutritional deficiencies, and nutritional deficiencies can produce a stress response. Because stress can alter the steady state of the body and challenge physiologic adaptive processes,[4,5] management of stress in cattle should involve removal of the cause of stress, and management of the physiologic changes observed in animals caused by stress. Theoretically, meeting nutrient requirements of calves should help them overcome the physiologic changes associated with stress. In contrast, it has become clear through several experiments that, after calves get sick, the economics of all subsequent segments of the beef industry are negatively affected.[6–12] These experiments have compared the economics and performance of cattle that become sick and require treatment with those that remain healthy throughout the growing and finishing phase. Results consistently show that, if an animal gets sick, the combination of mortality, medical costs, decreased performance, and poorer carcass quality results in decreased net returns for morbid calves compared with calves that remain healthy throughout the growing/finishing phase of production.

Calves of known origin and background or preconditioned calves, where health management practices (eg, dehorning, castration, vaccination, and weaning at least 30 days before transport) are known, have decreased risk for BRD compared with market-sourced calves with unknown history. Step and colleagues[13] reported that newly weaned calves shipped directly from a ranch to a receiving facility and maintained separately showed less morbidity, lower health cost, and greater daily gains than calves purchased from multiple sources and commingled before shipment. Health costs and daily gains from commingled groups made up of freshly weaned calves shipped immediately from the ranch and market-sourced calves were not different from market-sourced calves that were not commingled. However, compared with ranch calves weaned and then immediately shipped or market-sourced calves, this experiment indicated that weaning calves for 45 days on the ranch of origin before shipping resulted in less morbidity and lower medicine costs when they arrived at the receiving facility whether they were maintained separately or commingled with market-sourced calves.[13]

Preweaning interventions can also provide potential benefits. Creep feeding or limit feeding calves for 6 to 8 weeks before weaning seems to have economic benefits compared with a program in which calves are weaned and fed ad libitum for 4 weeks before marketing.[14] Whether ranch sourced, preconditioned, or market-sourced calves are purchased, the objectives of the receiving health and nutrition program are to assist the calf in recovering from stress, optimize the immune response, and shorten the time to begin productive weight gain during the next phase of production.

STRESS EFFECTS ON NUTRIENT METABOLISM

Inflammation resulting from BRD or other diseases or injury serves to protect tissues, which maintains homeostasis and supports animal survival. However, sustained stimulation of the inflammatory response impairs normal growth and development, and may prevent an animal from attaining its full genetic potential for growth and carcass merit. Direct interactions between proinflammatory molecules and muscle, fat, mammary, and intestinal epithelial cells result in modifications of their metabolic and anabolic functions. When viral and bacterial pathogens, trauma, or stress overcome host defenses, the innate immune system initiates a rapid and systemic acute phase response (APR). Molecules from pathogens are detected by toll-like receptors, which stimulate the production of proinflammatory cytokines (eg, tumor-necrosis factor-alpha, interleukin [IL]-1α, IL-1β, IL-6) and leads to an APR, fever, anorexia, muscle catabolism, coagulation, increased glucocorticoid hormone levels, changes in liver protein synthesis, and leukocytosis.[15–17] Although such a response is invaluable to the health of the animal, it can have consequences for growth and other physiologic outcomes. A sustained systemic immune response can increase risk of sepsis, organ failure, and mortality.[18,19]

The APR provides an early nonspecific defense against pathogen challenge through a process that involves metabolic changes.[20] As part of the early defense mechanism, acute phase proteins (APP) are produced in the liver.[21,22] APP production is initiated by proinflammatory cytokines.[23] In addition, Cooke and Bohnert[24] showed that increased circulating levels of cortisol resulted in increased levels of IL-6 and haptoglobin (Hp), indicating that the APR can be activated by systemic increases in the stress marker cortisol. As a component of the APR, the liver alters metabolism to increase or decrease the production of APP. The increased demand for amino acid (AA) for production of APP by the liver is likely supplied by muscle protein catabolism and subsequent AA uptake by the liver.[25] In addition, the liver provides energy substrates to the peripheral tissues in exchange for the AA substrates needed for protein synthesis. Whether the negative impact of BRD on growth could be prevented by supplying the proper array of AA and energy substrate to meet demands of the liver during inflammation needs further study.

It is unclear how or whether an APR can negatively affect long-term growth and carcass characteristics. Berry and colleagues[26] observed sustained increased Hp levels in calves requiring multiple treatments for BRD. Hp levels remained high for 28 days, indicating that calves receiving multiple treatments experience a sustained APR. In contrast, Burciaga-Robles and colleagues[27] showed a short APR in a BRD challenge model. There is limited information regarding APP levels or the APR throughout for multiple treatments for naturally acquired BRD and subsequent harvest. Because the APR can be stimulated by cortisol,[24] it might be difficult to distinguish between increased levels of APP in response to animal handling or other stressors versus increased levels caused by illness. It is clear that increased APP levels are associated with decreased daily gain,[28,29] and the APR and inflammatory responses, regardless of initiator, alter metabolic function in a variety of tissues.

Cattle are different from other species in that Hp and serum amyloid A (SAA) are the major APPs with levels that are observed to increase during infections.[16,17] Changes in Hp levels have been observed caused by several bacterial and viral infections, including M haemolytica and P multocida, BVDV, and BRSV, all of which are common BRD pathogens.[17,20] In addition, SAA is a second definitive positive APP in cattle and levels have been shown to be increased during acute inflammation and BRD.[30,31] The significant changes in protein synthesis that occur in the liver likely modify AA requirements for the host animal. Waggoner and colleagues[32] challenged beef steers with endotoxin, and plasma concentrations of isoleucine and leucine decreased 4 hours after infusion with lipopolysaccharide compared with unchallenged controls. Reeds and colleagues[33] compared the AA content of major APPs (C-reactive protein, fibrinogen,

α-glycerophosphate, α_1-antitrypsin, SAA, and Hp) and muscle protein and calculated that the demand for the aromatic AAs (ie, phenylalanine, tyrosine, and tryptophan) would lead to more than twice the amount of AA in skeletal muscle needed to be mobilized to accommodate APP synthesis. This need for specific AAs indicates the detriment that an APR may have on muscle in beef cattle with BRD. Future research is needed to describe changes in liver and peripheral tissue metabolism in calves affected by BRD and the immunologic signals that are responsible for long-term growth impairment and potential changes in carcass composition.

INFLUENCE OF NUTRITION ON BOVINE RESPIRATORY DISEASE

A consistent response in stressed calves that show clinical signs of BRD is a decrease in dry matter intake (DMI). In addition, technologies that allow the determination of feeding behavior have shown that changes in patterns of feeding behavior and DMI are good predictors of calves that will be treated for BRD.[34,35] Feed intake by light-weight stressed calves averages only 1.5% of body weight (BW) during the first 2 weeks after arrival to a feeding facility[36,37] (**Table 1**). In a summary of 18 experiments involving transit-stressed calves, 83.4% of morbid calves and 94.6% of healthy calves had consumed any feed by day 7 following arrival to the feedlot.[36] In addition, measured DMI of morbid calves was 58%, 68%, and 88% of healthy calves across days 1 to 7, 1 to 14, and 1 to 56, respectively. Similarly, Sowell and colleagues[38] observed that 94% of calves identified as healthy and 87% of morbid calves visited the feed bunk on the day of arrival, and 100% of healthy calves and only 91% of morbid calves had visited the bunk by day 3. In a second experiment,[38] only 13% and 10% of healthy and morbid calves, respectively, visited the feed bunk on day 1. All healthy calves had visited the bunk by day 4, but only 76% of morbid calves were observed at the feed bunk. In both experiments, healthy calves had more overall feeding events per day and spent more time at the bunk daily than morbid animals, both during the first 4 days and throughout the 32-day experiment. Total calves identified as sick were 52% in experiment 1 and 82% in experiment 2,[38] which likely explains the greater variation in feeding behavior. In both experiments, 80% of morbid calves were identified within 10 days of arrival.

It is apparent that newly received, highly stressed calves consume less feed than healthy calves exposed to fewer stress factors. As such, current recommendations are for nutritionists to increase the density of nutrients in diets of stressed calves so that animal requirements for nutrients are met even when intake is low.[39] In commercial settings, it is unclear whether disease causes decreased intake or decreased

Table 1
Dry matter intake (percentage of body weight) of newly arrived calves transported from Tennessee to Texas

Days After Arrival	Healthy Calves	Sick Calves
0–7	1.6	0.9
8–14	1.9	1.4
15–28	2.7	1.8
28–56	3.0	2.7

Data from Hutcheson DP, Cole NA. Management of transit-stress syndrome in cattle: nutritional and environmental effects. J. Anim. Sci. 1986; 62:555-560.

intake is responsible for disease incidence. After recovery, DMI may remain low or be similar compared with nontreated animals. However, there is evidence that, on recovery, morbid animals experience compensatory gain compared with nontreated animals. This compensation may be caused by recovering gastrointestinal fill or reduced competition for nutrients when cattle are moved from preconditioning pens to pasture[40] or are adapted to a finishing diet.[41] McBeth and colleagues[41] segregated heifers by the number of BRD treatments (0 or 1) administered during a 42-day preconditioning period and observed subsequent finishing performance. At the beginning of the finishing phase, no difference in BW between healthy and morbid steers existed. However, daily gain was increased 14.4% and 5.8% for treated heifers during day 0 to 28 and day 0 to 112, respectively. Although DMI was not different at any time during the 140-day finishing period, the increase in daily gain resulted in treated heifers being more efficient during the first 28 days on feed. An experiment by Holland and colleagues[42] showed that receiving-phase and overall (arrival to end) daily gain were 59% and 8.7% lower, respectively, for heifers treated 3 times for BRD compared with heifers that remained healthy throughout the feeding period. After the low growing phase gain by morbid animals, a compensatory response occurred in those animals, such that overall finishing-phase daily gain was similar across BRD treatment categories, and feed efficiency was improved. Therefore, segregation according to previous number of BRD treatments during finishing may result in a compensatory response in daily gain and improved feed efficiency for treated animals. Similar results were observed by Wilson and colleagues.[43] Although increased days on feed may be required to reach similar final BW and carcass characteristics, a restart program may be a viable alternative to realizing or railing animals treated multiple times for BRD.

ENERGY CONCENTRATION AND SOURCE

Energy deficiency in cattle can severely depress the immune system[44]; however, excess dietary energy can also have detrimental effects. Feedlot studies suggest that the incidence of BRD in market-transport stressed calves is increased when the diet contains more than 60% concentrate. Although it is unlikely that the energy concentration of the diet is excessive in most receiving diets, it is possible that an energy deficit could occur because of poor forage quality and/or an inadequate supply of forage. Lofgreen[45,46] reported that calves fed low-quality hay diets on arrival were not able to compensate for their lost early weight gain later in the feeding period.

A series of experiments with market-stressed calves was conducted to determine optimal dietary energy concentrations of receiving diets.[47] In experiment 1, diets with concentrations of 0.84, 1.01, and 1.10 Mcal/kg of net energy for gain (NE_g) (dry matter [DM] basis) were fed for 29 days followed by all treatment groups being fed the 1.01 Mcal/kg of NE_g diet for an additional 34 days. Calves received on the intermediate-energy and high-energy dietary treatments consumed more feed and gained more weight during the 29-day receiving period, with the calves consuming 1.10 Mcal/kg of NE_g gaining more than the intermediate-energy treatment group at similar DMI. Calves on the high-energy and low-energy diets had lower morbidity rates than calves on the intermediate-energy treatment. Given the outcome of this study, Lofgreen and colleagues[47] replaced the 0.84 Mcal/kg of NE_g diet with a 1.19 Mcal/kg NE_g diet to determine whether gain would increase further with increased dietary energy concentration. Intake decreased when the higher-energy diet was added and daily gain was not increased. In contrast with the previous study, calves on the 1.10 Mcal/kg of NE_g diet consumed more feed than calves on the 1.01 Mcal/kg of NE_g diet. Morbidity tended to increase with increasing energy concentration.

Fluharty and Loerch[48] fed corn silage–based diets with 1.15, 1.21, 1.25, or 1.30 Mcal/kg of NE_g to individually housed steers in a 28-day receiving study. There was a linear increase in DMI with increasing dietary energy concentration but there was no difference in daily gain, feed efficiency, or health status for the 28-day period. Similarly, DMI was improved and daily gain was not different between high-energy (1.17 Mcal/kg NE_g) and low-energy (1.01 Mcal/kg NE_g) diets in a 28-day preconditioning study conducted by Pritchard and Mendez.[49] Berry and colleagues[50] attempted to sort out the confounding effects of roughage and energy concentrations by feeding high-starch and low-starch concentrations within each of 2 dietary roughage concentrations. Energy concentration did not influence performance or overall morbidity, but morbid calves fed diets with the greater concentration had less shedding of P multocida and H somni than those fed the lower-energy diets. Dietary roughage concentration varied over a narrow range of 35% to 45% in the Berry and colleagues[50] study, and therefore comparison with results from experiments with greater variation in roughage/energy concentration is difficult. Rivera and colleagues[51] analyzed data to evaluate relationships between BRD and dietary roughage concentration in lightweight, stressed cattle. Diets ranged from all-hay to 75% concentrate. Morbidity (ie, percentage of calves treated for BRD using visual observation and rectal temperature) decreased as dietary roughage concentration increased [morbidity, % = 49.59 − (0.0675 × roughage, %); P = .003]. Average daily gain and DMI were decreased by increasing the dietary roughage concentration. In addition, economic analysis indicated that the slightly lesser morbidity noted with greater roughage concentrations would not offset the loss in profit resulting from decreased average daily gain. Rivera and colleagues[51] concluded that milled diets with greater levels of concentrate would provide the optimal receiving diet for lightweight, highly stressed, newly received cattle, with limited effects on BRD. Grain type used in receiving diets does not seem to affect calf health or performance.[39] Spore and colleagues[52] reported that limit feeding high-energy rations based on low-starch corn by-products such as Sweet Bran (Cargill Corn Milling, Blair, NE) resulted in greater feed efficiency without affecting health of newly received, stressed cattle. Limit feeding a high-energy diet (1.32 Mcal of net energy [NE]/kg of DM) containing 40% Sweet Bran during the receiving and growing phase improved feed efficiency by 22% compared with a low-energy diet (0.99 Mcal of NE/kg of DM) fed ad libitum.

PROTEIN CONCENTRATION AND SOURCE

Dietary protein requirements for beef cattle can be calculated using the National Academies of Sciences, Engineering, and Medicine (NASEM)[39] metabolizable protein model, which integrates BW and energy intake. Energy intake is the first-limiting nutrient involved with weight gain; therefore, protein deposited in gain largely depends on energy intake.[53] Because newly received stressed calves often have very low intakes during the first few days, protein requirements might be low. Requirements would then increase as energy intake increases.

Effects of various protein levels and sources for newly received calves have been characterized. Galyean and colleagues[54] fed 3 levels (12%, 14%, or 16%) of supplemental crude protein (CP) from soybean meal to 120 calves (185 kg) in a 42-day receiving experiment. Daily gain increased and DMI tended to increase linearly with increasing CP concentration. Morbidity was higher for calves fed the high-protein diet compared with the 14% CP diet. Fluharty and Loerch[55] conducted a series of experiments to access protein requirements of newly arrived cattle. In experiment 1, newly weaned Simmental × Angus crossbred (243 kg) steers were fed increasing

CP concentrations (12%, 14%, 16%, or 18%) from spray-dried blood meal or soybean meal. Feed efficiency improved linearly with increasing CP concentration for the first 7 days and for the entire 42-day feeding period. Daily gain increased linearly with increasing CP concentration during the first week after arrival. For the entire receiving period, calves fed the blood meal diets had a 7.4% increase in gain compared with calves fed the soybean meal diets. Similar to data reported by Galyean and colleagues,[54] morbidity also increased linearly with increasing CP concentration, with cattle on the 12%, 14%, 16%, and 18% CP diets experiencing 38%, 50%, 45%, and 68% morbidity, respectively. A second experiment was conducted in which 246-kg Simmental × Angus steers were fed 11%, 14%, 17%, 20%, 23%, or 26% CP diets with protein supplied by spray-dried blood meal or soybean meal.[55] DMI was not affected by CP concentration. Daily gain and feed efficiency both responded quadratically, with the 20% CP diet yielding the greatest performance. There were no differences in health status between treatment groups. In a summary of several experiments, Galyean and colleagues[56] noted that, as the protein concentration in receiving diets increased up to approximately 20% of DM, animal performance improved, but the incidence of BRD increased slightly. Cole[14,57] suggested that a CP concentration of approximately 14.5% is optimal for newly received calves and would meet their protein requirements.

Pritchard and Boggs[58] indicated that dried distiller's grains could effectively replace soybean meal as a protein supplement for incoming feedlot cattle. Morbidity rates in their study were very low (<3%). Van Koevering and colleagues[59] reported that replacing soybean meal with dried distiller's grains in a receiving supplement decreased performance but did not affect the incidence or severity of BRD.

In general, young calves have a limited capacity to use dietary urea. The NASEM[39] suggests that intakes of 30 g/d can be tolerated by stressed calves during the first 2 weeks of feeding. The use of ingredients high in ruminally undegraded protein (RUP) has been beneficial in some studies with calves on forage-based diets. It seems that RUP concentrations of 5.4% of dietary DM are generally adequate for stressed calves.[39]

MINERALS

Because of low feed intakes, the concentrations of most minerals need to be increased in receiving diets. However, with the possible exception of K, the mineral requirements (ie, grams per day) of stressed calves do not seem to be increased.[56]

Cu, Zn, and Se have been shown to be essential for optimal immune function. Although several studies have reported a beneficial effect of supplemental Cu, Se, and Zn on some indicators of immune function, data have been inconsistent, and few studies have shown a positive effect on animal health or performance when the control diet was not deficient in these minerals. In general, beneficial effects of supplementing these trace minerals on immunity or the incidence of BRD in beef calves would most likely occur in animals with marginal or deficient mineral status. Because the mineral status of calves is rarely known, it is advantageous to supplement with these minerals, especially because most forages are marginal or deficient in at least 1 of these minerals or contain increased concentrations of antagonists, such as Mo and S. However, feeding excessive quantities of the trace minerals may not be helpful and is potentially harmful. A good rule of thumb is to provide 50% or more of mineral requirements in the daily supplement.

Although some studies have reported improved immune responses when calves were supplemented with organic forms of Cu, Zn, Se, or Mn (proteinates, AA complexes, and so forth), other studies have reported no effect.[1,56] Garcia and colleagues[60] reported that varying level and source of trace minerals did not affect growth performance or morbidity in newly received cattle, and Ryan and colleagues[61] reported that source of Cu, Zn, and Mn had no effect on growth performance, morbidity, average antibiotic cost, plasma Cu and Zn concentrations, or antibody titer response to bovine viral diarrhea virus vaccination in shipping-stressed cattle over a 42-day to 45-day backgrounding phase. Supplying minerals in an AA-chelated form reduced the number of treatments required for morbid calves to recover from BRD compared with a complex mineral form, although morbidity and mortality did not differ.[62] In addition, an injectable trace mineral did not improve performance or morbidity when the incidence was low.[63]

The NASEM[39] noted that results of recent experiments indicate a need for supplemental Cr in some situations. Reports by Chang and Mowat[64] and Moonsie-Shageer and Mowat[65] indicated that BW gain by feeder calves was increased by supplements of 0.2 to 1.0 mg of Cr per kilogram of diet. The effect on morbidity was inconsistent. Bernhard and colleagues[66] fed 221-kg steers 0, 0.1, 0.2, or 0.3 mg/kg of Cr (DM basis) from Cr-propionate. Cr-supplemented steers had improvements in DMI, feed efficiency, and daily gain within the first 28 days of the experiment, when cattle would have been under nutritional and physiologic stress. Through the remainder of the experiment, Cr-supplemented steers maintained these advantages.

VITAMINS

Experiments with B-vitamin supplementation to newly weaned/received cattle have resulted in variable responses, with decreased morbidity and increased performance

Table 2
Recommended nutrient concentrations in diets for stressed calves (dry matter basis)

Nutrient	Concentration	Comments
Dry Matter (%)	80–85	Limit extreme high-moisture feeds
NE_m (Mcal/kg)	1.3–1.6	Higher first 7–14 d
NE_g (Mcal/kg)	0.8–0.9	Higher first 7–14 d
CP (%)	12.5–14.5	Limit urea to <30 g/d
Ca (%)	0.6–0.8	—
P (%)	0.4–0.5	—
K (%)	1.2–1.4	Avoid high Cl levels
Na (%)	0.2–0.3	Check water
Mg (%)	0.2–0.3	—
S (%)	0.15–0.25	Check water
Mn (ppm)	40–70	—
Co (ppm)	0.1–0.2	—
Cu (ppm)	10–15	Higher if high S or Mo
Fe (ppm)	100–200	—
Zinc (ppm)	75–100	—
Se (ppm)	0.1–0.2	—
Vitamin E (IU/d)	400–500	Concentrate if pelleted

Abbreviation: NE_m, net energy for maintenance.
Data from Refs.[14,39,57]

in some studies and little or no response in others.[14] In a review of several experiments, Cole[14] noted a 3% decrease in BRD morbidity, a 4.2% increase in BW gain, and a 5.1% improvement in feed efficiency with supplemental B vitamins.

Supplemental vitamin E in receiving diets seems to be beneficial for decreasing morbidity and improving performance. Several studies with feedlot diets suggest that feeding vitamin E in excess of requirements may be beneficial to animal health. In general, results have been better when vitamin E was fed than when it was injected.[14,57] In a summary of results of cattle feedlot receiving studies, Elam[67] noted that, as vitamin E supplementation increased from 0 to 2000 IU/d, BRD decreased 0.35% for every 100-IU increase in vitamin E intake. Results with supplementation of other fat-soluble vitamins have been inconsistent.[14]

Duff and Galyean[1] concluded that, with the possible exception of K, the stressors of weaning, marketing, transport, and disease do not seem to increase total nutrient requirements of calves. However, because of low feed intakes, the concentrations of nutrients in the diet need to be increased to meet the nutrient requirements of the animals (**Table 2**).[14,39,57]

SUMMARY

Nutritional management of newly received calves is key to recovery from stressors associated with weaning and marketing. Because of low initial intakes, nutrient deficiencies are difficult to meet and may limit the recovery process. More nutrient-dense diets should be formulated to aid calves in recovery, although it may take several days to return stressed calves to positive energy and protein balances. If deficiencies can be compensated for, energy and protein source seem to have minimal impact on health and performance of newly received, stressed calves. However, continued research in the area of nutrient requirements of calves facing immune challenges could prove beneficial in formulating nutritional management plans for stressed calves. This outcome would be especially beneficial for meeting nutrient/metabolic requirements during an APR, with potential consequences for long-term outcomes.

DISCLOSURE

The author has nothing to disclose.

REFERENCES

1. Duff GC, Galyean ML. Board-invited review: recent advances in management of highly stressed, newly received feedlot cattle. J Anim Sci 2007;85:823–40.

2. O'Conner AM, Sorden SD, Apley MD. Association between the existence of calves persistently infected with bovine viral diarrhea virus and commingling on pen morbidity in feedlot cattle. Am J Vet Res 2005;66:2130–4.

3. Loneragan GH, Thomson DU, Montgomery DL, et al. Prevalence, outcome, and health consequences associated with persistent infection with bovine viral diarrhea virus in feedlot cattle. J Am Vet Med Assoc 2005;226:595–601.

4. Frazer D, Ritchie JSD, Frazer AF. The term "stress" in a veterinary context. Br Vet J 1975;131:653–8.

5. Seyle H. The stress of life. New York: McGraw-Hill Book Company; 1976.

6. McNeill JW, Paschal JC, McNeill MS, et al. Effect of morbidity on performance and profitability of feedlot steers. J Anim Sci 1996;74(Suppl. 1):135.

7. McNeill JW. 1996-97 Texas A & M Ranch to Rail North/South summary Report. College Station (TX): Texas Agricultural Extension Service, Texas A & M University; 1997.
8. McNeill JW. 1997-98 Texas A & M Ranch to Rail North/South Summary Report. College Station (TX): Texas Agricultural Extension Service, Texas A & M University; 1998.
9. Montgomery TH, Adams R, Cole MA, et al. Influence of feeder calf management and bovine respiratory disease on carcass traits of beef steers. Proceedings: Western Section. J Anim Sci 1984;35:319–27.
10. Perino LJ. Overview of the bovine respiratory disease complex. Compend Contin Educ Pract Vet 1992;14(Suppl):3.
11. Gardner BA, Dolezal HG, Bryant LK, et al. Health of finishing steers: effects on performance, carcass traits, and meat tenderness. J Anim Sci 1999;77:3168–75.
12. Griffin D, Perino L, Whittum T. Feedlot respiratory disease: cost, value of preventives and intervention. Proceedings, Annual Convention – Am. Assoc. of Bovine Prac., vol. 27, San Antonio, TX. Am. Assoc. Bovine Prac., Rome, GA, July, 1995.
13. Step DL, Krehbiel CR, DePra HA, et al. Effects of commingling beef calves from difference sources and weaning protocols during a forty-two-day receiving period on performance and bovine respiratory disease. J Anim Sci 2008;86:3146–58.
14. Cole NA. Review of bovine respiratory disease: nutrition and disease interactions. In: Smith R, editor. Review of bovine respiratory disease – schering-plough animal health. Trenton (NJ): Veterinary Learning Systems; 1996. p. 57–74.
15. Gruys E, Toussaint MJM, Niewold TA, et al. Acute phase reaction and acute phase proteins. J Zhejiang Univ Sci 2005;6B:1045–56.
16. Cray C, Zaias J, Altman NH. Acute phase response in animals: a review. Comp Med 2009;59:517–26.
17. Eckersall PD, Bell R. Acute phase proteins: biomarkers of infection and inflammation in veterinary medicine. Vet J 2010;185:23–7.
18. De Maio A, de Lourdes Mooney M, Matesic LE, et al. Acute phase response in calves following infection with Pasteurella haemolytica, Ostertagia ostertagi and endotoxin administration. Res Vet Sci 1989;47:203–7.
19. Selzman CH, Shames BD, Miller SA, et al. Therapeutic implications of interleukin-10 in surgical disease. Shock 1998;10:309–18.
20. Peterson HH, Nielsen JP, Heegaard PMH. Application of acute phase protein measurements in veterinary clinical chemistry. Vet Res 2004;35:163–87.
21. Eckersall PD, Conner JG. Bovine and canine acute phase proteins. Vet Res Commun 1988;12:169–78.
22. Saini PK, Raiz M, Webert DW, et al. Development of a simple enzyme immunoassay for blood haptoglobin concentration in cattle and its application in improving food safety. Am J Vet Res 1998;59:1101–7.
23. Baumann H, Gauldie J. The acute phase response. Immunol Today 1994;15:74–80.
24. Cooke RF, Bohnert DW. Technical note: bovine acute-phase response after corticotrophin-release hormone challenge. J Anim Sci 2011;89:252–7.
25. Christ B, Nath A, Heinrich PC. Inhibition by recombinant human interleukin-6 of the glucagon-dependent induction of phosphoenolpyruvate carboxykinase and of the insulin-dependent induction of glucokinase gene expression in culture rat hepatocytes: regulation of gene transcription and messenger RNA degradation. Hepatology 1994;20:1577–83.

26. Berry BA, Confer AW, Krehbiel CR, et al. Effects of dietary energy and starch concentrations for newly received feedlot calves: II. Acute-phase protein response. J Anim Sci 2004;82:845–50.
27. Burciaga-Robles LO, Step DL, Krehbiel CR, et al. Effects of exposure to calves persistently infected with bovine viral diarrhea virus type 1b and subsequent infection with *Mannheima haemolytica* on clinical signs and immune parameters: Model for bovine respiratory disease via viral and bacterial interaction. J Anim Sci 2010;88:2166–78.
28. Qiu X, Arthington JD, Riley DG, et al. Genetic effects on acute phase protein response to the stresses of weaning and transportation in beef calves. J Anim Sci 2007;85:2367–74.
29. Cooke RF, Arthington JD, Austin BR, et al. Effects of acclimation to handling on performance, reproductive, and physiological responses of brahman-crossbred heifers. J Anim Sci 2009;87:3403–12.
30. Horadagoda NU, Knox KMG, Gibbs HA, et al. Acute phase proteins in cattle: discrimination between acute and chronic inflammation. Vet Rec 1999;144: 437–41.
31. Nikunen S, Härtel H, Orro T, et al. Association of bovine respiratory disease with clinical status and acute phase proteins in calves. Comp Immun Micro Inf Dis 2007;30:143–51.
32. Waggoner JW, Löest CA, Mathis CP, et al. Effects of rumen-protected methionine supplementation and bacterial lipopolysaccharide infusion on nitrogen metabolism and hormonal responses of growing beef steers. J Anim Sci 2009;87: 681–92.
33. Reeds PJ, Fjeld CR, Jahoor F. Do the differences between the amino acid compositions of acute-phase and muscle proteins have a bearing on nitrogen loss in traumatic states? J Nutr 1994;124:906–10.
34. Jackson KS, Carstens GE, Tedeschi LO, et al. Changes in feeding behavior patterns and dry matter intake before clinical symptoms associated with bovine respiratory disease in growing bulls. J Anim Sci 2016;94:1644–52.
35. Wolfger B, Schwartzkopf-Genswein KS, Barkema HW, et al. Feeding behavior as an early predictor of bovine respiratory disease in North American feedlot systems. J Anim Sci 2015;93:377–85.
36. Hutcheson DP, Cole NA. Management of transit-stress syndrome in cattle: nutritional and environmental effects. J Anim Sci 1986;62:555–60.
37. Galyean ML, Hubbert ME. Effects of season, health, and management on feed intake by beef cattle. In: Symposium: Intake by Feedlot Cattle. Okla. Agric. Exp. Sta. P-942. Pages 226-234. Oklahoma State Univ., Stillwater, September 11-13, 1995.
38. Sowell BF, Branine ME, Bowman JGP, et al. Feeding and watering behavior of healthy and morbid steers in a commercial feedlot. J Anim Sci 1999;77:1105–12.
39. National Academies of Sciences, Engineering, Medicine (NASEM). Nutrient requirements of beef cattle. 8th rev edition. Washington, DC: The National Academies Press; 2016. https://doi.org/10.17226/19014.
40. Montgomery SP, Sindt JJ, Greenquist MA, et al. Plasma metabolites of receiving heifers and the relationship between apparent bovine respiratory disease, body weight gain, and carcass characteristics. J Anim Sci 2009;87:328–33.
41. McBeth LJ, Gill DR, Krehbiel CR, et al. Effect of health status during the receiving period on subsequent feedlot performance and carcass characteristics. Okla Agric Exp Sta Res Rep 2001;986:30–3.

42. Holland BP, Burciaga-Robles LO, VanOverbeke DL, et al. Effect of bovine respiratory disease during preconditioning on subsequent feedlot performance, carcass characteristics, and beef attributes. J Anim Sci 2010;88:2486–99.

43. Wilson BK, Step DL, Maxwell CL, et al. Effect of bovine respiratory disease during the receiving period on steer finishing performance, efficiency, carcass characteristics, and lung scores. Prof Anim Sci 2017;33:24–36.

44. Nockels CF. The role of vitamins in modulating disease resistance. Vet Clin North Am Food Anim Pract 1988;4:531–42.

45. Lofgreen GP. Nutrition and management of stressed beef calves. In: Radostits OM, editor. Veterinary Clinics of North America: large animal practice, vol. 5. Philadelphia: W. B. Saunders; 1983. p. 87–101. No. 1.

46. Lofgreen GP. Nutrition and management of stressed beef calves: an update. In: Howard JL, editor. Veterinary Clinics of North America: food animal practice, vol. 4. Philadelphia: W. B. Saunders; 1988. p. 509–22. No. 3.

47. Lofgreen GP, Dunbar JR, Addis DG, et al. Energy level in starting rations for calves subjected to marketing and shipping stress. J Anim Sci 1975;41:1256–65.

48. Fluharty FL, Loerch SC. Effects of dietary energy source and level on performance of newly arrived feedlot calves. J Anim Sci 1996;74:504–13.

49. Pritchard RH, Mendez JK. Effects of preconditioning on pre- and post-shipment performance of feeder calves. J Anim Sci 1990;68:28–34.

50. Berry BA, Krehbiel CR, Confer AW, et al. Effects of dietary energy and starch concentrations for newly received feedlot calves: I. Growth performance and health. J Anim Sci 2004;82:837–44.

51. Rivera JD, Duff GC, Galyean ML, et al. Effects of graded levels of vitamin E on inflammatory response and evaluation of methods of delivering supplemental vitamin E on performance and health of beef steers. Prof Anim Sci 2003;19: 171–7.

52. Spore TJ, Montgomery SP, Titgemeyer EC, et al. Effects of a high-energy programmed feeding protocol on nutrient digestibility, health, and performance of newly received growing beef cattle. Appl Anim Sci 2019;35:397–407.

53. Galyean ML. Protein levels in beef cattle finishing diets: industry application, university research, and systems results. J Anim Sci 1996;74:2860–70.

54. Galyean ML, Gunter SA, Malcolm-Callis KJ, et al. Effects of crude protein concentration in the receiving diet on performance and health of newly received beef calves. Clayton Livestock Res Ctr Prog Rep 1993. No. 88. N.M. Agric. Exp. Sta., Las Cruces.

55. Fluharty FL, Loerch SC. Effects of protein concentration and protein source on performance of newly arrived feedlot steers. J Anim Sci 1995;73:1585–94.

56. Galyean ML, Perino LJ, Duff GC. Interaction of cattle health/immunity and nutrition. J Anim Sci 1999;77:1120–34.

57. Cole NA. Receiving nutrition and management for feedlots. Proc. XXV American Association of Bovine Practitioners Conference. St. Paul, MN, Aug 31-Sept 4, 1992. 2. p. 309-314. 1992.

58. Pritchard RH, Boggs DL. Use of DDGS as the primary source of supplemental crude protein in calf receiving diets. 2006 South Dakota Beef Report; 2006. p. 6–9.

59. Van Koevering MT, Gill DR, Owens FN. The effects of escape protein on health and performance of shipping stressed calves. Oklahoma State Univ. Anim Sci Res 1991;134:156–62.

60. Garcia ME, Oosthuysen E, Graves JR, et al. Effects of level and source of supplemental trace minerals on growth responses of beef calves received from New Mexico ranches. Proc West Sect Am Soc Anim Sci 2014;65:91–4.
61. Ryan AW, Kegley EB, Hawley J, et al. Supplemental trace minerals (zinc, copper, and manganese) as sulfates, organic amino acid complexes, or hydroxy trace mineral sources for shipping stressed calves. Prof Anim Sci 2015;31:333–41.
62. Goodall SR, Schuetze CJ. Complexed versus amino acid-chelated trace mineral programs in high-risk calves during receiving. Transl Anim Sci 2019;3:1636–40.
63. Roberts SL, May ND, Brauer CL, et al. Effect of injectable trace mineral administration on health, performance, and vaccine response of newly received feedlot cattle. Prof Anim Sci 2016;32:842–8.
64. Chang X, Mowat DN. Supplemental chromium for stressed and growing feeder calves. J Anim Sci 1992;70:559–65.
65. Moonsie-Shageer S, Mowat DN. Effect of level of supplemental chromium on performance, serum constituents, and immune response of stressed feeder steer calves. J Anim Sci 1993;71:232–8.
66. Bernhard BC, Burdick NC, Rounds W, et al. Chromium supplementation alters the performance and health of feedlot cattle during the receiving period and enhances their metabolic response to a lipopolysaccharide (LPS) challenge. J Anim Sci 2012;90:3879–88.
67. Elam NA. Impact of vitamin E supplementation on newly received calves. Proc. Colorado Nutr. Ft. Collins (CO): Roundtable, Colorado State Univ.; 2006.

How Does Housing Influence Bovine Respiratory Disease in Confinement Cow-Calf Operations?

Terry J. Engelken, DVM, MS

KEYWORDS

- Confined cow-calf • Bovine respiratory disease • Animal flow • Health management

KEY POINTS

- Confined cow-calf operations are a relatively new method of beef production. There is a learning curve associated with this type of production for owners and veterinarians.
- Recommendations for animal space and linear bunk allotment are still being defined in these operations. Limit-feeding offers an opportunity to decrease feed costs and improve efficiency.
- How animals are staged and moved through the operation during calving season will have a tremendous impact on the incidence of calf diarrhea and respiratory disease.
- Well-designed vaccination programs that consider disease risk, animal handling patterns, and the timing of vaccination need to be constructed with practitioner input.
- The maintenance of the pen environment in these buildings will have an effect on the expression of respiratory disease in the calves. Proper airflow and ventilation are required to reduce irritation to the respiratory tract of the animals housed in these building.

INTRODUCTION

Over the past decade, confined cow-calf operations have become more common in the US Corn Belt. There are multiple reasons for the development of this trend, with land costs and availability being primary. As the competition for tillable acres from row crop enterprises has increased, there has been a corresponding increase in the cost of pasture ownership. Even in areas of the Corn Belt where pasture acres are available to rent, these costs have increased rapidly as well. In addition, expanding urban development also competes for pasture acres and dramatically increases land costs. At a time when the next generation of young producers is moving back to the family farm, expansion or establishment of the cow herd via traditional grazing is

ᵃ Department of Veterinary Diagnostic and Production Animal Medicine, College of Veterinary Medicine, Iowa State University, 2438 Lloyd Veterinary Medical Center, Ames, IA 50011, USA
E-mail address: engelken@iastate.edu

Vet Clin Food Anim 36 (2020) 375–383
https://doi.org/10.1016/j.cvfa.2020.03.011
0749-0720/20/© 2020 Elsevier Inc. All rights reserved.
vetfood.theclinics.com

economically unfeasible. This situation has caused cow-calf producers to explore new methods of production that do not require such an extensive investment in land resources.

These types of operations vary tremendously in terms of how the cattle are confined, the way in which the breeding season is managed, the length of time and type of grazing incorporated into the production system, and the needed herd health protocols. Confinement may take place in dry lots with shelter for the cows, excess pen space at feed yards, or in a structure specifically designed to house cow-calf pairs. It is not uncommon to use short periods of grazing in the management of some of these operations. This grazing may occur during the summer, but in the Corn Belt, it is more common to place the animals on cornstalk or cover crop acres for a period of 90 days or less.[1] During the rest of the year, these operations depend on the delivery of stored feeds to maintain calf growth, cow condition, and reproduction.

Besides requiring less investment in land resources, there are other advantages to confined cow-calf production systems. With the herd confined in a relatively small area, it has been the author's observation that cow and calf docility improves greatly. This observation should not be surprising because the animals are in daily contact with the people working around them. This interaction improves animal welfare and decreases "wear and tear" on the facility. Assuming the building or dry lot is properly maintained, many of the environmental extremes that have a negative impact on feeding requirements, calf health, and female reproduction can be ameliorated. Weather events, such as extreme heat, cold, or snow accumulation, can be more easily managed in these types of facilities. This type of management has led to the use of the term "controlled environment" to describe these units.[2]

In addition, because these animals are in close proximity to the working facility, the use of reproductive technology is enhanced. Tools, such as estrus synchronization, artificial insemination, and embryo transfer recipient programs, are commonly used in these production units. This use of technology leads to a shorter calving season and better calf health outcomes because the age variation within calving groups is minimized. This shorter calving season also provides an opportunity to better organize and deliver the health program to suckling calves because they will be penned according to calving date and age. Although this type of production system does require increased labor, stored feed, and management ability, it can be a very sustainable model to maintain a beef enterprise on the farm.

HEALTH MANAGEMENT FOR CONFINED COW-CALF OPERATIONS

Because of the increased animal density in these operations, the potential for the rapid spread of pathogens is increased. Therefore, it is imperative that the practitioner evaluate the entire operation for disease risk and construct cost-effective intervention strategies. These strategies are especially important because many of these pathogens not only affect calf respiratory disease but also negatively affect cow reproductive performance. The goal of this type of evaluation is to prevent the introduction or reintroduction of infectious disease (biosecurity) and prevent or decrease the spread of a pathogen if introduced into the operation (biocontainment).[3,4]

Because most disease organisms are brought onto operations via newly added animals, it is imperative that contact be minimized between these animals and the resident herd.[3–5] If new animals are added, they should be held in isolation for a minimum of 30 days. This isolation recommendation will provide enough time for cattle stressed by movement to resolve their viremia and cover the incubation period of important infectious diseases. Protocols should be in place to make sure that needed samples for diagnostic screening are collected and submitted in a timely fashion. The results of these tests need to be compiled and interpreted before the animals leave isolation. Plans to prevent the spread of disease within the operation also need to be discussed, and protocols need to be implemented. This type of program that uses disease risk analysis, animal health records, and diagnostic testing offers the veterinarian a pivotal role to improve health programming and profitability.

Health management programs designed to prevent disease in calves must begin long before the calving season begins and extend beyond vaccination programs. Nutritional management of the pregnant female starting in late gestation is critical to minimizing dystocia, maximizing calf vigor, and optimizing passive transfer via colostrum.[6] Minimizing exposure to pathogens with adequate bedding, environmental cleanliness, and proper animal flow will decrease the incidence of calf diarrhea and respiratory disease during calving.[7] Finally, a comprehensive vaccination program for both the breeding herd and the suckling calves will prevent losses associated with respiratory pathogens during the suckling phase. This type of management will set the calf up for a successful weaning and productive lifespan.

Late Gestational Nutritional Management

Prepartum nutritional management is critical for the long-term health of the calf and reproductive performance in the cow.[6,8] Nutritional status of the cow at parturition will affect dystocia levels, calf birth weight, female colostrum production, calf morbidity, and weaning weight. Females need to be body-conditioned scored at pregnancy examination and approximately 60 days before the start of calving in order to build the needed supplementation programs to ensure they calve in moderate condition. **Table 1** illustrates the effect of body weight change during the last 100 days of gestation on calf birth weight, survival, scours morbidity, and weaning weight.[6] Research such as this clearly shows that nutritional mismanagement can play a central role in calf disease outbreaks and decreased growth performance. Therefore, the feeding program should always be reviewed before the start of calving and as part of any disease workup in beef herds.

There are special considerations for cows that are housed in confinement that differ substantially from grazing herds. It has been recommended that cows in late gestation through calf weaning be given 90 to 120 ft^2 per head.[7,9] Adequate space allows the cows to move freely, reduces musculoskeletal injuries, and provides a drier bedding pack. Adequate bunk space is critical in these operations, and it is recommended that cows be allowed 24 to 36 inches per animal.[9] The upper end of this range is certainly needed if cows are extremely large or if creep feeding is not used for the calves. Limit feeding in confined cow-calf operations is commonly used to take advantage of high forage diets and the efficiencies this practice provides.[10,11] Cows in these confinement systems may see a reduction in maintenance requirements of 20% because of their limited movement and increased diet digestibility associated with limit feeding.[11] Limiting adult animals to 2% of their body weight in dry matter is typically adequate to meet their maintenance requirements. Waterer space and flow are also critical to maintain feed intake and animal health.

Calving Season Management

Proper calving season management is of primary importance to the lifetime health and productivity of the newborn calves. The calving environment must be managed to maximize cow and calf comfort, minimize pathogen exposure, and ensure adequate

Table 1
Effect of prepartum energy levels on cow productivity

	Continuous Low-Energy Level	Elevated Energy Level Last 30 Days Prepartum
Level of energy		
Kilograms TDN first 70 d	2.1	2.1
Kilograms TDN last 30 d	2.1	4.82
Cow weight change		
First 70 d (kg)	−54.2	− 52.1
Last 30 d (kg)	−10.5	+42.2
Birth weight of calf (kg)	26.7	30.5
Calf survival		
At birth (%)	90.5	100
At weaning (%)	71.4	100
Calves treated for scours (%)	52	33.4
Cow milk production (kg/d)	4.1	5.45
Weaning weight (kg)	133.8	145.5
In estrus 40 d after calving (%)	37.5	47.6

Abbreviation: TDN, total digestible nutrients.
From Corah LR. Nutrition of beef cows for optimizing reproductive efficiency. Con Ed Pract Vet.1988;10:659-64; with permission.

colostrum intake by the calves; this is especially true for confined operations. In the first 3 weeks of life, the calf scours complex is typically the greatest health concern for newborn calves. Therefore, most of the producer's attention must be on those factors that affect the establishment of this disease. However, calf scours in beef herds has also been cited as a risk factor for the later development of respiratory disease in calves.[12] To this end, it is critically important that a complete preventative program be established to ensure calf survival and performance.

When managing calving in confined cow-calf operations, animal flow through the building during calving must be handled appropriately. The end goal of animal movement is to finish with pair pens that hold calves that are similar in age. This approach helps control subclinical infection and the multiplier effect of calf scours pathogens that lead to massive contamination of the calving area.[4] This age segregation also prevents pathogen spread from older calves to susceptible newborns. This end point is the same as described by the movement of pregnant cows associated with the Sandhills Calving System.[4,13] The difference is that the producer is moving pairs after they calve to fill an empty pen over a set period of days.

To begin this process, calving females are sorted into pens based on their expected calving date. The cows expected to calve first will be at the end of the building closest to the working facilities so that calving assistance may be rendered if needed. An empty pen is created at the opposite end of the building to serve as the first pair pen. After calving, calves nurse and bond with their dam, and then the pair is removed from the gestating pen. Any initial calf processing is done at this time, and the pair is moved to the empty pen at the other end of the building. This animal movement continues until the first pair pen reaches its capacity. At that point, pregnant cows are moved "forward" toward the working facility to create a new empty pen that is cleaned and rebedded. This new pen will receive the next group of pairs as they calve. This process continues through the end of the calving season. It is important to ensure that the age difference of the calves in any 1 pen does not exceed 10 days. This type of animal movement is referred to as a "snake" and is patterned after the way in which sow farms are managed in the swine industry (Chad Wilkerson, personal communication, 2018).[7] Besides improved calf health through the prevention of scours and respiratory outbreaks, there are other advantages to this type of animal movement. The first is that it prevents cross-nursing or mismothering of pregnant cows leading to the loss of their colostrum. In confined operations, it is common for calves to nurse multiple cows in the pen, especially when the females are at the feed bunk (**Fig. 1**). Moving young calves away from pregnant cows helps to ensure that all calves will receive colostrum. This system also simplifies the delivery of the animal health and reproductive management programs by having pairs in distinct pens.[7] Procedures, such as calf processing, cow prebreeding vaccination, and estrus synchronization, can be scheduled on a pen-by-pen basis, which improves scheduling and labor efficiency to ensure that calf health management practices are completed in a timely fashion.

Another critical area of calving season management is the environment inside the building. These operations use a bedding pack made of cornstalks, wheat straw, or even sawdust to provide an area for the cows to comfortably nurse their calf or lie down.[14] During the calving season, enough bedding needs to be added daily to ensure that the pack is firm and dry. Manure along the feed bunk should also be scraped daily during calving to decrease fecal contamination and water retention in the building. As calves get older, this frequency may be reduced to 3 times per week. Creep areas or "play pens" should be provided to allow calves their own area away from the cows. Construction of these areas will decrease musculoskeletal injuries in the calves and allow for the delivery of creep feed (**Figs. 2** and **3**). Creep feed should be offered within the first 7 days and contain an ionophore. It is imperative that these "play pens" receive increased attention so that they remain dry and comfortable.

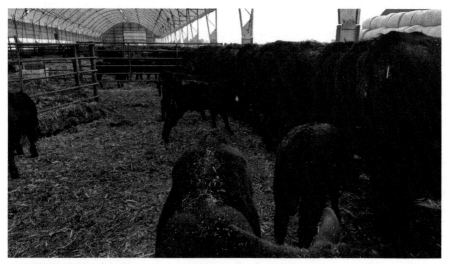

Fig. 1. Calf nursing behavior in a confined cow-calf operation. Nursing calves need to be separated from gestating cows to ensure that colostrum is not consumed through mismothering.

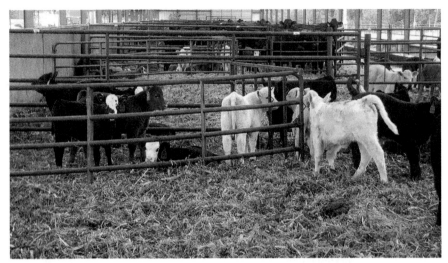

Fig. 2. Well-bedded calf creep area or "play pen" in a confined cow-calf operation. Calves can enter the area via the creep gate at the front of the pen. These areas allow a comfortable place for calves to lie down that is separate from the adult cows.

Suckling Calf Management

The management considerations for suckling beef calves in a confined unit are similar to traditional grazing operations. Like all operations, health programs have to consider disease risk, handling patterns, the presence of maternal antibody, and marketing options.[15,16] According to a recent Iowa State survey of confined cow-calf operations, producers cited calf scours, "pneumonia," coccidiosis, and "pinkeye" as the top health concerns in their suckling calves.[14] In calves less than 1 month of age, intranasal vaccines may offer the best opportunity to provide local immunity in the face of maternal antibody. These vaccines also prime the calf's immune system to generate an anamnestic response to later parenteral vaccination. Nebraska research would indicate that the timing of preweaning respiratory disease or "summer pneumonia" in confined suckling beef calves occurs at an age similar to grazing operations.[4,17] These results should emphasize the need to understand the risk factors for this complex present on the operation and the timing of respiratory vaccination. A well-designed vaccination program is still the cornerstone of respiratory disease prevention in these calves. Decisions concerning the strategic use of various antigen combinations, killed or modified-live virus vaccines, their route of administration, and timing of delivery need to be made with practitioner input.[16]

The buildings used to house confined operations normally rely on natural ventilation that is driven by buoyancy and wind.[9] Warm air is more buoyant and rises to the peak of the roof where it leaves the building through vents. This "chimney-like" movement of air is especially important for removing water vapor out of the building as well. Wind-driven ventilation is responsible for air movement across the cattle and can be controlled by the raising and lowering of a curtain. There may be a tendency among producers to keep the curtain raised for long periods of time to decrease wind speed during the cold months of the year. This practice can lead to increased moisture retention in the building and more cases of calf respiratory disease. As long as the cattle are dry, the waterers remain thawed, and moisture (rain or snow) is not blowing into the building, the curtain should remain open. Even when the curtain is positioned to

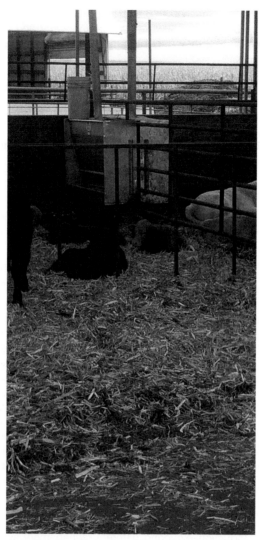

Fig. 3. Designated creep area that allows for calf comfort and protection. Note the presence of the metal creep feeder in the back of the pen. Commercially designed, pelleted rations that include an ionophore work well in these areas.

decrease wind speed, the building should be designed to allow a gap between the roof and the top of the curtain to allow some level of continuous air movement. Air movement is even more important in the summer heat. While bedding is being spread in these buildings, the curtain should be open for maximum airflow to allow for the dispersal of the dust and dirt that is invariably present in the bedding material, thus decreasing irritation to the respiratory tract of the calves and decreasing the potential for disease outbreaks.

As calves grow larger and approach weaning, there are additional management concerns that need to be considered to ensure calf health. Calves should have access to water at all times so mechanical waterers need to be constructed that allow calves to drink. It is recommended that a 4- to 6-inch lip be placed around the feed bunk and waterer to allow calves additional height to reach the water and feed.[9] By the time calves are 3 months of age, they may be consuming 1.0% of their body weight in dry matter.[10] Consumption will increase to 1.5% by the time the calves are ready for weaning so feed delivery will need to be adjusted. Typically, calves in confined operations are weaned between 120 and 150 days of age.[14] At this age, calves are readily eating from the bunk and consuming approximately 1 gallon of water per head per day. Calves of this size dramatically decrease the available space per head because they begin spending less time in the creep areas. It can also become a challenge to keep the pens dry because of the amount of urine and manure being produced by these calves.

SUMMARY

Confined cow-calf operations are a relatively new production model in the United States. As with any new technology, there will be a learning curve for producers and veterinarians as we attempt to optimize animal health and profitability. It is critical that cattle are managed properly in these units if disease issues are to be minimized. Allowing for adequate space in the pen and at the feed bunk is a critical factor affecting animal welfare, nutritional management, and disease transmission. Animal flow from outside and within the operation, along with proper maintenance of the pen environment, is the main driver affecting the incidence of calf diarrhea and respiratory disease. Going hand in hand with this type of management evaluation is a vaccination program designed to fit the characteristics of the operation. Practitioners have an opportunity to work with these units to help them understand the risk of disease and needed mitigation strategies.

DISCLOSURE

The confined cow/calf survey mentioned as reference 14 and cited in lines 279-281 was funded by Boehringer Ingelheim Animal Health. The name of the project was: A Survey of Production and Management Practices of Midwestern Confined Cow-Calf Operations.

REFERENCES

1. Iowa cow-calf production–exploring different management systems. Iowa State University Extension and Outreach, Iowa Beef Center. IBC 0131. 2019. Available at: http://www.iowabeefcenter.org/publications.html. Accessed January 23, 2020.

2. Redden MD, Bayliff CL, Spencer CM, et al. Energy use and efficiency of cow/calf management in controlled environment cattle systems. In: Proceedings, Dr. Kenneth & Caroline Eng Trust Fund Symposium on Cow-Calf Programs for Improved Efficiency, Sustainability, and Profitability. University of Nebraska-Lincoln. Lincoln, NE, October 5–6, 2016. pp. 85–91.

3. Huston C. Biosecurity and biocontainment for reproductive pathogens. In: Hopper RM, editor. Bovine reproduction. 1st edition. Ames (IA): John Wiley & Sons, Inc.; 2015. p. 259–66.

4. Smith DR. Health and management of confined cows and calves. In: Proceedings, Dr. Kenneth & Caroline McDonald Eng Foundation Cow-Calf Symposium. University of Nebraska-Lincoln. Lincoln, NE, September 12–13, 2013. pp. 15–22.

5. Engelken TJ, Dohlman TM. Beef herd health for optimum reproduction. In: Hopper RM, editor. Bovine reproduction. 1st edition. Ames (IA): John Wiley & Sons, Inc.; 2015. p. 347–52.
6. Corah LR. Nutrition of beef cows for optimizing reproductive efficiency. Compend Con Ed Pract Vet 1988;10:659–64.
7. Engelken TJ. Confined cow-calf operations. In: Proceedings, Academy of Veterinary Consultants Winter Meeting. Kansas City, MO, December 5–7, 2019. Available at: http://www.avc-beef.org/proceedings/default.asp. Accessed February 1, 2020.
8. Swecker W, Kasimanickam R. Effects of nutrition on reproductive performance of beef cattle. In: Younquist RS, Threlfall WR, editors. Current therapy in large animal theriogenology. 2nd edition. St. Louis (MO): Saunders Elsevier; 2007. p. 450–6.
9. Hayes M. Getting started in cow-calf confinement production. In: Proceedings, Midwest Cow-Calf Symposium. Omaha, NE, March 21–22, 2017. pp. 9–10.
10. Jenkins K. Nutritional management of confined production cows. In: Proceedings, Midwest Cow-Calf Symposium. Omaha, NE, March 21–22, 2017. pp. 27–34.
11. Redden MD, Bayliff CL, Spencer CM, et al. Energy use and efficiency of cow/calf management in controlled environment cattle systems. In: Proceedings, Midwest Cow-Calf Symposium. Omaha, NE, March 21–22, 2017. pp. 9–10.
12. Woolums AR, Berghaus RD, Smith DR, et al. A survey of veterinarians in six states in the US regarding their experience with nursing beef calf respiratory disease. In: Proceedings, 46th Annual Conference American Association of Bovine Practitioners. Milwaukee, WI, September 19–21, 2013. pp. 177–178.
13. Taylor JD. Health Management of Neonatal Calves Born in Confinement Systems. In: Proceedings, Dr. Kenneth &Caroline McDonald Eng Foundation Symposium, Innovations in Intensive Beef Cow Production, Care and Management. Oklahoma City, OK, September 17–18, 2015. pp. 87–98.
14. Engelken T. A survey on the production practices of confined cow/calf operations. In: Proceedings, 2020 Driftless Region Beef Conference. Dubuque, IA, January 30–31, 2020.
15. Windeyer MC, Gamsjäger L. Vaccinating calves in the face of maternal antibodies: challenges and opportunities. Vet Clin North Am Food Anim Pract 2019;35:557–73.
16. Stokka GL. Prevention of respiratory disease in cow/calf operations. Vet Clin Food Anim 2010;26:229–41.
17. Smith DR. Field epidemiology to manage BRD risk in beef cattle production systems. Anim Health Res Rev 2014;15:180–3.

How Does Housing Influence Bovine Respiratory Disease in Dairy and Veal Calves?

Theresa L. Ollivett, DVM, PhD

KEYWORDS

• Dairy calf housing • Group calf pens • Individual calf pens • Hutches

KEY POINTS

- Current literature is mixed in regard to the effect of penning strategy on calf health, although it appears as though smaller groups may impact respiratory health to a lesser degree than large groups.
- The lack of consistent definitions for quantifying and analyzing the impact of housing factors on the occurrence of respiratory disease in young cattle hinders the ability to make strong, evidence-based decisions regarding the best method to house calves.
- When designing, performing, and reporting studies in the future, researchers should adhere to the REFLECT and STROBE guidelines to improve the quality of randomized clinical trials and observational studies.

INTRODUCTION

Bovine respiratory disease (BRD) is a leading cause of morbidity and mortality in young cattle.[1] In the United States, most young dairy calves are housed individually, and there is increasing interest in group housing because of perceived improvements in labor efficiency, socialization, and potential health improvements.[2,3]

Conventional wisdom indicates that ventilation and poor air circulation are the primary reasons for excessive levels of respiratory disease in young cattle.[4,5] Clinically, ventilation is often the first risk factor addressed when trouble-shooting herd problems and is a critical consideration when designing calf barns. Nordlund and Halbach[5] have previously described an ideal calf barn design that considers sizing, ventilation requirements, and layout for maximal efficiency. Therefore, the primary objective of this article is not to describe how to build a calf barn, but to review how certain aspects of housing, such as rearing location and penning strategies, can impact respiratory health in young, predominately dairy, cattle. A secondary objective is to identify knowledge gaps and provide suggestions for future research investigating the link between housing and respiratory disease in young cattle.

Department of Medical Sciences, University of Wisconsin–Madison School of Veterinary Medicine, Room 2004, 2015 Linden Drive, Madison, WI 53706, USA
E-mail address: theresa.ollivett@wisc.edu

Vet Clin Food Anim 36 (2020) 385–398
https://doi.org/10.1016/j.cvfa.2020.03.012
0749-0720/20/© 2020 Elsevier Inc. All rights reserved.
vetfood.theclinics.com

LITERATURE REVIEW

A search of literature written in English from the past 40 years (1980–2020) was performed using the following combination of key words in Google Scholar (n = 131) and PubMed (n = 83) and yielded a total of 214 peer-reviewed results: ["bovine respiratory disease" and "housing" and "dairy" or "calf" not "feedlot" not "stocker"]. After removing duplicates, review articles, and articles that did not include preweaned dairy calf or veal housing, 34 studies remained. An additional 9 studies were excluded because respiratory disease was not specifically reported as an outcome (n = 5), study design precluded separation of housing and nutritional influences on the occurrence of BRD (n = 2), study was based solely on expert opinion (n = 1), and lack of access to full text (n = 1). Twenty-five studies were therefore included in this review and consisted of randomized controlled trials[6–13] (RCT; n = 8), observational studies[14–29] (n = 16), and 1 quasi-randomized study (qRCT).[30] Sixteen different sets of criteria were used to define respiratory disease, and 2 studies did not include any definition of disease (**Table 1**).

A statistically significant association between at least 1 housing factor and respiratory disease, as defined within each study, was identified in all 16 observational studies and 4 of the 8 RCT.[9,11–13] The single qRCT study suggested a significant association existed; however, pertinent statistical analysis was not included within the article.[30]

For the purpose of this article, penning strategy refers to the number of calves housed together in a single pen. Studies that investigate the effect of penning strategy might compare individual housing to group housing or they might assess the effect of group size. Throughout this article, group size refers to the number of calves per pen, not the physical size of the pen. The RCT compared penning strategies (n = 5),[6–10] hutch design (n = 2),[11,12] and indoor versus outdoor housing (n = 1).[13] Penning strategies, design characteristics, ventilation, air quality, bedding, and proximity to older cattle were commonly assessed in the observational studies (**Table 2**). Study characteristics, outcome measures, and results for the 25 studies included in this review are outlined in **Tables 3–5**.

Rearing Location

Although most bovine practitioners would likely agree that raising calves indoors comes with more challenges for the respiratory system than raising calves outside, there is little supportive evidence in the literature from the past 40 years. Only 1 study assessing the effect of housing calves indoors versus outdoors met the inclusion criteria for this review.[13] In this RCT, 90 calves were randomized to be reared in one of 3 groups: indoor group pen (n = 30), outdoor group pen with jackets (n = 30), or an outdoor group pen without jackets (n = 30). Although the investigators conclude that "the incidence of respiratory disease was higher in calves reared indoors" (see **Table 5**), a closer look at their data shows that nearly all calves (n = 26, 27, and 29 calves in outdoor-jacketed, outdoor–not jacketed, and indoor groups, respectively) were treated at least once for respiratory disease. The data actually indicate that more indoor-raised calves were treated 2 or more times (n = 29) compared with outdoor-reared calves (n = 18 and 16, for outdoor-jacketed, and outdoor-not jacketed calves, respectively).

Pen Strategy

Penning strategy was one of the more common factors evaluated in the 25 studies included in this review (see **Tables 3** and **4**). Four of the 8 studies that specifically

Table 1
Criteria used to define respiratory disease in clinical trials (n = 9) and observational studies (n = 16) that investigated the relationship between housing factors and respiratory health in young, preweaned cattle

Criteria	Fever	Publications
California Respiratory Score, total score $\geq$5	—	22,24,25
Caregiver-administered antibiotic for respiratory disease; criteria not specified	—	15
Hampered respiration, cough, nasal discharge (analyzed each component)	—	16
Any combination of nasal/ocular discharge, cough, RR > 45 bpm, adventitious lung sounds, depression, fever	>39.0°C	14
Increased resting RR, sound or effort and fever plus cough, nasal discharge, depression, inappetence, rough hair coat	>39.5°C	21,28
Coughing or sneezing accompanied by heavy breathing or nasal discharge for at least 2 d	—	9,17,19,20
Farm owner perception of their herd-level prevalence of respiratory disease (above or below 10%)	—	38
A subjective score of 1–4 (1 = no sign of respiratory symptom, and 4 = a clear sign of respiratory symptom)	—	30
UW Calf Health Scoring Chart, analyzed components; body temperature taken only if $\geq$2 on any health score category	>39.4°C	
UW Calf Health Scoring Chart, analyzed components	—	11,12
UW Calf Health Scoring Chart, total score >4	—	26
UW Calf Health Scoring Chart, total score $\geq$6	—	18
Difficult breathing, nasal discharge, cough (calves assessed in pairs, 1 sign in 1 calf = positive pair)	—	7
Respiratory disease, nasal discharge, cough, and fever	$\geq$39.5°C	6
Clinical signs of respiratory disease (moderate to severe respiratory distress on auscultation)	>40.0°C	13
Ultrasonographic lung consolidation $\geq$3 cm	—	23
Not defined	—	8,10

Abbreviations: RR, respiratory rate; UW, University of Wisconsin.
Data from Refs.[6–26,28,30,38]

compared individual and group housing showed that grouping was associated with more respiratory disease. Specifically, group housing was associated with greater odds of having a higher within-herd prevalence of ultrasonographic lung consolidation,[23] producers reporting greater than 10% incidence,[29] producer-reported treatments for respiratory disease,[20] and higher mean calf-level prevalence of BRD as defined by a California respiratory score $\geq$5.[24] For one of these studies,[20] group size was specified as 6 to 30 calves in an auto-feeder facility.

One of the remaining 4 studies showed a tendency for treatment incidence to increase when calves were housed in groups of 2 or 3 calves, compared with individually housed calves.[6] In the 3 studies that did not detect a difference in respiratory disease, individual housing was compared with either pair housing[7] or small groups of 5 to 6 calves.[8,10] In the 3 studies that specifically compared different sizes of multicalf

Table 2
Overview of housing factors assessed through observational studies (n = 16) that investigated the relationship between management and respiratory health in young cattle

Publication	Pen Strategy	Barn, Pen, or Hutch Design	Ventilation Type	Air Quality (Ammonia, ABC, Dust, Humidity, Temperature)	Flooring	Proximity to Older Cattle	Bedding	Shade
Pardon et al,[14] 2020	x	x	x	x	x	x	—	—
Dubrovsky et al,[15] 2019	—	x	—	x	—	x	x	x
Maier et al,[22] 2019	x	x	—	x	x	—	—	x
Buczinski et al,[23] 2018	x	—	—	x	—	—	x	—
Karle et al,[24] 2019	x	x	—	x	—	—	—	x
Louie et al,[25] 2018	—	—	—	x	—	—	—	—
Medrano-Galarza et al,[26] 2018	—	x	x	x	—	x	x	—
Jorgensen et al,[27] 2017	x	x	x	—	—	—	x	—

Study								
Windeyer et al,[28] 2014	—	x	x	—	x	x	—	—
Klein-Jöbstl et al,[29] 2015	—	—	—	—	—	—	x	x
Brscic et al,[16] 2012	—	x	—	x	x	x	x	x
Gulliksen et al,[17] 2009	—	x	x	x	—	—	—	x
Lago et al,[18] 2006	—	x	—	—	x	x	x	—
Lundborg et al,[19] 2004	—	x	x	—	x	—	x	—
Svensson et al,[20] 2003	—	—	—	—	—	—	—	x
Virtala et al,[21] 1999	—	—	x	—	—	—	—	x

Abbreviation: ABC, airborne bacteria count.
Data from Refs.[14–29]

Table 3
Peer-reviewed randomized controlled trials that investigated the effect of penning strategy on respiratory health in preweaned cattle

Publication	Location	DQS[35]	SSC	Class	Calves (n per Group)	Outcome Measure	Treatment Groups	P Value; Odds Ratio (95% CI)
Cobb et al,[6] 2014[a]	USA	13	—	Dairy	30	Incidence of treatments	1, 2, or 3 calves per pen	10%, 23%, 34%; P = .08
Jensen and Larsen,[7] 2014[b]	Denmark	14	—	Dairy	22	% of pairs with respiratory score = 1	Individual × 3 contact levels; paired early; paired late	NSD
Babu et al,[8] 2009[c]	India	12	—	Cross	18	Incidence of producer treatments	Individual Group	22.2%, 16.7%; NSD
Svensson and Liberg,[9] 2005[d]	Sweden	16	c	Dairy	Small: 297 Large: 595	Odds of producer-recorded clinical respiratory tract disease	6–9 calves per pen 12–18 calves per pen	0.69 (0.58–0.82)
Hanekamp and Smits,[10] 1994[e]	Netherlands	10	—	Beef	200	Respiratory disorders as percentage of initial no. of calves per 3 mo	Individual 5 calves	38.5% vs 60%; NSD

The DQS[35] was used to assess overall quality of the study with higher scores (max = 20) indicating higher quality studies. Sample size calculations (SSC) were described in 1 of the 5 studies.

Abbreviation: NSD, no significant difference.
[a] 2.50 m²/calf.
[b] 2.25 m²/calf.
[c] 2.3 to 2.6 m²/calf.
[d] 1.6 to 1.69 m²/calf.
[e] 1.07 to 1.20 m²/calf.
Data from Refs.[6–10]

Table 4
Peer-reviewed observational studies that investigated respiratory health and risk factors specifically related to preweaned penning strategy

Publication	Location	Design	SSC	Herds	Calves	Outcome Measure	Risk Factor	Comparison Group	P Value; Odds Ratio (95% CI)
Pardon et al,[14] 2020	Belgium	CS	+	128	—	Odds of detecting *M haemolytica* in a pooled non-endoscopic bronchoalveolar lavage fluid (nBALF) sample from 5 acutely ill calves per herd	5–10 calves per pen	<5 calves per pen	8.0 (1.4–46.9)
Buczinski et al,[23] 2018	Quebec	CS	+	39	608	Odds of having a higher within-herd prevalence of consolidated calves (≥3 cm)	Group housing	Individual housing	2.37 (1.06–5.29)
Karle et al,[24] 2019	USA	CS (calf)	+	100	4636	Mean BRD prevalence (%)	≥8 calves per pen Group pens Mixed material hutches Unpaved road	Individual housing hutches Single material hutches Paved road	P<.05 P<.05 P<.05 P<.05
Jorgensen et al,[27] 2017	USA	LCS	−	38	10,179	Odds of higher ear score Odds of higher eye score Odds of higher nasal score Odds of having a fever (T > 39.4°C)	Space per calf (m²/calf) Space per calf (m²/calf) Calves per pen No Positive Pressure Ventilation	— — — Positive Pressure Ventilation	0.90 (0.83–0.97) 0.92 (0.87–0.98) 1.01 (1–1.02); P = .04 1.81 (1.08–3.03)

(continued on next page)

Table 4
(continued)

Publication	Location	Design	SSC	Herds	Calves	Outcome Measure	Risk Factor	Comparison Group	P Value; Odds Ratio (95% CI)
Klein-Jöbstl et al,[29] 2015	Austria	Survey	—	1287	—	Odds of reporting respiratory tract disease incidence >10%	Individual and/or group	Individual only	1.97 (1.14–3.42)
Brscic et al,[16] 2012[a]	Europe	CS	—	174	—	Odds of having a higher prevalence of hampered respiration	>15 calves per pen	≤6 calves per pen	3.75 (1.48–9.52)
							No baby-box	Baby-box on arrival	1.94 (1.43–2.64)
						Odds of having a higher prevalence of nasal discharge	Space > 1.8 m²/calf	Space ≤1.8 m²/calf	1.87 (1.36–2.56)
						Odds of having a higher prevalence of cough	No baby-box	Baby-box	3.95 (1.18–13.20)
Gulliksen et al,[17] 2009	Norway	LCS	—	125	5101	Risk of producer treatment of respiratory disease	>8-wk age range in pen	≤8 wk	3.9 (1.8–8.2)[b]
							Near adults week 1	Separated from adults	16.7 (3.0–92.8)[b]
Lundborg et al,[19] 2004	Sweden	LCS	—	122	3081	Odds of producer treatment of respiratory disease (herd level)	Ammonia <6 ppm	Ammonia ≤6 ppm	2.39 (1.16–4.93)
Svensson et al,[20] 2003	Sweden	LCS (calf)	—	122	3038	Odds of producer treatment of respiratory disease (calf level)	6–30 calves per pen (autofeeder system)	Individual housing	2.2 (1.2–3.8)

Studies were performed using dairy breed calves and analyzed at the herd-level except where indicated by (calf) in the study design column. Study designs included cross-sectional (CS, n = 4), longitudinal cross-sectional (LCS, n = 4), and 1 online survey. SSC were described in 3 of the 9 studies (+).
[a] Veal.
[b] Hazard ratio (95% CI).
Data from Refs. [14,16,17,19,20,23,24,27,29]

Table 5
Peer-reviewed randomized clinical trials and observational studies that investigated the relationship between miscellaneous housing factors and respiratory health in young cattle

Publication	Location	Design	DQS[35]	SSC	Calves	Outcome Measures	Comparison	P Value; Odds Ratio (95% CI)
Calvo-Lorenzo et al,[11] 2016[a]	USA	RCT	14	—	20 per group	% observations with abnormal eye scores % observations with abnormal nasal scores	Increasing hutch space 1-3×	P = .05 P = .25
Peña et al,[12] 2016	USA	RCT	14	—	48 per group	Odds of abnormal eye scores Odds of abnormal ear scores Odds of abnormal nasal scores Odds of coughing Average rectal temperature	Plastic hutch in direct sun vs wire hutch with plywood shade	0.38 (0.16–0.92) 2.28 (0.92–5.66) 2.87 (1.24–6.66) 2.83 (1.12–7.18) 40.1 ± 0.28; 39.1 ± 0.22°C, P<.05
Earley et al,[13] 2004	Ireland	RCT	13	—	30 per group	Count of calves with ≥2 treatments	Indoor vs outdoor housing	P<.01
Maier et al,[22] 2019	USA	CS	NA	+	4636	Odds of positive CA respiratory score	Metal hutches vs wood only	11.19 (2.80–44.78)
Dubrovsky et al,[15] 2019	USA	C	NA	+	11,470	Hazard of caregiver treatment	Mixed material hutches vs wood only Never dust vs regularly dusty	1.24 (1.08–1.43)[b] 0.58 (0.39–0.85)[b]
Louie et al,[25] 2018	USA	C	NA	+	252	Odds; hazard of positive CA respiratory score	Max daily temperature (outside hutch) Max daily temperature (in hutch)	1.12 (1.03–1.22); 1.13 (1.05–1.21)[b] 1.20 (1.020–1.043);

(continued on next page)

Table 5
(continued)

Publication	Location	Design	DQS[35]	SSC	Calves	Outcome Measures	Comparison	P Value; Odds Ratio (95% CI)
Medrano-Galarza et al,[26] 2018	CA	LCS	NA	+	1488	Odds of greater prevalence of UW Calf Health Score >4 (within pen)	Max daily temperature humidity index (in hutch) Shared air: <4 mo vs >8 mo old More bedded space per calf (m²/calf)	1.12 (1.05–1.2)[b]; 1.07 (1.003–1.141)[b] 0.41 (0.19–1.01); $P = .05$ $P = .03$
Windeyer et al,[28] 2014	CA	C	NA	+	2874	Odds of producer treatment	Manual control of barn temperature vs automatic control	2.5% (SEM = 0.02) vs 39.3% (SEM = 0.26) $P = .05$
Lago et al,[18] 2006	USA	CS	NA	−	13 herds	Herd level prevalence, UW Calf Health Score ≥ 6	Mean pen airborne bacteria count Solid pen dividers lower prevalence Nesting score 3 lower prevalence	$P = .0027$ $P = .0016$ $P = .0031$
Virtala et al,[21] 1999	USA	C	NA	−	410	Odds of caregiver diagnosis Odds of veterinarian diagnosis	Caregiver: hutch housing veterinarian: housing near adults	0.4 (0.2–0.9) 1.9 (1.0–3.5)
Hillman et al,[30] 1992	USA	qRCT	NA	−	86	Average subjective score	Filtered air ventilation system	No statistical tests performed

The DQS[35] was used to assess overall quality of the RCT with higher scores (max 20) indicating higher quality studies. Study designs included RCT, cohort (C), CS, LCS, and 1 qRCT. SSC were described in 3 of the 11 studies (+).

Abbreviations: NA, not applicable; SEM, standard error of the mean.

[a] Conventional hutch: 1.23 m²/calf; Conv × 1.5: 1.85 m²/calf; Conv × 3: 3.71 m²/calf.
[b] Hazard ratio.

Data from Refs.[11–13,15,18,21,22,25,26,28,30]

groups, groups of 6 to 9 calves were associated with fewer producer-recorded cases of respiratory disease compared with groups of 12 to 18 calves,[9] groups of 5 to 10 calves were more likely to test positive for *Mannheimia haemolytica* compared with groups of less than 5 calves,[14] and groups of greater than 15 calves were more likely to have hampered respirations compared with groups of ≤ 6 calves.[16]

Surprisingly, there was not a clear benefit of increasing space per calf (m^2/calf) in the studies reviewed for this article. More space per calf was associated with better ear and eye scores[27] but a higher prevalence of nasal discharge[16] in studies of group-housed calves. Increasing space per calf was associated with a higher frequency of ocular discharge in calves housed individually in California-style wooden hutches.[11]

DISCUSSION

Although this review of the literature consisted of only 25 studies, it was extraordinarily difficult to report study results or compare the results from 1 study to another with any degree of confidence given the wide variety of disease definitions, analytical methods, and quality of reporting. For these reasons, study details have been provided to assist the reader in making their own assessment for each study (see **Tables 1–5**).

Disease Definitions and Outcomes Reported

Sixteen different sets of criteria were used to characterize respiratory disease, and outcomes were reported at the herd level, pen level, calf level, and individual clinical sign level. Previously published scoring systems were used in 8 of the studies (California, n = 3; Wisconsin, n = 5). All 3 studies using the CA score used the same cut-point to define positive (total score ≥ 5) and negative (total score <5) at the calf level.[22,24,25] For the 5 studies that used the WI score, cut-points of greater than 4[26] and ≥ 6[18] were used to designate positive and negative calves, whereas 3 studies[11,12,27] individually analyzed each component of the respiratory score instead of a totaled score. In the 9 studies that used a combination of clinical signs to define sick calves, four did not include fever in their definition. For the 5 studies that did include fever, 4 different temperature cut-points were used. Only 1 study used calf lung ultrasound to define BRD-affected calves.[23] Producer records were also used in a handful of these studies to classify BRD-positive and -negative calves. Both producer records and clinical scoring systems are known for their poor sensitivity for accurately identifying calves with respiratory disease. Classifying disease at the calf level by directly assessing lung health with ultrasound, instead of measuring individual abnormal clinical signs, will improve the quality of future studies.[31–34]

Quality of Reporting

Detsky quality scores (DQS)[35] were reported for the RCT reviewed in this article. For most of the RCT, the DQS were classified in the 10 to 14 range, which is well below the maximum score of 20. The low scores were driven by lack of blinding, lack of proper description of the randomization process, and failure to provide sample size or power calculations.

Sample size calculations were reported in only 9 of the 25 studies. More specifically, this calculation was reported by only 1 of the 8 RCT and 8 of the 16 observational studies. Sample size calculations should be driven by the primary outcome of interest for the study.[36] Failure to describe the calculation, which is inferred as a failure to calculate a sample size, or calculating it for the wrong outcome, can leave a study too underpowered to detect a difference between groups. This transparency becomes particularly important for studies that do not demonstrate a significant difference between groups.[7,8,10] Underpowered studies may fail to demonstrate important differences that actually exist. Underpowered studies may also lower the probability that an observed effect actually reflects a true effect.[37] Readers should be aware that the appearance of equal risk for disease in pair housed versus individually housed calves[7] does not guarantee that pair housing will not negatively impact calf health.

SUMMARY

Currently there is not enough evidence-based information available to confidently guide decision making when it comes to the best method to house calves to ensure exceptional respiratory health. The quality of information gained from future studies will benefit significantly by using highly sensitive tools, such as lung ultrasound, and appropriately designing studies to capture information about incident cases of disease. Besides implementing calf lung ultrasound, adhering to either the REFLECT guidelines for RCTs or the STROBE guidelines for reporting observational studies during the planning and design phase of a project will help to improve the quality of the data available. Sample size calculations are critical and must be considered with respect to the primary outcome of interest. We should refrain from investigating relationships that based on our sample size, and our study is too limited to have the power to limit type II error. When we declare something noninferior, we need to include confidence limits around our estimates so that the reader than can assess for themselves whether the study is underpowered.

DISCLOSURE

The authors have nothing to disclose.

REFERENCES

1. USDA. Dairy 2014. Fort Collins, CO: Natl Anim Heal Monit Syst; 2018.
2. Shivley CB, Lombard JE, Urie NJ, et al. Preweaned heifer management on US dairy operations: Part II. Factors associated with colostrum quality and passive transfer status of dairy heifer calves. J Dairy Sci 2018;101(10):9185–98.
3. Costa JHC, Von Keyserlingk MAG, Weary DM. Invited review: effects of group housing of dairy calves on behavior, cognition, performance, and health. J Dairy Sci 2016;99(4):2453–67.
4. Van Der Fels-Klerx HJ, Horst HS, Dijkhuizen AA. Risk factors for bovine respiratory disease in dairy youngstock in The Netherlands: the perception of experts. Livest Prod Sci 2000;66(1):35–46.
5. Nordlund KV, Halbach CE. Calf barn design to optimize health and ease of management. Vet Clin North Am Food Anim Pract 2019;35(1):29–45.
6. Cobb CJ, Obeidat BS, Sellers MD, et al. Group housing of Holstein calves in a poor indoor environment increases respiratory disease but does not influence performance or leukocyte responses. J Dairy Sci 2014;97(5):3099–109.
7. Jensen MB, Larsen LE. Effects of level of social contact on dairy calf behavior and health. J Dairy Sci 2014;97(8):5035–44.
8. Babu LK, Pandey H, Patra RC, et al. Hemato-biochemical changes, disease incidence and live weight gain in individual versus group reared calves fed on different levels of milk and skim milk. Anim Sci J 2009;80(2):149–56.
9. Svensson C, Liberg P. The effect of group size on health and growth rate of Swedish dairy calves housed in pens with automatic milk-feeders. Prev Vet Med 2006; 73(1):43–53.

10. Hanekamp WJA, Smits AC. Open versus closed barn and individual versus group-housing for bull calves destined beef production. Livestock Production Science 1994;37:261–70.

11. Calvo-Lorenzo MS, Hulbert LE, Fowler AL, et al. Wooden hutch space allowance influences male Holstein calf health, performance, daily lying time, and respiratory immunity. J Dairy Sci 2016;99(6):4678–92.

12. Peña G, Risco C, Kunihiro E, et al. Effect of housing type on health and performance of preweaned dairy calves during summer in Florida1. J Dairy Sci 2016; 99(2):1655–62.

13. Earley B, Murray M, Farrell JA, et al. Rearing calves outdoors with and without calf jackets compared with indoor housing on calf health and live-weight performance. Irish J Agric Food Res 2004;43(1):59–67.

14. Pardon B, Callens J, Maris J, et al. Pathogen-specific risk factors in acute outbreaks of respiratory disease in calves. J Dairy Sci 2020;103(3):2556–66.

15. Dubrovsky SA, Van Eenennaam AL, Karle BM, et al. Epidemiology of bovine respiratory disease (BRD) in preweaned calves on California dairies: the BRD 10K study. J Dairy Sci 2019;102(8):7306–19.

16. Brscic M, Leruste H, Heutinck LFM, et al. Prevalence of respiratory disorders in veal calves and potential risk factors. J Dairy Sci 2012;95(5):2753–64.

17. Gulliksen SM, Jor E, Lie KI, et al. Respiratory infections in Norwegian dairy calves. J Dairy Sci 2009;92(10):5139–46.

18. Lago A, McGuirk SM, Bennett TB, et al. Calf respiratory disease and pen microenvironments in naturally ventilated calf barns in winter. J Dairy Sci 2006;89(10): 4014–25.

19. Lundborg GK, Svensson EC, Oltenacu PA. Herd-level risk factors for infectious diseases in Swedish dairy calves aged 0-90 days. Prev Vet Med 2005. https:// doi.org/10.1016/j.prevetmed.2004.11.014.

20. Svensson C, Lundborg K, Emanuelson U, et al. Morbidity in Swedish dairy calves from birth to 90 days of age and individual calf-level risk factors for infectious diseases. Prev Vet Med 2003;58(3–4):179–97.

21. Virtala AMK, Gröhn YT, Mechor GD, et al. The effect of maternally derived immunoglobulin G on the risk of respiratory disease in heifers during the first 3 months of life. Prev Vet Med 1999;39(1):25–37.

22. Maier GU, Love WJ, Karle BM, et al. Management factors associated with bovine respiratory disease in preweaned calves on California dairies: the BRD 100 study. J Dairy Sci 2019;102(8):7288–305.

23. Buczinski S, Borris ME, Dubuc J. Herd-level prevalence of the ultrasonographic lung lesions associated with bovine respiratory disease and related environmental risk factors. J Dairy Sci 2018;101(3):2423–32.

24. Karle BM, Maier GU, Love WJ, et al. Regional management practices and prevalence of bovine respiratory disease in California's preweaned dairy calves. J Dairy Sci 2019;102(8):7583–96.

25. Louie AP, Rowe JD, Love WJ, et al. Effect of the environment on the risk of respiratory disease in preweaning dairy calves during summer months. J Dairy Sci 2018;101(11):10230–47.

26. Medrano-Galarza C, LeBlanc SJ, Jones-Bitton A, et al. Associations between management practices and within-pen prevalence of calf diarrhea and respiratory disease on dairy farms using automated milk feeders. J Dairy Sci 2018; 101(3):2293–308.

27. Jorgensen MW, De Passille AM, Rushen J, et al. Factors associated with dairy calf health in automated feeding systems in the upper Midwest United States. J Dairy Sci 2017;5675–86. https://doi.org/10.3168/jds.2016-12501.

28. Windeyer MC, Leslie KE, Godden SM, et al. Factors associated with morbidity, mortality, and growth of dairy heifer calves up to 3 months of age. Prev Vet Med 2014. https://doi.org/10.1016/j.prevetmed.2013.10.019.

29. Klein-Jöbstl D, Arnholdt T, Sturmlechner F, et al. Results of an online questionnaire to survey calf management practices on dairy cattle breeding farms in Austria and to estimate differences in disease incidences depending on farm structure and management practices. Acta Vet Scand 2015;57(1):1–10.

30. Hillman P, Gebremedhin K, Warner R. Ventilation system to minimize airborne bacteria, dust, humidity, and ammonia in calf nurseries. J Dairy Sci 1992;75: 1305–12.

31. Ollivett TL, Caswell JL, Nydam DV, et al. Thoracic ultrasonography and bronchoalveolar lavage fluid analysis in holstein calves with subclinical lung lesions. J Vet Intern Med 2015;29(6):1728–34.

32. Dunn TR, Ollivett TL, Renaud DL, et al. The effect of lung consolidation, as determined by ultrasonography, on first-lactation milk production in Holstein dairy calves. J Dairy Sci 2018;101(6):5404–10.

33. Cramer MC, Ollivett TL. Growth of preweaned, group-housed dairy calves diagnosed with respiratory disease using clinical respiratory scoring and thoracic ultrasound—a cohort study. J Dairy Sci 2019;102(5):4322–31.

34. Ollivett TL, Leslie KE, Duffield TF, et al. Field trial to evaluate the effect of an intranasal respiratory vaccine protocol on calf health, ultrasonographic lung consolidation, and growth in Holstein dairy calves. J Dairy Sci 2018;101(9):8159–68.

35. Detsky AS, Naylor CD, O'Rourke K, et al. Incorporating variations in the quality of individual randomized trials into metaanalysis. J Clin Epidemiol 1992;45:255–65.

36. Sargeant JM, Kelton DF, O'Connor AM. Randomized controlled trials and challenge trials: design and criterion for validity. Zoonoses Public Health 2014; 61(Suppl 1):18–27.

37. Button KS, Ioannidis JPA, Mokrysz C, et al. Power failure: why small sample size undermines the reliability of neuroscience. Nat Rev Neurosci 2013;14(5):365–76.

38. Klein-Jöbstl D, Iwersen M, Drillich M. Farm characteristics and calf management practices on dairy farms with and without diarrhea: a case-control study to investigate risk factors for calf diarrhea. J Dairy Sci 2014;97(8):5110–9.

Bovine Respiratory Disease Diagnosis

What Progress Has Been Made in Clinical Diagnosis?

Sébastien Buczinski, Dr Vét, MSc[a],*, Bart Pardon, DVM, PhD[b]

KEYWORDS

- Bronchopneumonia • Diagnosis • Gold standard • Accuracy

KEY POINTS

- Using the definition bovine respiratory disease complex may be a limitation for the progress of knowledge on infectious bronchopneumonia.
- The absence of an affordable gold standard for the definition of bovine infectious bronchopneumonia needs to be accounted for.
- Clinical and paraclinical diagnostic tests used in practice should be thoroughly validated in terms of repeatability/agreement as well as for their accuracy.

INTRODUCTION

Accurate diagnosis of bovine respiratory disease (BRD) is an ongoing challenge that impairs the ability to optimally treat and prevent BRD. This article focuses on the clinical diagnosis of infectious bronchopneumonia. The limitations of different diagnostic procedures are highlighted to indicate current strengths, potential pitfalls, and knowledge gaps. A companion article in this issue addresses causal diagnosis of infectious bronchopneumonia.[1]

IS BOVINE RESPIRATORY DISEASE TERMINOLOGY AN OBSTACLE FOR PROGRESS TOWARD A BETTER CASE DEFINITION?

The terminology BRD, and bovine respiratory disease complex, was initiated more than 5 decades ago[2] and mainly attempted to summarize the complexity of the

---

[a] Département des Sciences Cliniques, Faculté de Médecine Vétérinaire, Université de Montréal, 3200 Rue Sicotte, St-Hyacinthe, Québec J2S 2M2, Canada; [b] Department of Large Animal Internal Medicine, Faculty of Veterinary Medicine, Ghent University, Salisburylaan 133, Merelbeke 9820, Belgium
* Corresponding author.
E-mail address: s.buczinski@umontreal.ca

Vet Clin Food Anim 36 (2020) 399–423
https://doi.org/10.1016/j.cvfa.2020.03.004
0749-0720/20/© 2020 Elsevier Inc. All rights reserved.
vetfood.theclinics.com

interaction of respiratory tract infections with environmental and host-related risk factors in cattle. In those days, this definition meant progress in comprehension of respiratory diseases of cattle, but the individual case definition to initiate therapy has always remained poorly defined. Different scoring systems have been used in studies worldwide, which often did not distinguish between upper and lower respiratory tract disease, or between viral and bacterial infections, or, more clearly stated, between infections requiring antimicrobial treatment or not. Taking into account the worldwide pressure to reduce and rationalize antimicrobial use, the general or syndromic BRD concept may no longer cover the practical and scientific needs. It is surprising that only in food animal species such broad definitions of respiratory tract diseases, summarizing both infectious and noninfectious diseases into a single entity, are in use. In humans and companion animal species (small animals and horses), no such terminology is applied, for the obvious reason that respiratory tract infections are more clearly distinguished from dysregulated airway inflammation processes resulting in asthma or chronic obstructive pulmonary disease in these species. With the current pressure on antimicrobial use, food animal veterinarians must admit that they often treat a simple runny nose or noninfectious pneumonia as requiring antimicrobial therapy as much as life-threatening bacterial pneumonia, and recognize that they can no longer count on support for these practices.

In humans and companion animals, strictly viral pneumonias (eg, respiratory syncytial virus in humans or equine influenza virus) are diagnosed and primarily not treated with antimicrobials. Antimicrobials are used only if levels of a biomarker, such as C-reactive protein (commonly used in humans) are increased, indicating that bacterial superinfection is likely. In contrast, in food animals, clinicians often behave as if bacterial infection always follows viral pneumonia, indicating the need for antimicrobials in every case. On the one hand, this thinking has some merit. Ruminants are frequently exposed to adverse climatic conditions and accumulation of air pollutants that can breach innate immunity and aggravate the consequences of infection.[3] On the other hand, risk averseness in food animal species for economic and ethical reasons, together with pressure from the owners, might tempt clinicians to prioritize security more than risk and initiate antimicrobial therapy. The fact remains that the use of a single vague terminology to summarize the complexity of respiratory disease is oversimplified and dangerous, especially if the definition is linked to the initiation of antimicrobial use, which is currently still the main reason for any BRD case definition. This situation places us 180° in opposition between the current practices of bovine veterinarians and their clients, and societal demands, further challenging a market already under pressure for climate and animal welfare reasons. As recently shown in a review of antimicrobial trials for BRD using negative controls, there is a wide variation of relapse rates in nontreated cases, questioning the necessity of systematic use of antimicrobials and/or indicating case definition limitations.[4] It is stimulating to observe that practitioners are experimenting with strictly antiinflammatory options in early suspected pneumonia cases.[5] Especially in dairy cattle, this approach could also avoid unnecessary milk loss, although efficacy of such treatment must be confirmed to prevent negative welfare impacts of untreated pneumonia.

The evidence that the currently preferred metaphylactic antimicrobial therapeutic approaches in BRD are most efficient in terms of economics, animal welfare, and limiting antimicrobial resistance selection is, according to a recent meta-analysis, very weak.[6] The effects of metaphylaxis in reducing morbidity and mortality are not questioned, but the expense at which they are efficient is likely too great. For example, at an attack rate of 10%, the number needed to treat (an index allowing quantification of the treatment effect as the inverse of the absolute risk reduction) was 20, signifying that medicating 20 animals with antimicrobials was necessary to prevent/treat 1 new case of disease. This number becomes 7 from an attack rate of 20% onwards. Clearly, for human infants, these numbers to save individuals at the expense of the group would be generally accepted. In contrast, for calves or cattle, given the currently incompletely clarified but likely risk to human health, no such treatment to save a limited number of animals is likely to be supported by the general public. Although it is acknowledged that animal welfare and economics must be considered, these are the issues future bovine practitioners face, implying the need for a robust definition of antimicrobial treatment indication.

TOWARD NEW DEFINITIONS: DOES THE TERM BOVINE RESPIRATORY DISEASE STILL REFLECT THE NEEDS OF PRACTICE AND RESEARCH?

What definitions and terminology would better fit the current societal and scientific needs with regard to BRD? Some options are available from human and small animal medicine. One option is to distinguish upper respiratory tract infection (URTI) and lower respiratory tract infection (LRTI). This designation coincides with anatomic localization, differentiating rhinitis and pharyngitis from bronchitis and pneumonia. The advantage of this distinction is that it could provide clearer guidance regarding the need for antimicrobial treatment if it could be confirmed that URTIs generally do not require antimicrobials, whereas LRTIs often do. However, clinicians need tools to differentiate URTI from LRTI. This differentiation can partially be fulfilled by thoracic ultrasonography, as elaborated later, but the question of whether the infection is viral or bacterial remains. A critical issue is the turnaround time between sampling and availability of results. Understandably, practitioners and animal owners are not willing to postpone any treatment too long. Substantial progress has been made in the area of rapid diagnostics, described elsewhere in this issue.[1] However, any rapid test must be able to distinguish between bacterial contamination, colonization, and infection of the lower respiratory tract; these might be distinguished by concurrent identification of relevant bacteria and evidence of inflammation. Bovine medicine is currently constrained by these limits, and clinicians urgently need an exploration of better diagnostic tools for both causal identification and markers of inflammation to direct antimicrobial decision making. The strongest counterargument for the general use of this terminology is that URTI or LRTI does not inform clinicians of the clinical status of the animal, which is a prerequisite to initiating therapy. The clinical status, and whether the status results in economic losses or compromised animal welfare, needs to be taken into account when considering treatment.

In addition, airway inflammation with noninfectious causes has become a leading subject in human and horse respiratory health.[7] Many air pollutants, such as particulate matter, endotoxins, and ammonia, induce airway inflammation and hamper innate respiratory defense.[7] This process is characterized by influx of inflammatory cells; mucus accumulation; bronchoconstriction; and, chronically, airway remodeling.[7] This noninfectious inflammation facilitates secondary infection by opportunistic flora.[7] The relevance of such processes for the bovine lung has barely been explored. Altogether, definition of respiratory tract infection, respiratory tract disease, and in particular identifying animals requiring antimicrobial therapy is a major challenge currently seriously hampered by a lack of knowledge in the bovine species. Bovine infectious bronchopneumonia is nowadays the major reason for using antimicrobials in respiratory disease conditions.

CHALLENGES FOR THE DETERMINATION OF THE ACCURACY OF A NEW TEST

At present, the available information on diagnosis of respiratory tract infection mainly targets feedlot, dairy, and veal calves. The production context is important because the individual animal value may limit the cost of diagnostic test technology that can be used. In feedlot calves, an economic study on the impact of diagnostic test strategies for BRD has shown that the specificity of the diagnostic method was the most important driver in terms of costs.[8] The specificity is also important for avoiding unnecessary antimicrobial treatment. From a welfare perspective, sensitivity is important because delay in detection can be associated with animal suffering and increased risks of treatment failure. Recently, a review of the diagnostic tests used in feedlot diagnosis of BRD complex was also performed summarizing the key findings of practical diagnostic tests that can be used calf-side.[9]

Because of the complexity of infectious respiratory disease in cattle, a perfectly accurate and practical definition will never exist. The challenge for the determination of an accurate new diagnostic test (index test) must be fully understood in the light of this premise. Studies of diagnostic test accuracy have specific risks of bias that may falsely overestimate diagnostic test accuracy. The choice of the reference standard test to compare the index test results is also critically important because it will ultimately serve as a comparator to determine the index test sensitivity (ability of the new test to find affected animals) and specificity (ability of the new test to find nonaffected animals).

RISKS OF BIAS AND APPLICABILITY IN STUDIES OF DIAGNOSTIC TEST ACCURACY

Diagnostic test accuracy studies are particularly challenging because of their bivariate nature. Such studies include a mix between 2 different populations (affected vs nonaffected), in which test accuracy parameters (sensitivity and specificity) are derived. One of the most important risks of bias in diagnostic test accuracy study is the so-called 2-gate versus 1-gate design.[10] The difference between these types of design has been described for studies of thoracic ultrasonography for the diagnosis of respiratory disease in cattle.[11] Briefly, the 2-gate design is present when the inclusion criteria to define affected versus nonaffected animals are different (**Fig. 1**); in the 1-gate design, animals are identified by 1 mutually exclusive criterion. The 2-gate situation presents increased risk of overestimating test accuracy because the difference between affected and nonaffected cases is overestimated because of the study design. This study design is generally affected by the so-called spectrum bias, which means that the definition of affected animals tends to select more severely affected cases, for which the index test has higher chances of good performance (inflated test sensitivity). Because animals with unclear status tend to be rejected in selection of nonaffected cases, the specificity of the index test in this setting is also inflated. Other risks of bias that need to be known have been described extensively elsewhere[11,12] and are summarized in **Table 1**.

THE CHALLENGE OF THE ABSENCE OF AN AFFORDABLE AND PRACTICAL GOLD STANDARD

Classification bias is a common concern when assessing a new test for bovine infectious bronchopneumonia. If the reference standard test is not 100% accurate, there is a risk of underestimating index test accuracy if not accounting for this imperfect comparator. Necropsy could be considered a reasonable gold standard; however, using only this standard would make research on diagnostic test accuracy difficult,

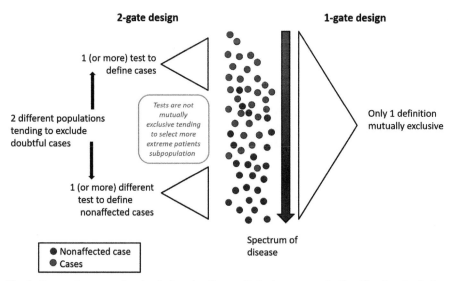

2-gate design

1 (or more) test to define cases

2 different populations tending to exclude doubtful cases

Tests are not mutually exclusive tending to select more extreme patients subpopulation

1 (or more) different test to define nonaffected cases

● Nonaffected case
● Cases

1-gate design

Only 1 definition mutually exclusive

Spectrum of disease

Fig. 1. Two-gate versus 1-gate designs in diagnostic test accuracy studies. The 2-gate design is similar to a case/control design. The case definitions of cases/noncases are not mutually exclusive, generally resulting in the exclusion of the doubtful animals and often resulting in overestimation of test accuracy because sensitivity and specificity are evaluated in artificially distinct populations. In the 1-gate design, there is only 1 mutually exclusive case/non-case definition, thus including doubtful cases. The accuracy obtained from these studies is generally closer to the expected accuracy that practitioners should expect in a practical setting.

because of the invasiveness of the gold standard and associated costs. Also, the necropsy needs to be performed as quickly as possible after use of the diagnostic test being investigated. This requirement highlights a weakness of the use of abattoir lung findings assessed long after testing, because lesions may have occurred or resolved since testing.

Experimental models of infection are an interestingly used alternative to obtain a gold-standard status for infected versus noninfected cattle, but they are generally limited to specific viral and bacterial challenge combinations. These challenges may not mirror naturally occurring infectious bronchopneumonia because they do not incorporate different stressors associated with natural disease. For this reason, the external validity of experimental models is limited.

In most natural infectious respiratory disease studies, imperfect case definition is the default for comparing a new diagnostic test. Using a composite reference standard test is an alternative. This approach uses a combination of different tests to define a positive or negative case.[13] Various case definitions can be developed using the "or" (at least 1 positive test to define an affected patient), "and" (all positive tests to define a patient), and "K" rules (at least K positive of tests out of a specific number of tests performed). However, concerns have been raised against this practice because (1) the risk of error increases if the index test (new test to assess) and tests included in case definition are correlated (ie, making the same types of errors), and (2) the accuracy of this case definition may vary depending on the true prevalence of the disease.[13]

The absence of a gold-standard diagnostic test is a problem in almost every medical field.[14] Recently, bayesian latent class methods have been applied for the

Table 1
Risk of bias and applicability concerns potentially affecting diagnostic test accuracy studies on bovine infectious bronchopneumonia

Risk of Bias	Explanation	Potential Impact
Spectrum bias	There are concerns that selection of affected animals or nonaffected animals is not representative of the full spectrum of the disease Eg, selecting affected animals if depressed increased respiratory score and abnormal auscultation vs nonaffected (not depressed, normal respiratory score and normal auscultation); this design would exclude animals with 1 or 2 abnormal inclusion criteria, therefore artificially inflating the difference between affected and nonaffected animals	Overestimation of test accuracy (eg, cases where the diagnosis is more difficult are excluded from this type of study)
Classification bias	The reference standard that serves as comparator for establishing index test accuracy is not 100% accurate Eg, determining thoracic ultrasonography accuracy in calves using an increased clinical score without accounting for imperfect accuracy of clinical score	Potential underestimation of index test accuracy because the reference standard is treated as a gold standard test
Diagnostic review and incorporation bias	Situations where the index test and reference standard test are not independent Eg, performing the reference standard test knowing the index test result. Eg, determination of ultrasonography accuracy for lung lesions detection (index test) using CT as a reference standard and concomitant knowledge of ultrasonography findings	In this case, the apparent accuracy of the index test could be affected in the way the radiologist would interpret the CT knowing the results of thoracic ultrasonography (potentially overinterpreting CT lesions in ultrasonography-positive animals, and underdetection of lesions in ultrasonography-negative animals)
Clinical review bias	This type of bias occurs when clinical information for the animals receiving the tests, as it would be in practice, is missing Eg, in a study assessing clinical signs associated with LRTI, not specifying, for example, the age and type of production (dairy, beef, veal) and minimal management practices could affect the accuracy of the test when further applied in practice	In this case, the interpretation of test results need a specific context. Eg, gut filling of the calves would not have the same meaning in a farm feeding dairy calves 2 L of milk per meal twice daily vs a farm feeding calves 3–4 L 3 times daily

Partial verification bias	The index test result has an impact on the probability of performing the reference standard test Eg, bias that can be found in a retrospective study where a test was more prescribed than another depending on a first test result. Eg, a study where thoracic radiographs were more commonly performed in animals where abnormal findings were suspected based on auscultation or ultrasonography	In this case, because most animals with normal index test results are not investigated further, the absence of reference standard test in that population could include bias in the apparent index test accuracy
Differential verification bias	This type of bias occurs when different reference standard tests are applied to the animals Eg, necropsy would be considered as a reference standard test for animals that have severe clinical signs of respiratory tract infection, but animals with no severe clinical signs are only followed with a clinical follow-up as a reference standard test	The accuracy of the 2 reference standard tests may differ and should be accounted for in the analyses of index test accuracy
Inconclusive results/ withdrawal bias	Some animals are withdrawn from the study because of either impossibility to perform or interpret the index test or the reference standard test Eg, animals that were not tractable enough to perform the index test safely (eg, BAL was excluded or some BAL samples were excluded from the analyses because of blood contamination)	This type of bias tends to inflate the apparent test accuracy, discarding animals or results where the index test could not be performed or interpreted

Abbreviations: BAL, bronchoalveolar lavage; CT, computed tomography.

determination of diagnostic test accuracy in bovine respiratory tract infection.[15–18] These flexible methods account for possible misclassification because of reference standard test imperfection and have been shown to give unbiased estimates of test accuracy. As with any bayesian methods, they are flexible and can account for prior information if reasonable knowledge is available. Specific guidelines for reporting these studies are also available.[19] Using these methods may be helpful for any study using an imperfect diagnostic test.[20] One of the criticisms of these techniques is that an objective definition of the latent status clinical meaning may be lacking, in the sense that they capture by essence some shared test characteristics on that specific disease (**Fig. 2**).

VALIDATION OF THE DIAGNOSTIC TEST, AND DISTINCTION BETWEEN SCREENING VERSUS CONFIRMATORY TEST

When using any new diagnostic test, it is critically important to know whether its conduct or results depend on the person performing the test (interoperator agreement/reliability) as well as whether that specific test conducted repeatedly by the same operator or laboratory would give an identical result (test-retest results). There are some discrepancies in the literature on the interpretation and calculation of agreement and reliability parameters. Reproducibility is a general term that addresses these 2 concepts.[21] As an example, the authors reported the agreement between 6 different raters scoring the same 50 video loops of thoracic ultrasonography images,[22] or agreement between raters scoring specific clinical signs in calves.[23] The reliability of a test is intended to determine how well patients' tests results can be distinguished from each other, accounting for test measurement error. In the previous study assessing thoracic ultrasonography, reliability indices (eg, intraclass correlation) were

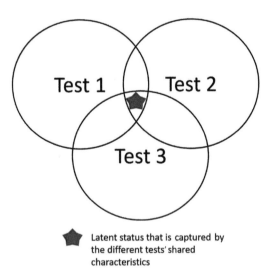

★ Latent status that is captured by the different tests' shared characteristics

Fig. 2. The latent class when using 3 different tests with imperfect accuracy. The concept of latent class may be challenging to represent using different tests for assessing the disease status. The latent class can be considered conceptually as the shared characteristics between the tests used. In a study focusing on clinical scoring, thoracic ultrasonography, and inflammatory blood markers, this latent class (*star*) can be represented as the shared characteristics between abnormal clinical score, lung lesions, and active inflammation, and could be a definition of infectious bronchopneumonia.

determined to report how reliable measurement of lung consolidation was when conducted by the different raters. Benchmarks have been recommended for determination of clinically relevant agreement and reliability indices.[24–26] However, it is important to recognize that there is no consensus on the best strategy for use of these different parameters in practice.[27] Using different types of complementary indices is useful to judge test agreement and reliability.[24]

Screening Tests

The application of diagnostic testing depends on the way tests are used in diagnosis. There are 2 different testing applications for investigation of infectious lower respiratory tract disease: screening and confirmatory testing. This terminology indicates the use of serial testing, with an easily accessible, performable, and preferably cheap screening test followed by a confirmation test only in animals positive in the screening test. Although debatable, screening tests generally are used rapidly and visually, such as clinical signs scoring or automatic detection of clinical signs/activity. Confirmation tests generally require deeper manipulation of the animal and/or a more expensive or time-consuming investigation. In epidemiology, a good screening test requires high sensitivity, to rule out the disease in negative cases, whereas the confirmation test should be highly specific to rule in positive cases. This process, inherently serial, results in higher specificity; this means clinicians are more confident of a positive test result. The outcome of such a strategy may be good for limiting unnecessary antimicrobial use but, given imperfect test sensitivity of the screening test, sick cattle may be missed. An alternative is to opt for parallel testing, with multiple tests on the same animal, and the animal considered positive when one of the tests is positive. Given imperfect test specificity, this approach increases the possibility of unnecessary treatment.

In addition, the clinical application of any diagnostic test also requires a good idea of the reason why it is performed. This context is particularly helpful to estimate the pretest probability of the disease, which can potentially be used to transform the test result to the probability that the patient has or does not have the disease.[28] An overview is given next on what tests are currently available, with their diagnostic accuracy, advantages, and limitations further summarized in **Table 2**.

Clinical sign assessment

Abnormal clinical signs or behavior have been historically used for day-to-day diagnosis of infectious bronchopneumonia. The infectious agents cause nonspecific clinical signs such as fever, anorexia, and depression, which are the response to cytokine release and downstream activations.[44] Clinical respiratory signs are then observed, such as abnormal or rapid breathing patterns, nasal discharge, or coughing.

Fever is a nonspecific sign of infectious bronchopneumonia that is observed secondary to experimental challenges for all major respiratory pathogens.[44] However, the duration of increased body temperature is variable depending on the settings and challenges. For example, following tracheal *Mannheimia haemolytica* challenge, fever is generally observed the day following challenge, then rapidly decreases despite evidence of ongoing infection.[44,45] This rapid change limits the ability to detect sick calves with fever if body temperature is not assessed at the correct time. In contrast, nonrespiratory or noninfectious (eg, heat stress) processes can be associated with increased body temperature. The accuracy of rectal temperature measurement depends on the thermometer used as well as on the technique used by the operator.[46] Continuous or automated monitoring of body temperature has been

Table 2
Summary findings of clinicoanatomic tests used for the diagnosis of infectious bronchopneumonia in cattle

Study	Study Summary	Test Under Investigation	Reference Standard Test	Were Possible Misclassifications of the Reference Standard Test Accounted For?	Sensitivity: 95% CI or BCI (%)	Specificity: 95% CI or BCI (%)	Comments
Clinical Scores							
Buczinski et al,[38] 2014	106 preweaned dairy calves in 13 dairy farms with thoracic auscultation, ultrasonography and clinical scoring	WRSC	Bilateral thoracic ultrasonography: positive if at least 1 site had consolidation depth $\geq$1 cm	No	55.4 (42–68)	58 (44–71)	Used $\geq$5 as a positivity threshold
Love et al,[33] 2014	2030 preweaned dairy calves with deep nasopharyngeal swab and WRSC	CRSC BRD3	Positive if: nasopharyngeal swab PCR positive for BRSV, IBR, or BVDV, or aerobic bacterial pathogen (or *Mycoplasma* spp) positive and WRSC $\geq$ 5)	No	89.4	90.3	Used BRD3 scoring system (score $\geq$ 5) further referenced as the CRSC (BRD1 and BRD2 score accuracy are also detailed)
Buczinski et al,[18] 2015	106 and 86 preweaned dairy calves in 2 different populations with thoracic ultrasonography and clinical scoring	WRSC	Bilateral thoracic ultrasonography: positive if at least 1 site had consolidation depth $\geq$1 cm	Reference standard uncertainty was accounted for using a bayesian latent class model	62.4 (47.9–75.8)	74.1 (64.9–82.8)	Used $\geq$5 as a positivity threshold vs negative if <5

	Sample	Score	Reference test	Reference standard	Se	Sp	Notes
Love et al,[34] 2016	536 calves from 5 premises in California, mixed enrollment criteria: animals suspected as sick (n = 135) by initial observation screening (depression, sunken eye, coughing, abnormal respiration) and a random selection of calves (n = 401)	CRSC BRD3	Bilateral auscultation and ultrasonography: positive if either abnormal auscultation or ultrasonographic evidence of multiple comet tails, consolidation of abscesses	No	SSe 46.8, DSe 72.6	87.4	Used ≥5 as a positivity threshold vs negative if <5, SSe estimated Se on randomly selected calves, DSe estimated Se on the suspected cases, specificity determined in all negative cases as classified by the reference standard test
Buczinski et al,[36] 2018	608 preweaned dairy calves in 39 dairy farms; clustering was accounted for using a random farm effect	Same clinical signs as in the WRSC and CRSC but updated weights for the clinical signs	Thoracic ultrasonography: positive if at least 1 site had consolidation ≥1 cm	Reference standard uncertainty was accounted for using a bayesian latent class model	81.6 (68.2–97.6)	71 (65.7–77.5)	Used ≥10 as a cutoff, various other cutoffs points with Se and Sp were also reported
Maier et al,[35] 2019	689 weaned dairy calves (89 with apparent signs of sickness, 600 randomly chosen)	6 different scores derived from Love et al,[33] 2014; adapted for postweaned calves (including body condition and diurnal temperature fluctuation)	Abnormal lung sounds or consolidation/abscesses ≥2 by 2 cm or any amount of pleural effusion	No	SSe 64.8–84.2, DSe from 76.9–100	45.7–76.7	Results from 4 different models obtained in a training sample (n = 515) tested in a new subgroup of 174 calves SSe: estimated Se on randomly selected calves, DSe estimated Se on the suspected cases, specificity determined in all negative cases as classified by the reference standard test

(continued on next page)

Table 2
(continued)

Study	Study Summary	Test Under Investigation	Reference Standard Test	Were Possible Misclassifications of the Reference Standard Test Accounted For?	Sensitivity: 95% CI or BCI (%)	Specificity: 95% CI or BCI (%)	Comments
Remote Early Disease Identification							
White et al,[37] 2016	Two feedlot population of 168 and 311 beef calves	REDI algorithm	Visual observation by the pen riders	Reference standard uncertainty was accounted for using a bayesian latent class model	81.3 (55.5, 95.8)	92.3 (88.2, 96.9)	1-gate study using 2 populations of feedlot calves followed during 30–37 d after arrival in the feedlots
Infrared Thermography							
Schaefer et al,[30] 2007	133 weaned beef calves	Absolute IRT value is equal to the orbital (eye) maximum value (best cutoff 38.1°C)	≥2 of the following symptoms: a core temperature of ≥40°C, a white blood cell count of <7 or >111,000/μL, a clinical score of ≥3, and neutrophil/lymphocyte ratio of <0.1 or >0.8. A true-negative animal had ≤1 of these signs or symptoms	No	67.6	86.8	2-gate study

Study	Population	Index test	Reference standard		Se	Sp	Comments
Schaefer et al,[31] 2012	65 beef Hereford Angus calves 220 kg BW	Infrared thermal value (FLIR-S60 camera) of the true-positive animals at peak temperature and true animals at their average maximum infrared thermal value (best cutoff 35.29°C)	≥3 of the following signs: a core temperature of >40 C, a white blood cell count of <7 or >111,000/µL, a clinical score of >3, or a neutrophil/lymphocyte ratio of 0.8 (neutrophilia). A true-negative had a score of 0 or 1	No	100	97.4	2-gate study design. The IRT value was based on serial measurements (typically >20 by day), the prevalence of truly affected calves was low (n = 9)
Thoracic Auscultation							
Buczinski et al,[38] 2014	106 preweaned dairy calves, thorax divided into 4 different areas	Thoracic auscultation positive if crackles, wheezes, or no sounds; otherwise negative	Bilateral thoracic ultrasonography: positive if at least 1 site had consolidation depth ≥1 cm	No	5.9 (from 0 to 16.7)	98.9 (from 97.3 to 100)	1-gate study design. Accuracy ranges based on the lung field examined
Buczinski et al,[39] 2016	209 dairy calves raised as veal calves, whole thorax auscultated	Thoracic auscultation	Bilateral thoracic ultrasonography: positive if at least 1 site had consolidation depth ≥1 cm	Reference standard uncertainty was accounted for using a bayesian latent class model	72.9 (50.1–96.4)	53.3 (43.3–64.0)	1-gate study design. Operator performing auscultation was blind to thoracic ultrasonography results
Pardon et al,[40] 2019	8–10 veal calves scored by 49 veterinary practitioners	Thoracic auscultation (normal vs abnormal based on veterinarian experience)	Bilateral thoracic ultrasonography: positive if at least 1 site had consolidation depth ≥1 cm	No	63 (20–100)	46 (0–100)	1-gate study design (range representing the spread of the results obtained by the 49 veterinarians, not CI)

(continued on next page)

Table 2
(continued)

Study	Study Summary	Test Under Investigation	Reference Standard Test	Were Possible Misclassifications of the Reference Standard Test Accounted For?	Sensitivity: 95% CI or BCI (%)	Specificity: 95% CI or BCI (%)	Comments
Computer-aided Auscultation							
Mang et al,[41] 2015	35 beef feedlot steers visually determined as sick, 35 steers not apparently sick	Whisper stethoscope (abnormal if score ≥2)	Pen-rider examination	Reference standard uncertainty was accounted for using a bayesian latent class model	92.9 (71–99)	89.6 (64–99)	2-gate design
Zeineldin et al,[42] 2016	24 feedlot steers with clinical signs of respiratory tract infection pen matched with 24 apparently healthy steers	Whisper stethoscope (abnormal if score ≥2)	Pen-rider examination	No	87.50	75	2-gate design
Thoracic Ultrasonography							
Rabeling et al,[29] 1998	18 calves up to 5 mo of age referred in a veterinary hospital with chronic lesions or arthritis	TUS (unit of interest is part of the lung field; 8 sites per calf)	Necropsy	No	85	98	Small case series of chronic cases, accuracy level at the site level not the calf, lung normal if well ventilated and not any lesion (vs abnormal)

Reference	Population	TUS criteria	Reference standard	Accounting for reference uncertainty	Sensitivity	Specificity	Notes
Ollivett et al,[43] 2015	25 dairy calves (1–12 wk old) with normal WRSC <5	TUS positive if any nonaerated lung visible	Necropsy	No	94 (69–100)	100 (64–100)	2-gate design calves were selected if normal WRSC and stratified by ultrasonography findings to be compared with necropsy
Zeineldin et al,[42] 2016	Feedlot calves 6–8 mo old, 24 cases and 24 matched control calves	TUS (7th–11th ICS) positive if heterogenous hyperechoic or echoic area	Pen-rider examination	No	70.8	87.5	2-gate design
Berman et al,[16] 2019	209 veal calves and 301 preweaned dairy calves	TUS positive if consolidation depth ≥3 cm not considering site cranial to the heart	WRSC and serum haptoglobin	Reference standards uncertainty was accounted for using a bayesian latent class model	89 (55–100)	95 (92–98)	1-gate design Other ultrasonographic thresholds including or not cranial sites accuracy are also mentioned

The sensitivity is the ability of the test to diagnose sick animals whereas the specificity is the ability of the test to diagnose nonsick animals.

Abbreviations: BCI, bayesian credible interval; BW, body weight; CI, confidence interval; CRSC, Californian respiratory scoring chart; CRSC BRD3, third model of the Californian respiratory scoring chart; DSe, diagnostic sensitivity; ICS, intercostal space; IRT, infrared thermography; PCR, polymerase chain reaction; REDI, remote early disease identification; Se, sensitivity; Sp, specificity; SSe, screening sensitivity; TUS, thoracic ultrasonography; WRSC, Wisconsin respiratory scoring chart.

Data from Refs.[16,18,29,31–42]

studied for the detection of BRD. For example, reticuloruminal boluses detected abnormal rumen temperature from 0.5 to 5.7 days before other respiratory signs were detected in 24 bulls.[47] Many episodes of increased ruminal temperature were not associated with any clinical sign, although they still negatively correlated with average daily gain.[47] As reviewed by Wolfger and colleagues,[9] infrared thermography (IRT) of the nasal planum surface is another way to monitor bovine body temperature. It can be helpful to detect fever when diagnosis of respiratory disease infection is made.[31,47] The technique has a good test-retest repeatability and a limited interoperator variability.[32,48] Standardization of the method is required for distance and weather, which can affect readings.[48] More recently, the use of nasal planum IRT has been used to detect respiratory rate,[49] which could be useful in the distance assessment of calves.

Several combinations of clinical signs have been used in past attempts to standardize BRD case definition at the farmer/producer level. Because diagnosis and treatment (at least in North America and in some European countries) is often not performed by a veterinarian but by animal caretakers based on veterinary-supervised protocols, standardized clinical assessment has also been used as a first-line diagnostic test. The Wisconsin scoring chart for dairy calves, initially intended to standardize treatment decisions among laypeople, resulted in international awareness of the importance of case definitions and standardization.[50] Other dairy calf scores have been reported, such as the Californian[33,34] scoring chart with a specific chart for postweaned calves[35] and a modified chart accounting for imperfect reference standard definition.[36] Despite its widespread use, the Wisconsin scoring chart was not initially created to accurately diagnose infectious bronchopneumonia but to standardize BRD treatment. Its accuracy was very different from other scoring approaches developed thereafter (sensitivity and specificity within the range of 60% to 80%; see **Table 2**). The 3 main limitations of the Wisconsin scoring system are (1) the 4-scale score per clinical sign, which can lead to limited inter-rater agreement, versus dichotomous (normal vs abnormal sign) notation[23]; (2) linear score increases, which assume that each 1-unit increase has the same effect on disease risk; and (3) the absence of specific weighting between clinical signs, which assumes that any clinical sign has the same strength of effect. Studies in California[33,35] and Quebec[36] have addressed these limitations. In feedlot calves, the diagnosis of respiratory tract infection by the pen rider generally uses a step-by-step approach (such as the DART [assessment for presence of depression, decreased appetite, respiratory signs, and increased temperature at the chute] approach[9,51]) or can use a less structured approach.[15,17] The detection of sick feedlot calves had been described as an art rather than a science,[52] which may explain why some pen riders are better than others, as well as the lack of specific consensus on case definition. In a systematic review using slaughterhouse lung lesions to determine the accuracy of clinical detection, the authors found wide heterogeneity between studies, which was at least partly attributed to various clinical definitions.[17]

The results concerning the accuracy of common combinations of clinical signs are reported in **Table 2**. However, little information is available concerning inter-rater agreement of these systems. The authors recently observed that, even after some teaching period, the agreement between 3 different scorers was slight to fair (using Cohen and Fleiss kappa statistics) when using 4-scale scoring per clinical sign included in the Wisconsin respiratory scoring chart.[23] These pitfalls of clinical scoring show the necessity of a structured teaching approach to achieve a level of agreement within and between different farms. This teaching opportunity would help standardize cases definitions even if imperfect.

Continuous monitoring of behavior and feeding
Visual monitoring of cattle is generally limited to short periods of observation. Although serial point measurements are hampered by the prey-animal nature of cattle, hiding clinical signs when observed by predators, continuous measurements by technology can overcome this. Several studies have shown that the progress of respiratory infection is accompanied by behavioral or feeding changes, such as increased lying time[45,53] or decreased standing time[54]; decreased feeding period, dry matter, or milk intake[53,55–60]; bunk feeding frequency[60,61]; and increased time to approach the feedbunk after feed delivery.[56] For sick preweaned calves, decreased drinking speed[58] and decreased suckling time for nonnutritive visits[53,58] were observed. It is beyond the scope of this article to review all parameters and algorithms used for disease diagnosis in cattle. In the field setting, one of the main advantages of these systems is the possibility to detect early changes before the human eye.[56,58,60] However, this comes with the limitation of false-positive risk with possible false alarms. Limited information is available to date on the usefulness of these observations as practical daily monitoring tools. For example, the use of daily feeding behavior in group-housed dairy calves fed with an automatic milk feeder was not accurate enough to predict sick animals.[58]

The major limitation of automatic systems is that all so far have been validated against a clinical definition, judged to be state of the art at the time of the particular study. However, it is now realized that there are limitations to many of the definitions. Therefore, an uncomfortable fact is that, in almost all field studies on automatic detection, the reference standard test was human clinical diagnosis. This situation could have biased the research finding toward the null, because any discrepancy between the test of interest and case definition would be interpreted as a test error. One exception is the remote early disease identification (REDI) system, which was evaluated through a bayesian latent class model (see **Table 2**).

In feedlot calves, the REDI system was based on real-time animal positional information.[37,62] The accuracy of REDI is higher than that of pen-rider visual observation when accounting for the absence of a gold standard to detect a clinical case (see **Table 2**).[37] Using this method for the detection of respiratory tract infection resulted in higher first-treatment success and lower average number of antimicrobial doses per animal without negative production impacts.[63] The future for incorporating these types of behavior monitoring systems is to be able to refine algorithms for sensitivity to detect early cases with an acceptable false-positive fraction. The specificity has been determined as the most important characteristic of a diagnostic test from a feedlot economic perspective.[8] This characteristic should also be developed in relation to welfare, production, and economic outcomes. Development of big-data and machine learning technology will potentially rapidly change the application of these tests because they can integrate many different dimensions of calf characteristics that the human eye cannot manage and thus filter animals that need to be monitored by a caretaker or veterinarian.

Confirmatory Tests

Confirmation diagnostic tests are generally used after an initial suspicion is raised by a screening test. Most of the confirmatory tests described here are more commonly used by veterinarians (except for computer-aided lung auscultation).

Thoracic auscultation
Historically, thoracic auscultation is the most frequently used confirmation test, as a way to assess for the presence of increased bronchial sounds or abnormal sounds

(eg crackles, wheezes, or absence of sound). However, the data concerning use of auscultation for disease assessment are surprisingly limited in veterinary and human medicine.[38–40] When using only abnormal respiratory sounds, the sensitivity to detect lung consolidation (diagnosed by ultrasonography) is low but very specific (see **Table 2**).[38] Adding increased bronchial sounds to the definition increased sensitivity and decreased specificity.[39] It should be remembered that auscultation as in human medicine is highly operator dependent. Recently the authors found a poor inter-rater reliability (Kripendorff alpha, 0.18; 95% confidence interval [CI], −0.01–0.38) between 49 Dutch practitioners.[40] The average sensitivity for lung auscultation to detect ultrasonographically defined lung lesions was 0.63 (from 0.2 to 1) and specificity was 0.46 (from 0 to 1). The variable accuracy has also been found in human medicine.[64] Using objective measurement of lung sounds to avoid inter-rater variability is therefore of interest and, recently, a computer-aided lung auscultation algorithm has been commercialized for feedlot calves, giving results after 8-second auscultation on a 1 to 5 step scale, with an abnormal score considered as greater than or equal to 2.[65] Currently available data concerning the accuracy of this stethoscope for the diagnosis of naturally occurring LRTI are limited to a case-control study[41,42] in which 35 steers with visual signs of disease were pulled with the same number of apparently healthy animals; assessment of the stethoscope found sensitivity and specificity of 92.9% (95% bayesian credible intervals [BCI] 71%–99%) and 89.6% (95% BCI, 64%–99%) respectively.[41] No information is available concerning its test-retest validation or use on cattle other than postweaned beef cattle (eg, calves around 250–300 kg).

Medical imaging of lung lesions

Medical imaging is another interesting way to confirm the presence of lung lesions associated with LRTI. Several imaging techniques have been used, including radiographs,[66–72] computed tomography,[66,73,74] and ultrasonography.[16,39,42,43,75–77] Ultrasonography especially has recently been studied more in depth because of its ease for use in field settings. The main findings on the accuracy of these imaging modalities are reported in **Table 2**.

Thoracic ultrasonography

The practical use of thoracic ultrasonography has recently been reviewed.[75] Available studies of the inter-rater agreement have shown that the presence of lung consolidation is a reliable parameter to monitor even if the operator does not have a strong expertise on medical ultrasonography use.[22,78] Diagnostic limitations associated with thoracic ultrasonography include the influence of the size of the animal and muscle development, which preclude the visualization of lung parenchyma cranial to the heart in large beef calves.[77] Also, it is not currently possible to distinguish active lung infection lesions that would benefit from treatment from lesions that are a sequela of previous disease for which treatment would not be beneficial. There is limited evidence that ultrasonography can be used for confirming infectious causes. Information obtained from thoracic ultrasonography assessment is therefore used to quantify lesions, which is associated with negative production outcomes.[79–82] Different recording systems exist to define normal versus abnormal findings.[75] Most available studies on lung lesion imaging are observational, and limited information is available concerning the added value of performing this test in terms of mitigating welfare or production outcomes. One of the main values of thoracic ultrasonography is to provide an imperfect but objective measurement to assess the effect of different interventions for infectious bronchopneumonia. Studies reporting ultrasonography accuracy results are described in **Table 2**.

Other imaging techniques
In the late 1980s, thoracic radiographs were mentioned as an interesting diagnostic technique to identify lung lesions in clinically healthy calves.[83] Specific findings associated with infectious bronchopneumonia have been further detailed in calves and cows.[66,67,69] Infectious pneumonia is characterized by tissue opacity (alveolar pattern) with or without air bronchogram.[66] Presence of cavitary lesions is generally associated with lung abscesses or emphysematous bulla.[67] Other patterns, such as bronchial pattern with thickened bronchial walls or interstitial patterns, can also be observed. One of the limitations of thoracic radiographs is the summation effect caused by superposition of three-dimensional structures in a two-dimensional image.[66] Moreover, the risk of exposure to radiation, and limited availability for practicing veterinarians working in purely food animal practice, have limited its field usefulness. Recently the authors compared thoracic radiographs with thoracic ultrasonography in 50 calves weighing less than 100 kg referred to a hospital, finding the tests to have similar accuracy compared with computed tomography.[84] Computed tomography has a strong potential to accurately detect slight to moderate lung changes and is used as a quasi–gold standard in human pneumonia studies.[85,86] However, because of the associated costs and necessity for sedation, it is of limited use in practice, but it can be used in referral or research imaging.

Blood markers for diagnosis of infectious bronchopneumonia
The systemic changes associated with infectious bronchopneumonia can be measured in different body fluids, but, from a practical standpoint, blood is predominantly used. White blood cell (WBC) changes have been well described in response to respiratory infection, but their discriminatory capacity is limited.[87] The basophil count, which was the most accurate white blood cell marker in the referenced study, had an area under the receiver operating characteristic curve (AUC) of 0.599, which indicates a low-accuracy test.[88] Comparable AUC ranges (0.5–0.6) were obtained from white blood cells and red blood cells analysis in feedlot calves with naturally occurring respiratory disease.[89] This finding confirms those of Wolfger and colleagues[9] that WBC findings are of limited practical use for infectious bronchopneumonia diagnosis.

Acute phase proteins (APPs) such as haptoglobin, fibrinogen, serum amyloid A, or C-reactive proteins have received attention for diagnosis of bovine respiratory tract infection and inflammation. The authors recently reviewed the diagnostic accuracy of these markers for naturally occurring respiratory infection.[90] The conclusion of this systematic review was that there was a high heterogeneity in reported test accuracy as well as sensitivity and specificity. Most of the studies reviewed were 2-gate (case-control) studies with patients at the end of the spectrum of disease, which, as discussed earlier, potentially biased the results toward inflated accuracy estimate of the APP tested. It was impossible to complete the meta-analysis because of the different study designs, settings, and case definitions. Thus, it is currently difficult to give a specific accuracy estimate of those markers for diagnosing infectious bronchopneumonia. Haptoglobin, which was the most commonly reported APP in this review, had sensitivity varying from 61% to 100% and a specificity from 80% to 100%. This finding contrasts with the recently reported sensitivity of 46% and specificity of 82% in a dairy calf study that also reported WBC accuracy.[87] Based on the ranges of reported accuracy and study limitations, it is difficult to give a practical recommendation on using only haptoglobin for a diagnosis in practice. Many other markers have been assessed but are not discussed further in this article because of limited field studies. Other tests, such as blood gas analysis, exhaled biomarkers, or analysis of respiratory secretion, are also not further detailed.

Necropsy

Necropsy is important in the investigation of respiratory tract problems. Necropsy not only serves to evaluate the lesions and identify specific pathogens but is also useful to monitor caretaker detection accuracy. Necropsy-based recording of the cause of death and percentage of calves that die of undiagnosed respiratory disease is a practical way to improve respiratory disease detection protocols. In a recent study of dairy calf mortality before 90 days of age, the agreement between the suspected cause of death based on treatments given versus gross necropsy or necropsy performed in a laboratory was slight to fair (Cohen kappa, 0.22 and 0.13, respectively).[91] In feedlot calves with lung lesions at slaughter, from 3% to 56% of these calves were detected as sick by the pen rider in 7 different studies included in a meta-analysis.[17]

SUMMARY

This article emphasizes different challenges inherent to BRD complex definitions, as well as limitations of clinical tests used for diagnosis. An important step to improve the case definition is to develop robust tests with high inter-rater and intrarater agreement and reliability, as well as to account for imperfection of case definition when determining diagnostic test accuracy. Maintaining health and welfare with decreased antimicrobial use would be a major benchmark allowing the veterinary profession to maintain its reputation and credibility in the One Health approach.

DISCLOSURE

S. Buczinski has received honoraria for acting as speaker or consultant as well as research grants for pharmaceutical companies (Zoetis, MSD, Hipra, and Ceva) and companies involved in commercialization of ancillary tests used in respiratory diseases (EI Medical Imaging, Geissler Corp). B. Pardon has received honoraria for acting as speaker or consultant for pharmaceutical (Zoetis, MSD, Vetoquinol, Dopharma, Boehringer Ingelheim, Dechra, Hipra, Ceva, Merial, and Elanco), agricultural (Algoet nutrition) and chemical (Proviron) companies, and nonprofit organizations (Boerenbond, AMCRA, DGZ-Vlaanderen).

REFERENCES

1. Pardon B, Buczinski S. BRD diagnosis: what progress have we made in infectious diagnosis? Vet Clin North Am Food Anim Pract 2020;36(2):425–44.
2. Lillie LE. The bovine respiratory disease complex. Can Vet J 1974;15:233–42.
3. Smith BP, Van Metre DC, Pusterla N. Large animal internal medicine. St-Louis (MO): Mosby; 2019.
4. DeDonder KD, Apley MD. A review of the expected effects of antimicrobials in bovine respiratory disease treatment and control using outcomes from published randomized clinical trials with negative controls. Vet Clin North Am Food Anim Pract 2015;31:97–111.
5. Mahendran S, Booth R, Burge M, et al. Randomised positive control trial of NSAID and antimicrobial treatment for calf fever caused by pneumonia. Vet Rec 2017; 181:45.
6. Baptiste KE, Kyvsgaard NC. Do antimicrobial mass medications work? A systematic review and meta-analysis of randomised clinical trials investigating

antimicrobial prophylaxis or metaphylaxis against naturally occurring bovine respiratory disease. Pathog Dis 2017;75.

7. Bond S, Léguillette R, Richard EA, et al. Equine asthma: Integrative biologic relevance of a recently proposed nomenclature. J Vet Intern Med 2018;32:2088–98.

8. Theurer M, White B, Larson R, et al. A stochastic model to determine the economic value of changing diagnostic test characteristics for identification of cattle for treatment of bovine respiratory disease. J Anim Sci 2015;93:1398–410.

9. Wolfger B, Timsit E, White BJ, et al. A systematic review of bovine respiratory disease diagnosis focused on diagnostic confirmation, early detection, and prediction of unfavorable outcomes in feedlot cattle. Vet Clin North Am Food Anim Pract 2015;31:351–65.

10. Rutjes AW, Reitsma JB, Di Nisio M, et al. Evidence of bias and variation in diagnostic accuracy studies. Can Med Assoc J 2006;174:469–76.

11. Buczinski S, O'Connor AM. Specific challenges in conducting and reporting studies on the diagnostic accuracy of ultrasonography in bovine medicine. Vet Clin North Am Food Anim Pract 2016;32:1–18.

12. Schmidt RL, Factor RE. Understanding sources of bias in diagnostic accuracy studies. Arch Pathol Lab Med 2013;137:558–65.

13. Schiller I, van Smeden M, Hadgu A, et al. Bias due to composite reference standards in diagnostic accuracy studies. Stat Med 2016;35:1454–70.

14. Rutjes AW, Reitsma JB, Coomarasamy A, et al. Evaluation of diagnostic tests when there is no gold standard. A review of methods. Health Technol Assess 2007;11:iii, ix-51.

15. White BJ, Renter DG. Bayesian estimation of the performance of using clinical observations and harvest lung lesions for diagnosing bovine respiratory disease in post-weaned beef calves. J Vet Diagn Invest 2009;21:446–53.

16. Berman J, Francoz D, Dufour S, et al. Bayesian estimation of sensitivity and specificity of systematic thoracic ultrasound exam for diagnosis of bovine respiratory disease in pre-weaned calves. Prev Vet Med 2019;162:38–45.

17. Timsit E, Dendukuri N, Schiller I, et al. Diagnostic accuracy of clinical illness for bovine respiratory disease (BRD) diagnosis in beef cattle placed in feedlots: A systematic literature review and hierarchical Bayesian latent-class meta-analysis. Prev Vet Med 2016;135:67–73.

18. Buczinski S, Ollivett TL, Dendukuri N. Bayesian estimation of the accuracy of the calf respiratory scoring chart and ultrasonography for the diagnosis of bovine respiratory disease in pre-weaned dairy calves. Prev Vet Med 2015;119:227–31.

19. Kostoulas P, Nielsen SS, Branscum AJ, et al. STARD-BLCM: Standards for the Reporting of Diagnostic accuracy studies that use Bayesian Latent Class Models. Prev Vet Med 2017;138:37–47.

20. McInturff P, Johnson WO, Cowling D, et al. Modelling risk when binary outcomes are subject to error. Stat Med 2004;23:1095–109.

21. de Vet HC, Terwee CB, Knol DL, et al. When to use agreement versus reliability measures. J Clin Epidemiol 2006;59:1033–9.

22. Buczinski S, Buathier C, Bélanger AM, et al. Inter-rater agreement and reliability of thoracic ultrasonographic findings in feedlot calves, with or without naturally occurring bronchopneumonia. J Vet Intern Med 2018;32:1787–92.

23. Buczinski S, Faure C, Jolivet S, et al. Evaluation of inter-observer agreement when using a clinical respiratory scoring system in pre-weaned dairy calves. N Z Vet J 2016;64:243–7.

24. Gwet KL. Handbook of inter-rater reliability: the definitive guide to measuring the extent of agreement among raters. Gaithersburg (MD): Advanced Analytics, LLC; 2014.

25. Cohen J. A coefficient of agreement for nominal scales. Educ Psychol Meas 1960;20:37–46.

26. Koo TK, Li MY. A Guideline of Selecting and Reporting Intraclass Correlation Coefficients for Reliability Research. J Chiropr Med 2016;15:155–63.

27. de Vet HC, Mokkink LB, Terwee CB, et al. Clinicians are right not to like Cohen's kappa. BMJ 2013;346:f2125.

28. Timsit E, Leguillette R, White BJ, et al. Likelihood ratios: an intuitive tool for incorporating diagnostic test results into decision-making. J Am Vet Med Assoc 2018; 252:1362–6.

29. Rabeling B, Rehage J, Dopfer D, et al. Ultrasonographic findings in calves with respiratory disease. Vet Rec 1998;143:468–71.

30. Schaefer AL, Cook NJ, Church JS, et al. The use of infrared thermography as an early indicator of bovine respiratory disease complex in calves. Res Vet Sci 2007; 83:376–84.

31. Schaefer AL, Cook NJ, Bench C, et al. The non-invasive and automated detection of bovine respiratory disease onset in receiver calves using infrared thermography. Res Vet Sci 2012;93:928–35.

32. Scoley GE, Gordon AW, Morrison SJ. Use of thermal imaging in dairy calves: exploring the repeatability and accuracy of measures taken from different anatomical regions1. Transl Anim Sci 2018;3:564–76.

33. Love WJ, Lehenbauer TW, Kass PH, et al. Development of a novel clinical scoring system for on-farm diagnosis of bovine respiratory disease in pre-weaned dairy calves. PeerJ 2014;2:e238.

34. Love WJ, Lehenbauer TW, Van Eenennaam AL, et al. Sensitivity and specificity of on-farm scoring systems and nasal culture to detect bovine respiratory disease complex in preweaned dairy calves. J Vet Diagn Invest 2016;28:119–28.

35. Maier GU, Rowe JD, Lehenbauer TW, et al. Development of a clinical scoring system for bovine respiratory disease in weaned dairy calves. J Dairy Sci 2019;102: 7329–44.

36. Buczinski S, Fecteau G, Dubuc J, et al. Validation of a clinical scoring system for bovine respiratory disease complex diagnosis in preweaned dairy calves using a Bayesian framework. Prev Vet Med 2018;156:102–12.

37. White BJ, Goehl DR, Amrine DE, et al. Bayesian evaluation of clinical diagnostic test characteristics of visual observations and remote monitoring to diagnose bovine respiratory disease in beef calves. Prev Vet Med 2016;126:74–80.

38. Buczinski S, Forté G, Francoz D, et al. Comparison of thoracic auscultation, clinical score, and ultrasonography as indicators of bovine respiratory disease in preweaned dairy calves. J Vet Intern Med 2014;28:234–42.

39. Buczinski S, Ménard J, Timsit E. Incremental Value (Bayesian Framework) of Thoracic Ultrasonography over Thoracic Auscultation for Diagnosis of Bronchopneumonia in Preweaned Dairy Calves. J Vet Intern Med 2016;30:1396–401.

40. Pardon B, Buczinski S, Deprez PR. Accuracy and inter-rater reliability of lung auscultation by bovine practitioners when compared with ultrasonographic findings. Vet Rec 2019;185:109.

41. Mang AV, Buczinski S, Booker CW, et al. Evaluation of a computer-aided lung auscultation system for diagnosis of bovine respiratory disease in feedlot cattle. J Vet Intern Med 2015;29:1112–6.

42. Zeineldin MM, El-Raof YMA, El-attar HA, et al. Lung ultrasonography and computer-aided scoring system as a diagnostic aid for bovine respiratory disease in feedlot cattle. Global Vet 2016;17:588–94.
43. Ollivett TL, Caswell JL, Nydam DV, et al. Thoracic ultrasonography and bronchoalveolar lavage fluid analysis in Holstein calves with subclinical lung lesions. J Vet Intern Med 2015;29:1728–34.
44. Grissett GP, White BJ, Larson RL. Structured literature review of responses of cattle to viral and bacterial pathogens causing bovine respiratory disease complex. J Vet Intern Med 2015;29:770–80.
45. Eberhart NL, Storer JM, Caldwell M, et al. Behavioral and physiologic changes in Holstein steers experimentally infected with Mannheimia haemolytica. Am J Vet Res 2017;78:1056–64.
46. Naylor JM, Streeter RM, Torgerson P. Factors affecting rectal temperature measurement using commonly available digital thermometers. Res Vet Sci 2012;92:121–3.
47. Timsit E, Bareille N, Seegers H, et al. Visually undetected fever episodes in newly received beef bulls at a fattening operation: occurrence, duration, and impact on performance. J Anim Sci 2011;89:4272–80.
48. Montanholi YR, Lim M, Macdonald A, et al. Technological, environmental and biological factors: referent variance values for infrared imaging of the bovine. J Anim Sci Biotechnol 2015;6:27.
49. Lowe G, Sutherland M, Waas J, et al. Infrared Thermography-A Non-Invasive Method of Measuring Respiration Rate in Calves. Animals (Basel) 2019;9 [pii: E535].
50. McGuirk SM. Disease management of dairy calves and heifers. Vet Clin North Am Food Anim Pract 2008;24:139–53.
51. Griffin D, Chengappa MM, Kuszak J, et al. Bacterial pathogens of the bovine respiratory disease complex. Vet Clin North Am Food Anim Pract 2010;26:381–94.
52. Portillo T. Pen riding and evaluation of cattle in pens to identify compromised individuals. In: Proceedings of the 47th Annual Conference of the American Association of Bovine Practitioners, Albuquerque, New Mexico, September 18-20, 2014. p. 5–8.
53. Hixson CL, Krawczel PD, Caldwell JM, et al. Behavioral changes in group-housed dairy calves infected with Mannheimia haemolytica. J Dairy Sci 2018;101:10351–60.
54. Hanzlicek GA, White BJ, Mosier D, et al. Serial evaluation of physiologic, pathological, and behavioral changes related to disease progression of experimentally induced Mannheimia haemolytica pneumonia in postweaned calves. Am J Vet Res 2010;71:359–69.
55. Toaff-Rosenstein RL, Gershwin LJ, Tucker CB. Fever, feeding, and grooming behavior around peak clinical signs in bovine respiratory disease. J Anim Sci 2016;94:3918–32.
56. Jackson KS, Carstens GE, Tedeschi LO, et al. Changes in feeding behavior patterns and dry matter intake before clinical symptoms associated with bovine respiratory disease in growing bulls. J Anim Sci 2016;94:1644–52.
57. Swartz TH, Findlay AN, Petersson-Wolfe CS. Short communication: Automated detection of behavioral changes from respiratory disease in pre-weaned calves. J Dairy Sci 2017;100:9273–8.
58. Knauer WA, Godden SM, Dietrich A, et al. The association between daily average feeding behaviors and morbidity in automatically fed group-housed preweaned dairy calves. J Dairy Sci 2017;100:5642–52.

59. Sowell BF, Branine ME, Bowman JG, et al. Feeding and watering behavior of healthy and morbid steers in a commercial feedlot. J Anim Sci 1999;77:1105–12.

60. Kayser WC, Carstens GE, Jackson KS, et al. Evaluation of statistical process control procedures to monitor feeding behavior patterns and detect onset of bovine respiratory disease in growing bulls. J Anim Sci 2019;97:1158–70.

61. Wolfger B, Schwartzkopf-Genswein KS, Barkema HW, et al. Feeding behavior as an early predictor of bovine respiratory disease in North American feedlot systems. J Anim Sci 2015;93:377–85.

62. White BJ, Amrine DE, Goehl DR. Determination of value of bovine respiratory disease control using a remote early disease identification system compared with conventional methods of metaphylaxis and visual observations. J Anim Sci 2015;93:4115–22.

63. White B, Goehl D, Theurer M, et al. Determining health, performance, and economic value of using a remote early disease identification system compared to conventional method for diagnosis of bovine respiratory disease. J Anim Health Behav Sci 2017;1:2.

64. Hafke-Dys H, Breborowicz A, Kleka P, et al. The accuracy of lung auscultation in the practice of physicians and medical students. PLoS One 2019;14:e0220606.

65. Noffsinger T, Brattain K, Quakenbush G, et al. Field results from Whisper(R) stethoscope studies. Anim Health Res Rev 2014;15:142–4.

66. Fowler J, Stieger-Vanegas SM, Vanegas JA, et al. Comparison of thoracic radiography and computed tomography in calves with naturally occurring respiratory disease. Front Vet Sci 2017;4:101.

67. Masseau I, Fecteau G, Breton L, et al. Radiographic detection of thoracic lesions in adult cows: a retrospective study of 42 cases (1995-2002). Can Vet J 2008;49: 261–7.

68. Tegtmeier C, Arnbjerg J. Evaluation of radiology as a tool to diagnose pulmonic lesions in calves, for example prior to experimental infection studies. J Vet Med B Infect Dis Vet Public Health 2000;47:229–34.

69. Farrow CS. Bovine pneumonia. Its radiographic appearance. Vet Clin North Am Food Anim Pract 1999;15:301–58.

70. Jones GF, Feeney DA, Mews C. Comparison of radiographic and necropsy findings of lung lesions in calves after challenge exposure with Pasteurella multocida. Am J Vet Res 1998;59:1108–12.

71. Jung C, Bostedt H. Thoracic ultrasonography technique in newborn calves and description of normal and pathological findings. Vet Radiol Ultrasound 2004;45: 331–5.

72. Shimbo G, Tagawa M, Matsumoto K, et al. Three-legged radiographic view for evaluating cranioventral lung region in standing calves with bovine respiratory disease. J Vet Med Sci 2019;81:120–6.

73. Lubbers BV, Apley MD, Coetzee JF, et al. Use of computed tomography to evaluate pathologic changes in the lungs of calves with experimentally induced respiratory tract disease. Am J Vet Res 2007;68:1259–64.

74. Ohlerth S, Augsburger H, Abe M, et al. Computed tomography of the thorax in calves from birth to 105 days of age. Schweiz Arch Tierheilk 2014;156:489–97.

75. Ollivett TL, Buczinski S. On-farm use of ultrasonography for bovine respiratory disease. Vet Clin North Am Food Anim Pract 2016;32:19–35.

76. Braun U, Gerspach C, Brammertz C. The frequency of abnormal ultrasonographic findings in the lungs of 129 calves with bronchopneumonia. Schweiz Arch Tierheilk 2018;160:737–41.

77. Rademacher R, Buczinski S, Edmonds M, et al. Systematic thoracic ultrasonography in acute bovine respiratory disease of feedlot steers: impact of lung consolidation on diagnosis and prognosis in a case-control study. Bovine Pract 2014; 41:1–10.
78. Buczinski S, Forté G, Bélanger AM. Short communication: ultrasonographic assessment of the thorax as a fast technique to assess pulmonary lesions in dairy calves with bovine respiratory disease. J Dairy Sci 2013;96(7):4523–8.
79. Dunn TR, Ollivett TL, Renaud DL, et al. The effect of lung consolidation, as determined by ultrasonography, on first-lactation milk production in Holstein dairy calves. J Dairy Sci 2018;101:5404–10.
80. Teixeira AG, McArt JA, Bicalho RC. Thoracic ultrasound assessment of lung consolidation at weaning in Holstein dairy heifers: Reproductive performance and survival. J Dairy Sci 2017;100:2985–91.
81. Adams EA, Buczinski S. Short communication: Ultrasonographic assessment of lung consolidation postweaning and survival to the first lactation in dairy heifers. J Dairy Sci 2016;99:1465–70.
82. Timsit E, Tison N, Booker CW, et al. Association of lung lesions measured by thoracic ultrasonography at first diagnosis of bronchopneumonia with relapse rate and growth performance in feedlot cattle. J Vet Intern Med 2019;33:1540–6.
83. Pringle J, Viel L, Shewen P, et al. Bronchoalveolar lavage of cranial and caudal lung regions in selected normal calves: cellular, microbiological, immunoglobulin, serological and histological variables. Can J Vet Res 1988;52:239.
84. Berman J, Masseau I, Fecteau G, et al. Comparison between thoracic ultrasonography and thoracic radiography for the detection of lung lesions in dairy calves using a two stage Bayesian approach. In: Annual Convention of the American Association of Bovine Practitioners, St-Louis, MO, September 12-14, 2019.
85. Self WH, Courtney DM, McNaughton CD, et al. High discordance of chest x-ray and computed tomography for detection of pulmonary opacities in ED patients: implications for diagnosing pneumonia. Am J Emerg Med 2013;31:401–5.
86. Cortellaro F, Colombo S, Coen D, et al. Lung ultrasound is an accurate diagnostic tool for the diagnosis of pneumonia in the emergency department. Emerg Med J 2012;29:19–23.
87. Moisá SJ, Aly SS, Lehenbauer TW, et al. Association of plasma haptoglobin concentration and other biomarkers with bovine respiratory disease status in preweaned dairy calves. J Vet Diagn Invest 2019;31:40–6.
88. Gardner IA, Greiner M. Receiver-operating characteristic curves and likelihood ratios: improvements over traditional methods for the evaluation and application of veterinary clinical pathology tests. Vet Clin Pathol 2006;35:8–17.
89. Fontenot LR. Hematological variables as predictors of bovine respiratory disease in newly received cattle fed in confinement. Texas A&M; 2017. p. 83.
90. Abdallah A, Hewson J, Francoz D, et al. Systematic review of the diagnostic accuracy of haptoglobin, serum amyloid A, and fibrinogen versus clinical reference standards for the diagnosis of bovine respiratory disease. J Vet Intern Med 2016; 30:1356–68.
91. McConnel CS, Nelson DD, Burbick CR, et al. Clarifying dairy calf mortality phenotypes through postmortem analysis. J Dairy Sci 2019;102:4415–26.

Bovine Respiratory Disease Diagnosis

What Progress Has Been Made in Infectious Diagnosis?

Bart Pardon, DVM, PhD[a],*, Sébastien Buczinski, Dr Vét, MSc[b]

KEYWORDS

- Bronchoalveolar lavage • Calves • MALDI-TOF • PCR
- Next-generation sequencing

KEY POINTS

- Diagnostic tests to identify pathogens involved in respiratory diseases of cattle are increasingly used, predominantly driven by the need to rationalize antimicrobial use.
- Several methods to sample the respiratory tract are available, of which a deep nasopharyngeal swab, transtracheal wash, and nonendoscopic bronchoalveolar lavage best fit practice. Each technique has advantages and disadvantages, and consensus regarding the best choice is not yet reached.
- Next to microbial culture, for microbiologic diagnosis polymerase chain reaction is especially popular. Promising techniques for a rapid diagnosis are matrix-assisted laser desorption/ionization time of flight mass spectrometry and next-generation sequencing, which will become widely available in coming years.
- It is still difficult to interpret identification of opportunistic pathogens, both at the individual and herd level. More research is needed before evidence-based guidelines can be developed.

INTRODUCTION

In 2012, Fulton and Confer[1] warned that the speed of development of new laboratory diagnostics has outpaced clinicians' ability to properly interpret test results. A range of diagnostic tests is now available, ranging from culture to polymerase chain reaction (PCR) to next-generation sequencing (NGS). However, there is still doubt regarding the clinical significance of some pathogens detected, and how to interpret a diagnostic test result depending on what sample was tested. In contrast to this is the

[a] Department of Large Animal Internal Medicine, Faculty of Veterinary Medicine, Ghent University, Salisburylaan 133, Merelbeke 9820, Belgium; [b] Département des Sciences Cliniques, Faculté de Médecine Vétérinaire, Université de Montréal, 3200 rue Sicotte, St-Hyacinthe, Québec J2S 2M2, Canada
* Corresponding author.
E-mail address: Bart.Pardon@UGent.be

Vet Clin Food Anim 36 (2020) 425–444
https://doi.org/10.1016/j.cvfa.2020.03.005
0749-0720/20/© 2020 Elsevier Inc. All rights reserved.

increasing pressure on antimicrobial use and the need for veterinarians and farmers to use antimicrobials more rationally.[2] The use of diagnostic support by laboratory analysis is one of the frequently mentioned cornerstones of antimicrobial stewardship programs.[3] However, scientifically reasoned, the evidence that systematic use of laboratory diagnostics, especially the antibiogram, would result in selection of a different first-choice therapy compared with an empiric decision preferably following (evidence-based) guidelines, is limited, especially in cattle. Antimicrobial resistance in respiratory tract bacteria from cattle is present and varies highly between systems. Resistance levels are generally lower in closed dairy and beef herds, substantially higher in feedlots, and most worrisome in veal calf operations, where oral mass medication is frequently used.[4,5] Although there is no doubt of the presence of resistance, and multiresistance, in respiratory bacteria from cattle, to what extent this results in therapy failure when following guidelines for antimicrobial therapy is poorly documented. In recent years, guidelines specifying first-line, second-line, and third-line antimicrobial choices for the different cattle diseases have been initiated in several European Union countries, including the Netherlands, Belgium, Denmark, Sweden, and Germany.[2,6,7] However, the amount of literature reporting the clinical benefit of every antimicrobial-bacteria combination in highly variable field settings is currently very limited. Therefore, these guidelines mainly include the spectrum of the antimicrobial, pharmaceutical leaflet recommendations and follow classification of the importance of antimicrobials for human medicine of the World Health Organization.[8] In contrast with human medicine, to the authors' knowledge there are no extensive, sufficiently detailed, and large-scale studies available on therapy failure caused by antimicrobial resistance in cattle.

Regardless of the limitations mentioned earlier, diagnostics are more and more frequently used when addressing bovine respiratory disease (BRD). This increased use is understandable, because antimicrobial decision making for BRD still often involves a decision to use group therapy, and, in the current climate, mass medicating without any evidence of the need for this therapy will increasingly be criticized. The authors fully acknowledge the complexity of advising on the implementation and interpretation of diagnostic tests for BRD, given the huge gaps in the current knowledge.[9] However, the need is urgent, and therefore this article provides a framework to assist practitioners and clinicians in their everyday decision-making process. This reasoning may not withstand time; this article does not represent a consensus of all leading experts, nor is the objective to provide a complete literature overview. This discussion reflects on the body site sampled, the test used, and the pathogen detected.

TYPES OF SAMPLES AND SAMPLING PROCEDURES

The selected sampling site of the respiratory tract is of great importance for interpretation of the test result. **Table 1** provides an overview of available sampling techniques, with their advantages and drawbacks. Descriptions of these techniques are available elsewhere (eg, deep nasopharyngeal swabs [DNSs] and nonendoscopic bronchoalveolar lavage [nBAL],[10] transtracheal aspiration [TTA]/transtracheal wash [TTW],[11] and endoscopic bronchoalveolar lavage [BAL][12]; **Fig. 1**).

Nasal swabs, predominantly sampling the cutaneous part of the nose, are generally considered of limited value for infectious diagnostics. In contrast, DNSs sample the respiratory and associated lymphoid epithelium of the nasopharynx and return more meaningful samples. However, the biggest issue with nasopharyngeal swabs is the large number of polymicrobial samples recovered (>80%),[10] which heavily compromises clinical interpretation when only opportunistic pathogens are retrieved.

Table 1
Overview of available sampling techniques of the respiratory tract of calves and cattle, with advantages and disadvantages

	Nasopharyngeal Swab	Transtracheal Wash or Transtracheal Aspirate	Nonendoscopic Bronchoalveolar Lavage	Endoscopic Bronchoalveolar Lavage
Sampling Site	Nasopharyngeal mucosa	Tracheal bifurcation	Individual random lung lobe	Individual (or multiple) targeted lung lobes
Use	Single use, disposable	Single use, disposable, or multiple use, sterilizable	Multiple use, sterilizable	Multiple use, sterilizable
Representative for Lower Airways	±	Yes	Yes, but controversial	Yes
Sampled Surface	<0.5 cm^2	5–10 cm^2	>10 cm^2	>10 cm^2
Procedure Costs	–	++	+	+++
Estimated Procedure Time per Animal, Including Preparation (min)	<1	10	1–10	10
Contamination Risk from Nasal Passage	High	Absent	Moderate (protective sleeve or agar plug possible)	Low (protective sleeve or agar plug possible)
Difficulty of the Technique	–	+	+	++
Possible Complications	• Nasal hemorrhage • Fracture of the swab shaft	• Subcutaneous emphysema • Wound infection • Local hemorrhage • Accidental tearing of the catheter by retraction over the needle and intratracheal loss of the remaining part • Respiratory distress caused by insufficient aspiration of instilled fluid	• Nasal hemorrhage • Intrapulmonary hemorrhage • Airway perforation (rigid catheter only) • Respiratory distress caused by insufficient aspiration of instilled fluid	• Nasal hemorrhage • Respiratory distress caused by insufficient aspiration of instilled fluid

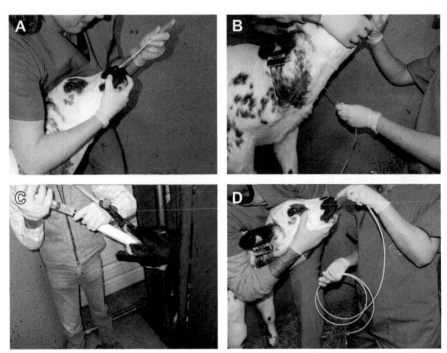

Fig. 1. Overview of accessible sampling methods of the airways in cattle. (*A*) DNS, (*B*) TTW, (*C*) nBAL through the mouth under visual control; (*D*) nBAL performed blindly through the nose.

Contamination can be reduced by rinsing the nares (with a single-use paper towel or a gauze with alcohol) or by using a guarded DNS. However, studies specifically focusing on the effect of guarded swabs to reduce nasal contamination are, to the authors' knowledge, not available in cattle. Recent reports on the respiratory microbiome in cattle also put the idea of contamination at that sampling site into another perspective, given the large variation in bacterial species normally present.[13,14] The largest disadvantage of DNSs is that they do not directly sample the lower respiratory tract. Despite some conflicting results, previous studies overall showed that, for most pathogens, an association between DNS results and TTW or BAL is present.[10,15–17] In addition to cotton swabs, brush swabs also exist, which cause more intensive swabbing of the mucosa (although possibly also blood staining of the sample), presumably with higher detection rates. No evidence on their benefit for use in cattle is currently available. Complications of DNS are rare and included nasal hemorrhage and fracture of the shaft of the swab. The latter is without any harmful consequence because the animal evacuates the remaining part of the swab either by sneezing or swallowing.

To overcome the issue of nasal contamination, transtracheal sampling techniques relying on perforation of the trachea with a needle or catheter after surgical preparation of the skin have been developed. Historically, transtracheal swabs have been used,[18] but the transtracheal aspirate and wash are now common. Although an aspirate (TTA) only involves aspiration of mucus present in the respiratory tract, a wash (TTW) requires fluid instilment and immediate aspiration. Despite the terminology TTA being frequently used in the field, the technique usually used is a TTW. Most frequently, for TTW in cattle, TTW kits (Large Animal Trans-Tracheal Wash Kit, MILA International, Inc, Florence, KY), or human central venous catheters (eg. Centracath 75, Vygon,

Ecouen, France) are used, which are commercially available and sterile packed for single use. Alternatively, a male dog urinary catheter can be used in combination with a 12-G catheter/needle to perforate the trachea in between 2 tracheal rings.[19]

In veterinary medicine, the common thinking is that the TTW is preferred for bacteriology and BAL to study inflammation (cytology). However, this recommendation generally comes from horse medicine, and seems to be expert opinion rather than supported by substantial peer-reviewed studies.[20] In humans, TTW is generally not used for ethical reasons. The general idea is that the bronchial bifurcation is the site where the efflux of the mucociliary system of the whole of the lung comes together. Hence sampling there would be representative for the whole of the lung.[20] However, there are some counterarguments for this reasoning. First, the mucociliary system can be heavily impaired by pneumonia. Second, microbial aspiration from the nasopharynx into the upper trachea is likely frequent. Third, normal pathogenesis involves gradual descent of bacteria down the respiratory tree toward the lung. Taking the second and third arguments into account, a positive TTW culture might equally represent a bacterial tracheitis or even an insignificant colonization or upper airway contamination, resulting in false positive diagnosis of infectious bronchopneumonia. Advantages are that a new disposable catheter can easily be used for each animal, and sampling is theoretically achievable within a predictable time frame given that no active cooperation of the animal is required, in contrast with BAL. However, sedation of the animal and local anesthesia of the puncture site can be done to improve animal comfort during the procedure.

In a BAL procedure, a BAL catheter or flexible endoscope is introduced through the nose and trachea into the lower airways until it wedges into a larger (or smaller depending on catheter diameter) bronchus. Next, while holding in this wedged position, a volume (usually 60 mL in calves, if necessary followed by a second or third injection) of sterile saline is injected and immediately aspirated. Classically, as in human medicine, a BAL is performed by endoscopy. The major advantage is that a specific lung lobe, previously shown to be affected on radiology or ultrasonography, can be sampled. Also, protective sheets or agar plugs can be used to reduce the risk of nasal contamination. The major disadvantage of the endoscope is the high operating costs and risk for equipment damage in the farm setting. Also, sampling multiple animals becomes difficult because time to resterilize the endoscope between animals is needed (15–20 minutes minimum).

To overcome the cost and risks of endoscopic BAL, nBAL techniques have been developed. In nBAL, a BAL catheter is blindly introduced through the nose, larynx, and trachea until the wedged position in a large bronchus is reached. Next, a volume of saline is injected and gently aspirated. The volume used varies substantially between studies (30–250 mL[16,17]), but a trend to reduce the volume for welfare/comfort reasons is present.[21] On average, 33.5% of the volume (12.0%–73.8%) can be recovered in nBAL, which is substantially larger than in a TTW procedure.[21] It is important to realize that sedation not only suppresses the required responses (coughing, curving of the nose, and extroversion of the tongue) to ensure an intratracheal position but also causes systematic sampling of the diaphragmatic lung lobes, which are less likely to be affected.[22] Good restraint of the calf with the head fixed with the nose pointing upward as much as possible is advisable to ease blind introduction of the tube into the trachea. Alternatively, the calf might be surprised into allowing the tube to be advanced into the airways by placing the head in a horizontal position, and introducing the catheter on inspiration visible by the opening of the nostrils. Overall, in 80% of animals, nBAL sampling can be completed within minutes. For the remaining 20%, the practical advice is to select another animal to sample when undertaking group diagnosis, rather than spending excessive time and causing prolonged irritation to a reluctant animal. Alternatively, a technique where a double-guarded BAL catheter is orally introduced into the larynx through a PVC (polyvinyl chloride) speculum has been described for calves that are at least 3 to 4 months old, where the guarded catheter is inserted through the larynx under visual control.[23]

The use of BAL samples (especially nBAL) for bacteriology is still highly controversial, mainly because of the risk of nasal contamination. Although contamination is far less than with DNS, 20.8% of nBAL samples were still polymicrobial.[10] A large influence of the sampler seems to be present,[10] likely depending not only on differences in hygienic sample handling but also on skills to swiftly introduce the catheter without touching too much of the nasopharynx. However, it is important to realize that hard evidence on substantial nasal contamination by using nBAL catheters is currently not available in any species. The only available study on this matter showed pure culture and negative results in 29.2% and 40.3% of the nBAL samples, even though DNS samples of the same animals were polymicrobial.[10] Further, the currently most extensive study on sample method comparison showed very good agreement for bacteriology between DNS, TTW, and nBAL.[17] Interestingly, in human medicine, there are growing efforts toward the use of a mini-BAL procedure for bacterial diagnosis in ventilator-assisted pneumonia.[24] Overall, sample contamination should be avoided and, in the case of nBAL, this can be done by adequate training or visualization of the larynx by a video speculum (Ivetscope, Dairymac Limited, Hampshire, United Kingdom) or endoscopic cameras intended for plumbers or auto mechanics. These devices are available at much lower prices than traditional endoscopes.

Next to the site of the respiratory tract sampled (upper or lower airway), the cultural perception of the effect of the sampling technique on animal welfare also plays an important role in what technique is currently preferred in a given country/region. No studies on the effect of respiratory tract sampling on stress or pain have yet been conducted in calves. A Master of Science thesis showed that both animals sampled by DNS or nBAL spent less time walking compared with the unsampled control group, whereas lying or eating were unaffected.[25] For TTW as well as nBAL, the required volume of saline to be instilled is unclear; it is also unclear whether the volume instilled influences bacteriology results, as it does for cytology.[26]

In summary, sampling techniques for the field need to be economically feasible both in terms of equipment/disposables cost and also invested time. The DNS, TTW, and nBAL best suit this profile and are currently most frequently used in the field. Differences in use exist between countries, which mainly originate from historical or cultural preference.

AVAILABLE DIAGNOSTIC TESTS FOR THE CAUSAL DIAGNOSIS OF BOVINE RESPIRATORY DISEASE

An overview of available diagnostic tests for pathogen identification in respiratory diseases in cattle is shown in **Table 2**. It is beyond the scope of this article to provide a complete overview of all tests possible. The focus is on the most frequently used tests and the most promising future tests likely to become widely available for practice within the next 5 years. In the current international context, the pressure to reduce antimicrobial use has become the main driver of diagnostic test performance for causal diagnosis of BRD. A crucial aspect for field efficacy is a short turnaround time (TAT), the time between sampling and availability of the test result. In order to be able to use the diagnostic test result to target therapy or initiate control measures TAT needs to be as short as possible, ideally less than a day. However, having test

Table 2
Advantages and disadvantages of available diagnostic tests to detect bacterial pathogens involved in respiratory disease in live cattle

	Use	Turnaround Time*	Advantages	Disadvantages
Microbial Culture	Live bacteria detection	• 24 h to 3 d for Pasteurellaceae • >5 d for Mycoplasmata	• Cheap • Evidence of live pathogen • Quantification possible • Antibiogram possible	• Live organisms needed • More time consuming • Lower sensitivity • Fastidious growers (eg, *Histophilus somni*) more easily overgrown (false-negatives) • Specific media needed for certain pathogens (eg, mycoplasmata)
PCR	DNA detection (specific genomic region)	• 24 h	• Very high sensitivity • No live organisms required • Limited effects of contaminated samples • Pooling of samples possible • Quantification possible (qPCR)	• Possible detection of insignificant quantities or dead bacteria (high sensitivity) • Possible detection vaccine antigen (false-positive) • More expensive
Serology (Antibody ELISA)	Antibody detection	• Variable (24 h to 1 wk) depending on laboratory routine • 3 wk for paired sera	• Longer time frame for pathogen detection • Both infection as vaccination status	• Indirect evidence of infection • Variable, but generally lower sensitivity and specificity • Results require 3 wk (paired sera) • No differentiation vaccine induced antibodies from natural infections
Culture-enriched Direct MALDI-TOF	Live bacteria detection	• 6 h for Pasteurellaceae • 3 d for Mycoplasmata	• Cheap (cost comparable with culture) • Rapid • Antibiogram possible with MBT-ASTRA	• MALDI-TOF required • Lower diagnostic accuracy in polymicrobial or mixed culture samples
Nanosequencing	DNA detection (whole genome)	• Possible within 1–2 d	• All possible pathogens simultaneously detected and quantified • Strain typing possible	• No classic antibiogram possible • More expensive

* Turnaround time is the time between arrival in the laboratory and availability of the test result. Reported times are in optimal conditions.
Abbreviations: ELISA, enzyme-linked immunosorbent assay; MALDI-TOF, matrix-assisted laser desorption/ionization time of flight; MBT-ASTRA, MALDI Biotyper Antibiotic Susceptibility Test Rapid Assay; qPCR, quantitative PCR.

results the next morning might also be workable for most outbreaks. Also, the use of cow-side testing for a causal diagnosis of BRD has great potential to reduce TAT. However, to the authors' knowledge, no such tests are currently commercially available. Hence, attention should be given to ensuring proper and timely transport to the laboratory. At refrigerator temperature (4°C–8°C), the isolation rate of *Mannheimia haemolytica* and *Pasteurella multocida* was not reduced for 24 hours, whereas a transport temperature of more than 30°C resulted in reduced isolation as soon as 2 hours later.[27]

Serology

Serologic tests are useful to target vaccination programs, to determine protective status, and to evaluate infection dynamics at larger scale. However, they are not suitable to direct immediate therapy because they have a TAT of 3 weeks (required time for seroconversion) and only provide indirect evidence of infection. Also, for the opportunistic Pasteurellaceae family, maternal immunity smoothly shifts to acquired immunity, without any signs of disease or seroconversion.[28] Another important issue is that sensitivity and specificity can be highly variable between different antibody enzyme-linked immunosorbent assays (ELISAs), hampering clinical interpretation and their use for individual animal decisions (eg, culling or purchase).[29] For targeting therapy, direct identification of the pathogen is needed, and this can be achieved by microbial culture, matrix-assisted laser desorption/ionization time of flight (MALDI-TOF) mass spectrometry (MS), PCR, or NGS/third-generation sequencing.

Microbial Culture

Microbial culture is most frequently used for identification of bacteria. Next to low operating costs, the possibility of antimicrobial susceptibility testing is an important advantage of culture. For mycoplasmata, specific media are required,[29] and fastidious growers, especially *Histophilus somni*, are easily overgrown, resulting in false-negative results.[10,30] Sensitivity and specificity of microbial culture have not been determined for most of the bacteria involved in BRD. A recent study using bayesian latent class analysis showed that *Mycoplasma bovis* culture on solid medium containing Tween 80 is 70.7% (95% bayesian credible intervals [BCI], 52.1 to 87.1) sensitive and 93.9% (95% BCI, 85.9–98.4) specific.[31]

Matrix-Assisted Laser Desorption/Ionization Time of Flight Mass Spectrometry

In the last decade, MALDI-TOF MS, which identifies bacteria by their unique protein profiles, has revolutionized routine diagnostics. It is primarily used for identification of bacteria after culturing, including *Mycoplasma* species.[32] However, MALDI-TOF MS can also be applied directly on the sample after a very short period of enhanced growth in a liquid medium. Relative to classic microbial culture, these culture-enriched direct MALDI-TOF MS techniques allow correct bacterial identification in 73% of the samples (sensitivity = 59.1%; 95% confidence interval [CI], 47.2–71.0; specificity = 100% [100–100]) within 6 hours.[33] The technique performed less well in polymicrobial samples and in samples with mixed infection. Also for *M bovis*, a culture-enriched direct MALDI-TOF MS technique was developed, which was 86.6% (95% BCI, 54–99) sensitive and 86.4% (95% BCI, 80–96) specific in a bayesian latent class model including PCR and microbial culture on solid agar.[31] TAT was reduced from more than 5 days to less than 3 days.[31] In addition, different MALDI-TOF MS methods are available for antimicrobial susceptibility testing. By means of MBT-ASTRA (MALDI Biotyper Antibiotic Susceptibility Test Rapid Assay), oxytetracycline resistance in *P multocida* could be identified with high accuracy (Se = 95.7%;

95% CI, 86.3–100.6; Sp = 100%; [95% CI, 100–100]) in as little as 3 hours, outperforming the disc diffusion antibiogram.[34] The MBT-ASTRA technique can be designed for every bacterium-antibiotic combination, but logistical changes are needed to create a good intralaboratory workflow. The costs of MALDI-TOF procedures are generally low, in line with microbial culture.

Polymerase Chain Reaction

PCR for the causal diagnosis of BRD is now very popular. The main reasons are that multiplex PCR or multiple single PCRs allow detection of multiple bacteria and viruses, providing practitioners with a more extended view of the pathogens involved and hence more options to better target therapy, control, and prevention. Fastidious and metabolically active viable but unculturable viruses and bacteria can be detected, in contrast with standard microbial culture.[35] However, in contrast with sequencing techniques, specific primers are needed, and the pathogen of interest needs to be determined beforehand. In this way, the diagnostics are potentially biased and possibly lead to false-negative results. Another problem is that viral genomes evolve rapidly and primers might become outdated, limiting the efficient detection of the pathogens of interest. PCR is generally not cheap, but, by pooling samples (DNS, TTW, or BALs), a group diagnosis can be reached and costs are decreased. In available studies, pools of samples from 5 animals were shown to improve diagnostic accuracy at the group level.[36,37] The largest disadvantage of PCR is interpretative difficulty, because PCR can identify dead pathogens, opportunists currently not involved in infection, and contaminants, none of which signify a clinically meaningful test result. This disadvantage was shown, for example, for H somni.[19] The use of quantitative PCR is more informative because the pathogen load, especially in the respiratory disease complex, is important to consider. For this reason, quantitative PCR is increasingly used in veterinary laboratories, although interpretative questions remain. Especially, when multiple pathogens are detected, determining the attributable fraction of each pathogen to the clinical presentation remains very difficult.[38]

Next-Generation and Third-Generation Sequencing

NGS technologies are now becoming more widely available because of the democratization of the technologies, and because platforms such as MinION (Oxford Nanopore Technologies, Oxford, UK) allow decentralized sequencing experiments. The first studies using NGS (metagenomics) to detect viruses involved in BRD in feedlots are already reported; these detected known pathogenic viruses as well as previously unknown or incompletely understood viruses (eg, influenza D virus).[39,40] Hence, the advantage of NGS is that all pathogens can be simultaneously detected, without prior selection of which pathogens to test for. Also, semiquantitative results can be reported because, for most viruses, the number of reads corresponds to the initial load of the pathogen present.[41] Not only viruses but also whole genomes can be recovered at a scale that is constantly increasing. Eventually, direct sequencing of bacteria will allow detection of virulence genes, phylogenetic clustering of strains during outbreaks, and ultimately prediction of antimicrobial resistance based on single nucleotide polymorphisms or resistance genes. A high total bacterial burden and low bacterial community diversity were associated with positive culture results in classic microbial culture.[35] NGS is the basis for microbiome studies, which are discussed elsewhere in this issue.[42] Disadvantages are that NGS is costly and requires a long TAT under the current conditions using the most accurate devices (eg, Illumina, San Diego, CA). However, with nanopore sequencing platforms (eg, MinION) a higher throughput and shorter TAT can be achieved. This long-read technology has been commercially available since 2014 and has made tremendous improvements in output and accuracy. In humans and pigs, MinION has been used to characterize pathogens in different types of samples, even at the site of disease outbreaks, because data analysis can be done in the field on portable hardware.[43,44] On human lower respiratory tract samples, within 6 hours of sampling, a result was given at a sensitivity of 96.6%.[45] However, in order to achieve wide implementation in veterinary practice, the cost, the ability to correctly interpret, and setup of an actionable logistic chain will be essential. Therefore, this technology is another case in which analysis of pooled samples from multiple animals to obtain a group diagnosis of primary pathogens will be the most likely application.

INTERPRETATION OF DIAGNOSTIC TEST RESULTS AND SAMPLING STRATEGY

Clinical interpretation of a diagnostic test result to determine the infectious cause of a respiratory tract disease requires information on the pathogen identified, the site of the respiratory tract sampled, the diagnostic test used, the clinical condition of the animal, and whether the sample originates from a single animal or is pooled. There is no current consensus on the way to sample the respiratory tract or to interpret diagnostic test results in humans and many other species. Based on the available research, it is unlikely that an evidence-based consensus on respiratory tract sampling method, diagnostic testing, and interpretation of results in cattle can be reached. Hence, this article assists readers to properly interpret results of testing by providing information not only on current recommendations but especially on the drawbacks and research gaps.

Detection of Primary Pathogens

The first point to consider is the nature of the pathogen retrieved, whether it is a primary or secondary pathogen. A primary or obligate pathogen (when present), per definition, induces damage to the respiratory tract, mostly followed by an inflammatory response. However, depending on the infectious dose and host immunity, infection might result in clinical disease or not. Also, certain primary pathogens can chronically and even asymptomatically infect animals, resulting in carriers: for example, *Salmonella* spp or *M bovis*. Most primary pathogens weaken innate immunity of the airways, facilitating superinfection by opportunistic bacteria. Some, such as bovine respiratory syncytial virus, bovine herpesvirus type 1 (BHV-1), and potentially also others (**Table 3**), are able to induce life-threatening disease without bacterial superinfection. Despite still being controversial in some scientific communities or countries, *M bovis* is generally considered a primary pathogen.[46] Detection of a primary pathogen can, with some caution, be interpreted straightforwardly. The primary pathogen should normally not be present, and, depending on its virulence, it can, either as a sole agent or in combination with other agents, be held responsible for the clinical picture. Also, detection from any site of the respiratory tract is meaningful. For animal welfare reasons and following the pathogenesis, which starts with nasal infection, DNS samples might be sufficient and even most appropriate to detect primary pathogens. However, detection rates at the different sites of the respiratory tract differ between pathogens. For bovine coronavirus, DNS was more frequently positive than samples from the lower respiratory tract, whereas the inverse was true for bovine respiratory syncytial virus.[17] For BHV-1, DNS is recommended given that the infection most frequently remains limited to the upper airways. The true interest of any diagnostic effort lies in extrapolation of test results from the sampled animals to the whole group. Detection of primary pathogens in some animals makes involvement of the same pathogen in the cohoused animals very likely.[47] Hence, to improve sensitivity of the group diagnosis,

Table 3
Overview of viruses and bacteria commonly isolated from samples of the respiratory tract in cattle

Pathogen	Primary or Secondary Pathogen	Remarks	Reference
Bovine adenovirus	Primary, but controversial	Widespread, but generally mild disease, except immunocompromised calves (types 3, 4, and 7) Type 10 associated with lethal enteritis	58–61
Bovine coronavirus	Primary, but controversial	As a sole agent, experimentally only able to induce mild disease. Outbreaks with single viral infection resulting in severe morbidity and mortality described in calves and adult cattle	62,63
BHV-1	Primary	Limited to the nasal cavity, pharynx, and trachea. Immunosuppression by hampering function and number of white blood cells. Potentially lethal as a single agent	62
Bovine rhinitis virus A and B	Likely apathogenic	—	39
Bovine respiratory syncytial virus	Primary	As a single viral agent, able to cause lethal bronchopneumonia. In older animals frequently subclinical	52,62
Bovine viral diarrhea virus	Primary	Mainly immunosuppression by hampering function and number of white blood cells. Potentially lethal as a single agent	62,64
Parainfluenza virus type 3	Primary	As a single agent, generally mild disease	52,62
Influenza D virus	Controversial, likely primary	As a sole agent, experimentally only able to induce mild disease. Epidemiologically linked with disease	39,65
Bibersteinia trehalosi	Secondary	Occasionally isolated from cattle. More pathogenic role attributed to this bacterium in sheep	66
Histophilus somni	Controversial, likely secondary	Part of the resident flora. Septicemia is a lethal complication resulting in myocarditis, polyserositis, and thrombotic meningoencephalitis. Risk factors of septicemia unclear	52
Mannheimia haemolytica	Controversial, likely secondary	Part of the resident flora, differences in strain virulence described possibly resulting in some primary pathogenic strains. Other studies show cattle to become ill from their own resident strain on exposure to other pathogens and/or risk factors	11,49,52
Chlamydia psittaci	Controversial, likely primary	Natural infections result in mild or subclinical disease	75

(continued on next page)

Table 3
(continued)

Pathogen	Primary or Secondary Pathogen	Remarks	Reference
M bovis	Primary	Extended immunosuppressive effect on white blood cells combined with immune-evasive mechanisms resulting in chronicity. Clonal spread of a strain limited in time and space is the general rule	46,47
Mycoplasma bovirhinis	Apathogenic	—	19
Mycoplasma dispar	Controversial, likely apathogenic	Recently shown to be more part of the microbiome of feedlot cattle classified as healthy	14,19,67
Moraxella bovis/ovis	Secondary	Primary eye pathogen, occasionally isolated in pure culture from animals with bronchopneumonia	68
Pasteurella multocida	Secondary	Part of the resident flora. Strain virulence differences exist, and some disease presentations (eg, septicemia or peritonitis) have been linked to certain strains	52,69
Salmonella spp	Primary	Primary site of infection of most Salmonella spp is the gastrointestinal tract. Localization in the respiratory tract is possible, most likely after septicemic spread	70
Trueperella pyogenes	Secondary	Involved in purulent processes. Often regarded as characteristic for chronicity. However, naturally resistant to fluoroquinolones	71
Escherichia coli, Gallibacterium anatis, Enterobacter hormaechei, staphylococci, streptococci, fungi	Secondary	Single reports on cattle-specific strains isolated in pure culture in an outbreak of pneumonia in calves	52,72–74

Multiple other bacterial species can be detected in the bovine respiratory tract. This table is limited to either known primary pathogens or frequently isolated pathogens, currently assumed to have a pathogenic significance.
Data from Refs.[11,14,19,39,46,47,49,52,58–74]

the use of PCR on a pooled sample (up to 5 animals) can be considered.[36,37] A pitfall when working with PCR to detect primary pathogens is that vaccine antigen can be detected up to 14 days after intranasal vaccination with a live vaccine, resulting in false-positives.[48]

Detection of Secondary Pathogens

A secondary or opportunistic pathogen can be part of the normal respiratory micro-biome, without inducing inflammation. In general, breaching of innate immunity, either by another pathogen or a noninfectious cause, is needed before the opportunistic pathogen invades tissues and induces inflammation. Interpretation of detection of an opportunistic pathogen is more difficult, given that they can be present in healthy animals.[10,16,19] Therefore, simply detecting the pathogen cannot be seen as evidence of its involvement. The Pasteurellaceae family and a range of other bacteria (eg, *Streptococcus* spp and *Trueperella pyogenes*) are generally considered secondary pathogens. Although there seems to be little discussion of *P multocida*, scientific opinions on the potential primary role and differences in strain virulence of *M haemolytica* and *H somni* vary greatly.[11,49] It is outside the scope of this article to review or take a position on this matter. Similarly, in other species, including humans, this issue of opportunistic pathogens exists. When interpreting a positive culture result, a differentiation between contamination, colonization, and infection needs to be made. Contamination is defined as the presence, usually in low numbers, of bacteria in a sample that are not expected to be present in the sampled site. Colonization can be defined as the presence of a micro-organism in a host, with growth and multiplication of the organism, but without interaction between host and organisms, hence no inflammatory reaction, immune response, or clinical expression occurs.[50] Similarly, infection is isolation of a high number of bacteria from a site of the respiratory tract, but in the presence of inflammation of the mucosa, presenting either clinically or subclinically.[50] Hence, simply picking a suspected colony from an agar plate, to confirm the cause of the respiratory disease, and subsequently using an antibiogram based on this single colony may be misleading. More information can be derived from culture results if quantitative descriptions and at least the degree of contamination are described. A possible way to better describe culture results, previously used for research purposes,[10,33] is presented in **Table 4**. It is also important to realize that using selective media for Pasteurellaceae, as, for example, by adding bacitracin, ensures better growth and detection of these opportunistic pathogens, but information on the amount of pathogens and degree of contamination of the sample will be lost.[5,51]

Pasteurellaceae are part of the normal respiratory flora, and can even be abundantly present in the nasal cavity of healthy animals.[52] An association between the presence of a *Pasteurella* species in the nose and its presence in the lower respiratory tract is described.[10,15,16] However, interpretation of DNS results for opportunistic pathogens remains very difficult, especially because the composition of the nasopharyngeal microbiota seems to be heavily influenced by bioaerosols from the agricultural environment.[53] Loss of biodiversity and overgrowth of opportunistic pathogens occurs in the pathogenesis of BRD, resulting in higher odds that Pasteurellaceae can be cultured from nasal swabs in larger quantities in ill animals.[10,35,54] However, with current knowledge on the interpretation of DNS results at the individual or group level, samples of the lower respiratory tract are likely a better option to evaluate potential involvement of opportunistic pathogens. Interpretation of detection of opportunists in lower respiratory tract samples remains difficult, even in ill animals, because, even with very strict clinical case definitions, Pasteurellaceae can also be cultured from the lower airways in healthy animals.[10,14] Previously explored ways to overcome the issue of interpreting detection

Table 4
Overview of possible culture results for respiratory samples from cattle

Observation	Interpretation	Explanation
	Negative culture	No growth
	Pure culture	Abundant growth of a single bacterial species
	Dominant culture	Abundant growth of 1 bacterial species combined with a limited number of colonies from other bacteria (contaminants)
	Mixed culture	Equal growth of 2 bacterial species (primary or secondary pathogens)
	Polymicrobial culture	Growth of multiple bacterial species (and possibly molds), of which the most dominant ones are considered apathogenic for the host (contaminants or apathogenic flora)

All cultures are on Columbia blood agar and derived from nonendoscopic bronchoalveolar lavage samples.
Images courtesy of Dr. L. Van Driessche, PhD, Merelbeke, Belgium.

of opportunistic pathogens in humans and other species are the use of quantitative cultures or cytologic evidence of inflammation. Quantitative culture is derived from the assumption that, in case of a severe infection, the opportunistic pathogen will be present in larger numbers.[50] Cutoffs such as greater than 10^3 colony-forming units per milliliter of BAL fluid have been suggested in dogs and horses.[20,55] However, pathogen burden builds up, and sampling early in the disease process could mean that much lower numbers are detected despite the pathogen being involved in the inflammatory process.[56] Another option is derived from the assumption that a bacterial infection will result in a massive airway neutrophilia.[55] However, clear cutoff percentages for neutrophilia differentiating a bacterial infection from a viral one or a strictly noninfectious airway inflammation have not been determined in calves. Given that some BAL techniques result in a larger contribution of the bronchial component in the total BAL fluid, the neutrophil percentage is increased compared with a larger volume of mainly alveolar lavage fluid.[21] Primary insights in calf BAL fluid analysis show that cytologic parameters coincide poorly with clinical or ultrasonographical findings or culture results for opportunistic pathogens, at least when using nBAL.[57] The presence of phagocytosis by bacteria in neutrophils or macrophages may be helpful to differentiate active infection versus simple presence of the bacteria.[57] Although interpreting culture results for opportunistic pathogens is already difficult, interpretation of PCR results is even more so. Not only can insignificant quantities or even dead bacteria result in a positive PCR, the nasal passages also pick up bacterial DNA, making the lower respiratory tract sample positive. Quantitative PCR might overcome this issue, but, to the authors' knowledge, no guidelines on how to interpret these results are currently available in the bovine species.

Sampling Strategy

Although laboratory costs are fixed, the return on investment of an analysis greatly depends on selection of appropriate animals to sample and on the technical sampling skills of the veterinarian. An animal in the first days of the disease, not previously treated with antimicrobials and not displaying severe respiratory signs, is first choice. By sampling in the acute phase of the disease, the odds of detecting the viral component are higher. By avoiding previous antimicrobial treatment and by sampling early in the disease course, the probability that the antibiogram derived is useful for empiric therapy increases. By avoiding sampling animals in heavy respiratory distress, the odds of aggravation of disease or even mortality can be decreased.

In addition, in spite of all reasoning made earlier, veterinarians still make decisions at an individual animal level. When sampling an individual, the main interest is usually to make a decision representing the group, and to judge the utility of the diagnostic test to support this group decision. Different epidemiologic approaches are possible to determine an appropriate sample size. The goal is more a detection of disease approach (being 95% confident that the pathogen was detected when present) rather than determining the prevalence of the pathogen in a group of animals. In the field, sample size is currently more driven by practical reasons such as available time to sample or maximum samples allowed to pool for economic reasons. For example, performing PCR on pools of 5 animals increases sensitivity without diluting the sample too much. **Fig. 2** provides an overview on the risk of not finding a positive animal in 2 scenarios, 1 related to 100% prevalence of the pathogen in the diseased population and 1 scenario with a pretest probability that 70% of sick calves are affected by the pathogen (ie, where multiple pathogens are involved and can cause the same clinical disease). Results of a test with 70% sensitivity (ie, detects the pathogen in 7 of 10 infected calves) and 100% specificity (no false-positive calves) are presented. Using this test in a scenario with 70% of the affected animals being positive for the pathogen, after 5 calves not finding a positive, will misclassify only 3.5% of the herds (the 2 scenarios assume that the pooled tests' accuracy is the same as the individual test). In the case of opportunistic pathogens, given that they can be found in healthy or subclinical animals, at this time it might be most prudent to only sample animals with evidence of clinical bronchopneumonia by using a combination of clinical scoring and thoracic ultrasonography.[57] Focusing on bacterial isolation to direct intervention strategies, without taking the clinical status into account, holds great danger for overtreatment with antimicrobials.

CONCLUDING REMARKS

Knowledge of respiratory health is rapidly evolving in animals, following new developments in humans. In particular, better insights into the role of the respiratory microbiome and the interaction of the airway inflammatory response with different

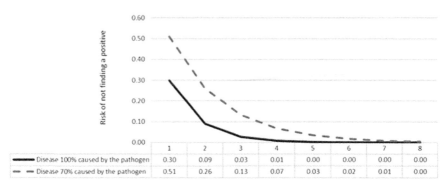

	1	2	3	4	5	6	7	8
Disease 100% caused by the pathogen	0.30	0.09	0.03	0.01	0.00	0.00	0.00	0.00
Disease 70% caused by the pathogen	0.51	0.26	0.13	0.07	0.03	0.02	0.01	0.00

Fig. 2. Risk (probability ranging between 0 and 1) of not finding a positive animal for a given pathogen according to sample size (x axis) in a scenario where 100% (*solid line*) and 70% (*dashed line*) of affected animals are positive for a given pathogen. The graph represents a test with 70% sensitivity and 100% specificity. It assumes that there are no false-positive results (ie, when the test indicates that the pathogen is present, this is a true-positive result). In the example where the pathogen is causing the disease in 100% of affected calves, the risk of not finding an infected animal after sampling n cases is $(1\text{-}Se)^n$, where Se is the test sensitivity. In the alternative scenario where only 70% of cases are caused by the pathogen (ie, in 30% of cases, this is another cause), the probability of not finding a case is $(1\text{-}0.7*Se)^n$.

organisms and air pollutants are likely to change how the diagnostic tests discussed in this article are interpreted. The authors hope that the information, tools, and provisional advice provided can aid the large group of cattle veterinarians, already having to make rational treatment decisions today.

DISCLOSURE

B. Pardon has received honoraria for acting as speaker or consultant for pharmaceutical (Zoetis, MSD, Vetoquinol, Dopharma, Boehringer Ingelheim, Dechra, Hipra, Ceva, Merial, and Elanco), agricultural (Algoet nutrition), and chemical (Proviron) companies and nonprofit organizations (Boerenbond, AMCRA, DGZ-Vlaanderen). S. Buczinski has received honoraria for acting as speaker or consultant as well as research grants for pharmaceutical companies (Zoetis, MSD, Hipra, and Ceva) and companies involved in commercialization of ancillary tests used in respiratory diseases (El Medical Imaging, Geissler Corp.).

REFERENCES

1. Fulton RW, Confer AW. Laboratory test descriptions for bovine respiratory disease diagnosis and their strengths and weaknesses: gold standards for diagnosis, do they exist? Can Vet J 2012;53:754–61.
2. FVE (Federation of Veterinarians of Europe). FVE guidelines for responsible use of antibiotics. Available at: https://wwwfveorg/cms/wp-content/uploads/FVE_sheet_vet_doctor_dentist_EN_november_2014_webpdf 2019.
3. de With K, Allerberger F, Amann S, et al. Strategies to enhance rational use of antibiotics in hospital: a guideline by the German Society for Infectious Diseases. Infection 2016;44:395–439.
4. Catry B, Dewulf J, Maes D, et al. Effect of antimicrobial consumption and production type on antibacterial resistance in the bovine respiratory and digestive tract. PLoS One 2016;11:e0146488.

5. Timsit E, Hallewell J, Booker C, et al. Prevalence and antimicrobial susceptibility of *Mannheimia haemolytica, Pasteurella multocida*, and *Histophilus somni* isolated from the lower respiratory tract of healthy feedlot cattle and those diagnosed with bovine respiratory disease. Vet Microbiol 2017;208:118–25.

6. AMCRA. Classification of antimicrobials: methods. 2019. Available at: https://formularium.amcra.be/classification.php.

7. KNMVD. Procedures for the development of formularies for responsible antimicrobial use. 2015. Available at: https://www.knmvd.nl/app/uploads/sites/4/2018/09/150209-procedure-opstellen-formularia-definitief.pdf.

8. WHO (World Health Organization). Critically important antimicrobials for human medicine, 6th revision. 2019. Available at: https://apps.who.int/iris/bitstream/handle/10665/312266/9789241515528-eng.pdf?ua=1.

9. Buczinski S, Pardon B. BRD diagnosis: what progress have we made in clinical diagnosis? Vet Clin North Am Food Anim Pract 2020;36(2):399–423.

10. Van Driessche L, Valgaeren BR, Gille L, et al. A deep nasopharyngeal swab versus nonendoscopic bronchoalveolar lavage for isolation of bacterial pathogens from preweaned calves with respiratory disease. J Vet Intern Med 2017;31:946–53.

11. Timsit E, Christensen H, Bareille N, et al. Transmission dynamics of *Mannheimia haemolytica* in newly-received beef bulls at fattening operations. Vet Microbiol 2013;161:295–304.

12. Viso M, el Jaraki MR, Espinasse J, et al. A sequential broncho-alveolar washing in non-anaesthetized normal bovines: method and preliminary results. Vet Res Commun 1985;9:213–9.

13. McMullen C, Orsel K, Alexander TW, et al. Comparison of the nasopharyngeal bacterial microbiota of beef calves raised without the use of antimicrobials between healthy calves and those diagnosed with bovine respiratory disease. Vet Microbiol 2019;231:56–62.

14. Timsit E, Workentine M, van der Meer F, et al. Distinct bacterial metacommunities inhabit the upper and lower respiratory tracts of healthy feedlot cattle and those diagnosed with bronchopneumonia. Vet Microbiol 2018;221:105–13.

15. Godinho KS, Sarasola P, Renoult E, et al. Use of deep nasopharyngeal swabs as a predictive diagnostic method for natural respiratory infections in calves. Vet Rec 2007;160:22–5.

16. Allen JW, Viel L, Bateman KG, et al. The microbial flora of the respiratory tract in feedlot calves: associations between nasopharyngeal and bronchoalveolar lavage cultures. Can J Vet Res 1991;55:341–6.

17. Doyle D, Credille B, Lehenbauer TW, et al. Agreement among 4 sampling methods to identify respiratory pathogens in dairy calves with acute bovine respiratory disease. J Vet Intern Med 2017;31:954–9.

18. Heckert HP, Rohn M, Hofmann W. Sample collection for diagnostics of bovine respiratory diseases. Prakt Tierarzt 1997;78:1056.

19. Angen O, Thomsen J, Larsen LE, et al. Respiratory disease in calves: microbiological investigations on trans-tracheally aspirated bronchoalveolar fluid and acute phase protein response. Vet Microbiol 2009;137:165–71.

20. Hodgson JL. Collection and interpretation of tracheal wash and bronchoalveolar lavage for diagnosis of infectious and non-infectious lower airway disorders. In: Proceedings of the 9th International Congress of WEVA. Marrakech, Morocco, 2006. p. 71–7.

21. van Leenen K, Van Driessche L, De Cremer L, et al. Factors associated with lung cytology as obtained by non-endoscopic broncho-alveolar lavage in group-housed calves. BMC Vet Res 2019;15:167.

22. Van Driessche L, Valgaeren B, De Schutter P, et al. Effect of sedation on the intrapulmonary position of a bronchoalveolar lavage catheter in calves. Vet Rec 2016;179.

23. Allen TH, Johnson EG, Edmonds MD, et al. Influence of tilmicosin on quantified pulmonary concentrations of three bacterial pathogens in calves with naturally-occurring bovine respiratory disease. Bovine Pract 2013;47:65–72.

24. Lavigne MC. Nonbronchoscopic methods [Nonbronchoscopic Bronchoalveolar Lavage (BAL), Mini-BAL, Blinded Bronchial Sampling, Blinded Protected Specimen Brush] to investigate for pulmonary infections, inflammation, and cellular and molecular markers: a narrative review. Clin Pulm Med 2017;24:13–25.

25. Roelants B. Comparison of deep nasopharyngeal swab, bronchoalveolar lavage and transtracheal wash for the diagnosis of infectious bronchopneumonia in calves: which one is most animal friendly? Master students thesis. Ghent University; 2018. Available at: https://lib.ugent.be/catalog/rug01:002481486.

26. Orard M, Depecker M, Hue E, et al. Influence of bronchoalveolar lavage volume on cytological profiles and subsequent diagnosis of inflammatory airway disease in horses. Vet J 2016;207:193–5.

27. Van Driessche L. It's about time. Rapid detection and susceptibility testing of Pasteurellaceae causing respiratory disease in cattle by MALDI-TOF MS [PhD thesis]. Merelbeke (Belgium): Ghent University; 2019. p. 1–279.

28. Prado ME, Prado TM, Payton M, et al. Maternally and naturally acquired antibodies to Mannheimia haemolytica and Pasteurella multocida in beef calves. Vet Immunol Immunopathol 2006;111:301–7.

29. Parker AM, Sheehy PA, Hazelton MS, et al. A review of mycoplasma diagnostics in cattle. J Vet Intern Med 2018;32:1241–52.

30. Quinn PF, Carter ME, Markey B, et al. Haemophilus species. In: Quinn PJ, editor. Clinical veterinary microbiology35. London: Mosby International Limited; 1994. p. 121–8.

31. Bokma J, Van Driessche L, Deprez P, et al. Rapid identification of mycoplasma bovis from bovine bronchoalveolar lavage fluid with MALDI-TOF MS after enrichment procedure. J Clin Microbiol 2020. [Epub ahead of print].

32. Spergser J, Hess C, Loncaric I, et al. Matrix-assisted laser desorption ionization-time of flight mass spectrometry is a superior diagnostic tool for the identification and differentiation of Mycoplasmas isolated from animals. J Clin Microbiol 2019; 57 [pii:e00316-19].

33. Van Driessche L, Bokma J, Deprez P, et al. Rapid identification of respiratory bacterial pathogens from bronchoalveolar lavage fluid in cattle by MALDI-TOF MS. Sci Rep 2019;9:18381.

34. Van Driessche L, Bokma J, Gille L, et al. Rapid detection of tetracycline resistance in bovine Pasteurella multocida isolates by MALDI Biotyper antibiotic susceptibility test rapid assay (MBT-ASTRA). Sci Rep 2018;8:13599.

35. Dickson RP, Erb-Downward JR, Prescott HC, et al. Analysis of culture-dependent versus culture-independent techniques for identification of bacteria in clinically obtained bronchoalveolar lavage fluid. J Clin Microbiol 2014;52:3605–13.

36. O'Neill R, Mooney J, Connaghan E, et al. Patterns of detection of respiratory viruses in nasal swabs from calves in Ireland: a retrospective study. Vet Rec 2014;175:351.

37. Pardon B, Callens J, Maris J, et al. Pathogen-specific risk factors in acute outbreaks of respiratory disease in calves. J Dairy Sci 2020;2556–66.

38. Deloria Knoll M, Fu W, Shi Q, et al. Bayesian estimation of pneumonia etiology: epidemiologic considerations and applications to the pneumonia etiology research for child health study. Clin Infect Dis 2017;64:S213–27.

39. Mitra N, Cernicchiaro N, Torres S, et al. Metagenomic characterization of the virome associated with bovine respiratory disease in feedlot cattle identified novel viruses and suggests an etiologic role for influenza D virus. J Gen Virol 2016;97:1771–84.

40. Zhang M, Hill JE, Fernando C, et al. Respiratory viruses identified in western Canadian beef cattle by metagenomic sequencing and their association with bovine respiratory disease. Transbound Emerg Dis 2019;66:1379–86.

41. Conceicao-Neto N, Zeller M, Lefrere H, et al. Modular approach to customise sample preparation procedures for viral metagenomics: a reproducible protocol for virome analysis. Sci Rep 2015;5:16532.

42. Timsit E, McMullen C, Amat S, et al. Respiratory bacterial microbiota in cattle: from development to modulation to enhance respiratory health. Vet Clin North Am Food Anim Pract 2020;36(2):297–320.

43. Quick J, Grubaugh ND, Pullan ST, et al. Multiplex PCR method for MinION and Illumina sequencing of Zika and other virus genomes directly from clinical samples. Nat Protoc 2017;12:1261–76.

44. Theuns S, Vanmechelen B, Bernaert Q, et al. Nanopore sequencing as a revolutionary diagnostic tool for porcine viral enteric disease complexes identifies porcine kobuvirus as an important enteric virus. Sci Rep 2018;8:9830.

45. Charalampous T, Kay GL, Richardson H, et al. Nanopore metagenomics enables rapid clinical diagnosis of bacterial lower respiratory infection. Nat Biotechnol 2019;37:783–92.

46. Maunsell FP, Woolums AR, Francoz D, et al. *Mycoplasma bovis* infections in cattle. J Vet Intern Med 2011;25:772–83.

47. Timsit E, Arcangioli MA, Bareille N, et al. Transmission dynamics of *Mycoplasma bovis* in newly received beef bulls at fattening operations. J Vet Diagn Invest 2012;24:1172–6.

48. Timsit E, Le Drean E, Maingourd C, et al. Detection by real-time RT-PCR of a bovine respiratory syncytial virus vaccine in calves vaccinated intranasally. Vet Rec 2009;165:230–3.

49. Klima CL, Alexander TW, Hendrick S, et al. Characterization of *Mannheimia haemolytica* isolated from feedlot cattle that were healthy or treated for bovine respiratory disease. Can J Vet Res 2014;78:38–45.

50. Dani A. Colonization and infection. Cent European J Urol 2014;67:86–7.

51. Catry B, Haesebrouck F, Vliegher SD, et al. Variability in acquired resistance of Pasteurella and Mannheimia isolates from the nasopharynx of calves, with particular reference to different herd types. Microb Drug Resist 2005;11:387–94.

52. Griffin D, Chengappa MM, Kuszak J, et al. Bacterial pathogens of the bovine respiratory disease complex. Vet Clin North Am Food Anim Pract 2010;26:381–94.

53. Mbareche H, Veillette M, Pilote J, et al. Bioaerosols play a major role in the nasopharyngeal microbiota content in agricultural environment. Int J Environ Res Public Health 2019;16 [pii:E1375].

54. Stroebel C, Alexander T, Workentine ML, et al. Effects of transportation to and co-mingling at an auction market on nasopharyngeal and tracheal bacterial communities of recently weaned beef cattle. Vet Microbiol 2018;223:126–33.

55. Peeters DE, McKiernan BC, Weisiger RM, et al. Quantitative bacterial cultures and cytological examination of bronchoalveolar lavage specimens in dogs. J Vet Intern Med 2000;14:534–41.

56. Ackermann MR, Gallup JM, Zabner J, et al. Differential expression of sheep beta-defensin-1 and -2 and interleukin 8 during acute Mannheimia haemolytica pneumonia. Microb Pathog 2004;37:21–7.

57. van Leenen K, Van Driessche L, De Cremer L, et al. Comparison of bronchoalveolar lavage fluid bacteriology and cytology in calves classified based on combined clinical scoring and lung ultrasonography. Prev Vet Med 2020;176:104901.

58. Vaatstra BL, Tisdall DJ, Blackwood M, et al. Clinicopathological features of 11 suspected outbreaks of bovine adenovirus infection and development of a real-time quantitative PCR to detect bovine adenovirus type 10. N Z Vet J 2016;64:308–13.

59. Pardon B, De Bleecker K, Dewulf J, et al. Prevalence of respiratory pathogens in diseased, non-vaccinated, routinely medicated veal calves. Vet Rec 2011;169:278.

60. Narita M, Yamada M, Tsuboi T, et al. Bovine adenovirus type 3 pneumonia in dexamethasone-treated calves. Vet Pathol 2003;40:128–35.

61. Yamada M, Narita M, Nakamura K, et al. Apoptosis in calf pneumonia induced by endobronchial inoculation with bovine adenovirus type 3 (BAV-3). J Comp Pathol 2003;128:140–5.

62. Grissett GP, White BJ, Larson RL. Structured literature review of responses of cattle to viral and bacterial pathogens causing bovine respiratory disease complex. J Vet Intern Med 2015;29:770–80.

63. Ellis J. What is the evidence that bovine coronavirus is a biologically significant respiratory pathogen in cattle? Can Vet J 2019;60:147–52.

64. Larson RL. Bovine viral diarrhea virus-associated disease in feedlot cattle. Vet Clin North Am Food Anim Pract 2015;31:367–80, vi.

65. Ferguson L, Olivier AK, Genova S, et al. Pathogenesis of Influenza D virus in cattle. J Virol 2016;90:5636–42.

66. Hanthorn CJ, Dewell RD, Cooper VL, et al. Randomized clinical trial to evaluate the pathogenicity of Bibersteinia trehalosi in respiratory disease among calves. BMC Vet Res 2014;10:89.

67. McMullen C, Orsel K, Alexander TW, et al. Evolution of the nasopharyngeal bacterial microbiota of beef calves from spring processing to 40 days after feedlot arrival. Vet Microbiol 2018;225:139–48.

68. Catry B, Boyen F, Baele M, et al. Recovery of Moraxella ovis from the bovine respiratory tract and differentiation of Moraxella species by tDNA-intergenic spacer PCR. Vet Microbiol 2007;120:375–80.

69. Catry B, Chiers K, Schwarz S, et al. Fatal peritonitis caused by Pasteurella multocida capsular type F in calves. J Clin Microbiol 2005;43:1480–3.

70. Rings DM. Salmonellosis in calves. Vet Clin North Am Food Anim Pract 1985;1:529–39.

71. Catry B, Croubels S, Schwarz S, et al. Influence of systemic fluoroquinolone administration on the presence of Pasteurella multocida in the upper respiratory tract of clinically healthy calves. Acta Vet Scand 2008;50:36.

72. Wang Z, Duan L, Liu F, et al. First report of Enterobacter hormaechei with respiratory disease in calves. BMC Vet Res 2020;16:1.

73. Contrepois M, Dubourguier HC, Parodi AL, et al. Septicaemic Escherichia coli and experimental infection of calves. Vet Microbiol 1986;12:109–18.

74. Van Driessche L, Vanneste K, Bogaerts B, et al. Isolation of drug-resistant Gallibacterium anatis from calves with unresponsive bronchopneumonia, Belgium. Emerg Infect Dis 2020;26(4). https://doi.org/10.3201/eid2604.190962.

75. Osterman C, Rüttger A, Schubert E, et al. Infection, disease, and transmission dynamics in calves after experimental and natural challenge with a Bovine Chlamydia psitacci isolate. Plos One 2013;8(5):e64066.

Details to Attend to When Managing High-Risk Cattle

John T. Groves, DVM

KEYWORDS

- Systems thinking • Complex adaptive system • Husbandry
- Bovine respiratory disease • Biocontainment

KEY POINTS

- Beef cattle production is North America is a complex adaptive system that is essential to understand and appreciate before long-term and sustainable improvements can be made to the management of high-risk cattle.
- Biocontainment and biosecurity strategies are often overlooked, but are high leverage opportunities to advance the management of high-risk cattle.
- The development of efficient vaccination and treatment protocols require well-informed veterinary expertise and a systems-level understanding of the business models of operations managing high-risk cattle.

INTRODUCTION

Beef cattle production has evolved over time to capture economic efficiencies into a large, complex, and adaptive system that can be difficult to understand and appreciate. North America in particular has a very diverse and broad industry that is fundamentally segmented. The segmented nature of the beef production model is an important structural feature and a critical reason that high-risk cattle exist. Ranches and cow–calf operations produce calves on a semiseasonal schedule with most calves born in the spring, although a significant number of calves are born throughout the rest of the year. However, cattle finishing by feedlots is essentially constant throughout the year, to efficiently meet consumer demand and thus the needs of the meat packing industry. One of the critical roles of the stocker industry is to manage the discontinuity of the supply chain of feeder calves that exists between cow–calf operations and feedlot operations.[1] The stocker segment of the industry has advanced over time not only to act as a holding point to absorb excess and irregular capacity of calf product, but also to add value to the feeder calf in ways that make it more fit for movement to the feeding/finishing sector.[2] Many calves produced in North America are unfit to move directly to the feeding segment from many standpoints, such as immunologic naivete, weaning status, lot size, nutritional status, weight, age, and

Livestock Veterinary Service, PO Box 353, 917 South Aurora Street, Eldon, MO 65026, USA
E-mail address: john@livestockvetservice.com

Vet Clin Food Anim 36 (2020) 445–460
https://doi.org/10.1016/j.cvfa.2020.02.005
0749-0720/20/© 2020 Elsevier Inc. All rights reserved.

sexual status. Both cultural and economic drivers can motivate cow–calf operations to market calves to meet cash flow demands at a point before they can be prepared adequately.

Because of these production model structures, many calves are marketed as un-weaned, immunologically naïve, and sexually intact through sales auctions and are commingled into groups.[3] Because of their inclination for higher treatment rates for bovine respiratory disease (BRD), they are managed as high-risk calves. Populations of high-risk calves are routinely purchased in production models (both stocker and feedlot) designed specifically to address the challenges of increased BRD rates. Concomitant with addressing the increased health risk is the increased cost of pro-duction. The additional costs associated with these production models are borne pre-dominately by the seller of the calves in the form of a discount at the time of sale.[4] The dynamic between the level of discounts in the marketplace and the additional costs (financial, opportunity, and societal) associated with handling high-risk calves pro-duces some unintended consequences over time that can be self-perpetuating. As veterinarians and producers more economically and efficiently manage the increased risk for BRD in these cattle populations, a vicious cycle is initiated in which the oper-ations are motivated to buy ever larger numbers of high-risk calves over time and un-intentionally contribute to escalating BRD risk even more.[5] The systems-thinking causal flow diagram (**Fig. 1**) illustrates the relationship between effectively managing BRD risk in the short term and producing the long-term and delayed unintended consequence of increasing BRD risk by purchasing greater numbers of calves to

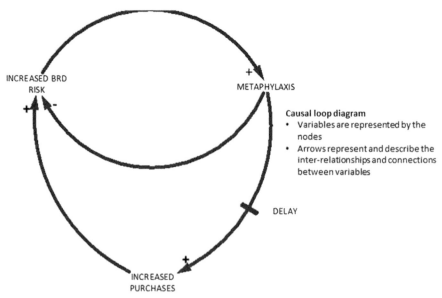

Fig. 1. This causal loop diagram illustrates how an effective solution in the short-term cre-ates unintended consequences for the long-term behavior of the system and could result in the need for more solutions.

manage with the same resources. In the example in this article, increased BRD risk is mitigated by implementation of antimicrobial metaphylaxis, which in the short term is a successful strategy; however, as the operation becomes adept at using this tool, producers are motivated to purchase more calves. Over time and as more calves enter the operation, BRD risk insidiously escalates. Awareness of these systems-level adaptations and changes are key details relevant to sustainable and long-term management strategies[5] for high-risk calves. Veterinarians and producers aware of these relationships are better able to address the fundamental issues in their production models, rather than just symptomatically addressing problems as they arise.

DEFINING SUCCESS IN MANAGING HIGH-RISK CALVES

Operations handling high-risk calves fulfill a systems-level requirement to produce high-quality feeder cattle for the finishing sector. Owing to this aspect of their business model, it is important to look beyond traditional close-out metrics when defining success. Traditionally, health and management approaches have been assessed by performance and health metrics linked to 45- to 60-day close-out reports similar to finishing operations. Owing to the multifaceted nature of operations that handle high-risk calves, a more comprehensive methodology is appropriate. Fundamentally, these operations must provide calves to the finishing sector with low variability, robust protective immunity across a broad range of pathogens, and in quantities sufficient to meet the feedlot's demand over time. The development of robust protective immunity against the pathogens and challenges encountered upon placement in the feedlot lies at the foundation of the function of these operations. Calves leaving these operations require levels of protective immunity sufficient to overcome the challenges of transitioning to the feeding and finishing sector. As the beef feeding and finishing sector currently exists, long hauls and additional commingling are often required. Cattle not sufficiently prepared for this transition will be challenged with additional BRD risk.

Balance and diligence are required in managing the short-term and long-term health expectations so they do not become mutually exclusive. High-risk calves managed with the sole goal of minimizing BRD morbidity and mortality during the first 60 days can sometimes have difficulty and delays in addressing the need to strengthen immunity in the long term. Conversely, operations focusing on quickly establishing high levels of immunity often have to deal with increased BRD morbidity and mortality early in the receiving period. Successful management strategies are those that correctly balance both short-term and long-term challenges surrounding high-risk cattle in a way that are sustainable and adaptable over time. Without discipline and effective communication with the management team, it is possible to focus so much effort and attention on the short-term health challenges of an operation that it hinders management's ability to properly address long-term health challenges[5] (**Fig. 2**). Because of how health metrics are measured in the feeding and finishing sector, many operations that handle high-risk cattle focus their resources on short-term strategies to such an extent that it becomes difficult to impossible to devote the effort needed to fundamentally address the long-term health program that usually requires more time to implement and reap benefits.

BIOCONTAINMENT STRATEGIES AND DISEASE DYNAMICS IMPERATIVE TO SUSTAINABILITY IN STOCKER OPERATIONS

Predictably, the veterinary and scientific communities have expended tremendous effort investigating and better understanding a myriad of variables contributing to

Shifting the Burden

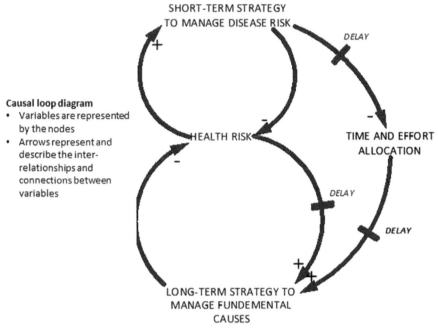

Fig. 2. This causal loop diagram illustrates how effort to manage short-term strategies can insidiously over time lead to an unintended reduction in the time and effort allocated to long-term fundamental strategies, which often require more effort and time to reap measurable paybacks.

increased risk of untoward health outcomes in feeder cattle systems. Traditionally most scientific effort has focused on 3 main areas:

1. Risk factors inherent to the calf – immune status and function, age, weight, breed, weaning status, nutritional status, genetic considerations, sexual status, and so on.[6,7]
2. Risk factors inherent to pathogens – virulence mechanisms, mutations, copathogen synergies, mechanisms of immune system evasion, and so on.[7]
3. Risk factors inherent to marketing channels – commingling, social stress, nutritional stress, transportation stress, and so on.[7]

Not to diminish the critical importance of better understanding health risk in these traditional ways, but this is only a partial understanding of what contributes to the health risks in high-risk cattle populations. Many professionals working in feeder cattle production systems would recognize the health status of the resident receiving population as having the greatest impact on the health outcomes of the incoming cattle.[8] Operations managing high-risk cattle are in a precarious and somewhat unique situation. The populations of cattle moving into these operations are typically healthy, and the resident population they are entering is often experiencing or recovering from an epidemic of BRD. This type of scenario is a fundamental detail of managing high-risk cattle that is difficult to measure and appreciate. Because of their very nature, many stocker operations enter a vicious cycle of disease propagation that is unmanageable. Healthy, immunologically naïve cattle enter cattle facilities at regular intervals and serve as powerful amplifiers of the pathogens being circulated by the existing population, and, if left unchecked, uncontrollable disease will occur.[8] Although many practitioners and producers are conceptually and observationally aware of this, health outcomes deteriorate over time when dealing with populations of high-risk calves, because nearly all efforts have been directed at dealing with and managing all the traditional risk factors being studied by the scientific community and available in the literature. In the late 1990s and early 2000s, insightful recommendations were made for practical applications of biocontainment principles that effectively mitigated the cycle of disease inherent to many high-risk cattle production models.[8]

Key Biocontainment Principles

- Understanding the business models of the operations—unlike other segments of the cattle industry, stocker operations have developed diverse and adaptable business models. If not practical for the operation, biocontainment efforts will not be adopted.
- Understanding current disease status of existing cattle population—although many feeder cattle operations operate with limited professional veterinary input, those that use modern veterinary services as part of their management strategy have more insight into pathogen dynamics over time and are best positioned to use impactful biocontainment interventions.
- Effect of pen size on disease dynamics—as pen size increases, the risk and severity of epidemic disease increases. Mitigating disease risk by reducing pen size can be a powerful management technique.[9]
- Cattle flow—placement of immunologically naïve cattle in pens near or adjacent to cattle in the peak of a BRD epidemic provides opportunity for disease propagation and pathogen amplification. Strategically separating naïve and susceptible populations from epidemic and endemic populations is the foundation of biocontainment efforts.[8]
- Mitigating pathogen spread through use of common facilities such as hospital and treatment recovery pens.

Well-managed operations implementing biocontainment strategies in innovative ways have been able to grow their operations' size and profitability, while at the same time reduce antibiotic use and improve health. Some large diversified operations will use contract and cooperating producers to capitalize on the benefits of biocontainment in an all-in/all-out basis.

DATA, INFORMATION, AND KNOWLEDGE

The multiplicity of business models in the stocker segment, as well as the relatively fast pace of cattle flow, have outstripped management's ability to maintain up-to-date and relevant records in many operations handling high-risk cattle. Furthermore, metrics important to the success of 1 particular business model may not be applicable or as important in other models. Feedlot style health and production records work well in small and seasonal operations, but tend not to function well in large, diversified, and continuous flow operations that operate multiple business models simultaneously and regularly sort and blend cattle at certain points in the production chain.

Foundational to modern production medicine and production management is the concept that relevant information derived from observed and collected health and production data drive knowledgeable health and management protocols and decisions. Handicapping many operations handling high-risk cattle is the inherent and apparent information risk that arises from underdeveloped information structures. Correcting this inadequacy is often one of the highest leverage interventions a veterinary professional can contribute.

Groups of cattle often move through stocker systems quickly, which is not intuitive to those lacking experience with large adaptive stocker systems. Moreover, this rapid movement of populations, and the delays associated with many programs used for records analysis, make it difficult to acquire and maintain relevant numbers for analysis. Many successful operations have found innovative ways to address challenges associated with delays and operational segmentation. Dedicated data collection for defined stages of production, electronic reporting of events, tracking important metrics over time on process control type charts, and developing up-to-date dashboard reporting templates are all examples of adapting record systems to be more practical and functional.

Archiving data historically and using practical applications of epidemiologic principles allows operations and the veterinary professionals to collectively learn over time and address fundamentally the long-term challenges facing their production approach. Having the ability to learn, adapt, and improve over time are essential characteristics for sustainability.

PROCUREMENT

The structure of the marketing channels for feedlot cattle in North America is well-established and responsive to changes in market forces. As the value proposition available in the market place changes over time, perceptive cattle buyers and cattle buying organizations have the capability of assessing, with some degree of precision, the innate health risk of purchased cattle populations and can adjust their buying parameters.[4] Because of both market conditions and health considerations, buyers may elect to procure very high-risk cattle for a business model; conversely, they have the opportunity to buy cattle with less inherent health risk. Notably, many operations use this strategy in their overall BRD management program.

Although market forces often drive most decisions regarding the health risk of purchased cattle, an area often overlooked is the inadequacies of market facilities with regard to basic husbandry and access to hay and water. Managing BRD in high-risk calves is only made more difficult when calves do not receive reasonable basic husbandry care as they move through market facilities. Astute operators are aware of the animal care habits of different market facilities and make specific purchasing decisions based on that knowledge.

Owing to constraints surrounding lot size, market trends, and transportation logistics, many auction-derived and privately purchased high-risk calves move to commingling and shipping facilities for a short period of time. Historically, these facilities have increased the overall health risks associated with the cattle by compromising the quality of husbandry, extending the duration of stress, and providing a profound break in biocontainment that is difficult to overcome. Anecdotally, many of the worst health outcomes have been associated with these gathering facilities and the mass use of antimicrobials in an effort to maintain the health status of the population before shipping. However, many of these facilities still exist and have developed good husbandry and biocontainment practices that have allowed them to remain as important components to marketing channels.

TRANSPORT

The North American beef industry has evolved in a way that has made the logistics of cattle transportation a significant part of the system. It is important to consider, study, and manage the risks attributable to transport, and how those risks impact our ability to manage BRD. Traditionally, the cost and risks associated with transporting cattle have been borne by basis adjustments in price and accounted for in break-even estimates. Although cattle buyers have long understood the direct implications on hauling cattle, efforts to document and quantify more scientifically the long-term impact of cattle transport have only recently been undertaken.[10] Understanding which factors associating with cattle transport are most impactful to long-term health outcome are important details in managing BRD in high-risk cattle.[11] Chronicity of stress, dehydration, fasting, weather exposure (heat, cold), physical exhaustion, and physical injuries are obvious contributors to negative health outcomes, and their negative impact should be mitigated and managed when possible.[12] Pathogen exposure is an often-overlooked risk factor associated with long-haul cattle.[13]

Because the risks associated with transport are so great, operations that can procure and receive cattle with less transport risk may be able to manage high-risk cattle more effectively with regard to BRD. Industry observations indicate that over the past 15 years much of the management of high-risk calves has moved away from the High Plains to large diversified stocker operations in the Southeast and Midwest. Operations located regionally near the herds of origin for the high-risk calves are adventitiously positioned to receive cattle before stress becomes chronic. Many operations in the Midwest can purchase, transport, process, and place high-risk cattle populations in less than 24 hours, mitigating and avoiding many of the risks associated with long hauls.

ARRIVAL MANAGEMENT

Inadequate receiving facilities are common on operations that purchase high-risk cattle because of the nature of these operations as opportunity buyers. Having facilities designed to fit the particular needs of the operation is an important detail in the management of BRD in high-risk cattle. Historically, arrival facilities developed as a set of pens designed to hold cattle before processing. However, some progressive veterinarians and producers realized arrival facilities are a critical control point for biosecurity and biocontainment. Small operations and seasonal operations generally avoid many of the complexities of managing an arrival facility, but larger and more diverse operations need to understand the importance of maintaining biocontainment at arrival. Key components to biocontainment in arrival barns are as follows.

- Ensure adequate pens and space are available to keep purchase cohorts together, minimizing the need to resort cattle after receiving.
- Avoid carry-over population, that is, processed calves that remain in the arrival facility as new groups of calves arrive, between purchased groups. Do not keep resident populations in the arrival barn. Incubation times can be relatively short for many respiratory pathogens.[14] All-in/all-out management methods minimize the cross-contamination of pathogens between groups over time.

Pens in arrival facilities need to be well-shaded and well-ventilated and kept clean, dry, and dust free. Cattle received during the summer months are adversely affected by the increased temperatures, resulting in reduced performance, decreased animal comfort, and death.[15] Thus, provisions for heat abatement are important details during the summer months. The impacts of mud on feeder cattle are also substantial.[16] Cattle in mud have a tendency to eat less while at the same time have higher nutritional demands owing to heat loss.[17] Natural surfaces allow for better footing and are more conducive to low-stress handling techniques. A clean and ample water supply is critical so calves can correct their hydration status.[18,19] Because many high-risk calves have never previously consumed water from a tank or automatic waterer, many producers find it beneficial to manage watering equipment that takes advantage of natural cattle behavior and encourages calves to drink, such as:

- Place the waterer on the fence line, so calves are more likely to find it as they explore their pen;
- Allow enough waterer space, so that multiple calves can drink simultaneously; and
- Allow water to recirculate or overflow in a way that produces the sounds of running water.

Free choice grass hay is offered in the arrival pens at many operations and is helpful in promoting and maintaining rumen function.

In addition to the general functions of arrival facilities, many operations enhance arrival pens to meet their more specific needs. Operations that receive long-haul cattle that have endured chronic stress find it beneficial to build sufficient facilities that allow enough space to rest and recover before any health or management protocols. Many operations will develop a set of criteria that fits their production model to set the amount of time the calves are given to recover. Some operators will observe the cattle closely at arrival and when they see the return of some natural behaviors such as eating, drinking, and investigating their environment, they will consider handling the calves again.

It should be noted that some production systems benefit from making a decision at arrival to delaying receiving vaccination protocol for up to 30 days after arrival, until the calves are more physiologically recovered from the stress of marketing and transport.[20] Veterinarians and producers need to carefully consider the potential biocontainment impact on the operation and make provisions to minimize any unintended consequences.

RECEIVING HEALTH PROTOCOLS

Health programs at arrival are traditionally where most veterinarians devoted their time. The scientific community has published volumes on the topic; practitioners have used observation, clinical experience, and insight into production models to develop protocols; and individual operations have used trial and error to design their own programs. Unfortunately, because of the diversity that exists in the industry, no one master protocol would be appropriate for all production situations. There is tremendous opportunity in the industry for producers and veterinarians to work together and make rational, scientifically based, and systemically sustainable decisions to build health protocols that work.

Important tactical considerations in developing a receiving health protocol include the following.

- Physiologic state of the calves at arrival and duration of stress: we have known for a long time that stress impacts immune function and is an important risk factor for BRD. It has been conventional wisdom among many in the veterinary profession that immune suppression associated with stress, although important, was not enough in itself to warrant not vaccinating cattle at arrival. Current scientific work would suggest stress not only causes cattle to react poorly to vaccine, but there is mounting evidence that giving certain vaccines may be harmful under chronic stress conditions and produce negative impacts on health outcomes.[21,22]

- What is known about the risk status of the population of arriving calves?
- What is known about the current health status and health risks associated with the resident population?
- How many times can the calves be handled within the constraints of the business model to execute the health protocol?
- What is the overall business model of the operation and goal of health program?

VACCINATION FOR RESPIRATORY PATHOGENS

In North America, there are numerous approved and licensed preparations aimed at strengthening immunity and assisting in managing BRD, although there is surprisingly little literature describing the efficiency and safety of these products in different production systems, including the use of modified live virus vaccines in high-risk cattle.[23] Important viral pathogens such as bovine viral diarrhea virus (BVDV)-1, BVDV-2, BHV-1, and PI3V can all be addressed in vaccination protocols with a wide variety of products including both killed virus, modified live virus, and combination killed and modified live products available for both parenteral and intranasal administration. Multiple bacterin and toxoid products are available to combat the bacterial pathogens *Manheimia haemolytica*, *Pasteurella mutocida*, and *Histophilus somni*. Bacterial antigens are offered in combination with other antigen and as stand-alone products. Additionally, there are conditionally licensed and autogenous products available for other pathogens known to be involved with the BRD complex. Understanding potential unintended sequelae from vaccination, as well the impact of timing of vaccination on efficacy, are important when designing vaccination protocols.

Veterinary professionals working closely with high-risk cattle operations are valuably positioned to develop an understanding of the role individual pathogens and combinations of pathogens play as contributors to endemic and epidemic disease in specific production systems, and they should play the key role in designing vaccine protocols. Outside expertise and consultation is often very productive when making vaccine decisions owing to the rapidly evolving knowledge base surrounding BRD, vaccinology, and immune function.

Endotoxin-containing products should be used prudently in high-risk cattle.[23] Endotoxins are known to elicit high fevers, and cattle with altered immune function may be more susceptible to the negative effects of endotoxin.[24] Interactions from multiple simultaneous endotoxin-containing products, as well the interactions with other various animal health products, is not well-studied or well-understood.

METAPHYLAXIS

The use of metaphylactic antimicrobials at arrival has become nearly standard operating procedure for many large operations managing high-risk cattle.[25] Metaphylaxis seems to have a more profound role than simply treating cases of BRD already in progress. When the treatment is applied, epidemics are not merely delayed for the time corresponding with the period the antimicrobial is active, but there is also a significant decrease in the overall morbidity.[26] Since its inception in the mid-1990s, metaphylaxis has driven systems-level changes in the cattle industry and allowed some production models to expand. Despite growing concern regarding the use of antimicrobials in beef production,[27] metaphylaxis remains currently an efficient and effective short-term tool in managing BRD in high-risk cattle.[28] Conscientious use of this technology from a systems-level approach would also dictate that, as an industry, we must maintain a primary focus on continued progress in the development of long-term fundamental and sustainable solutions addressing the root causes of BRD. A wide variety of compounds are approved for metaphylactic use in the United States, and multiple factors drive decisions regarding selection and use. Knowledge regarding current disease status and sensitivity data of bacterial isolates from resident cattle populations, risk factors associated with arriving cattle, and efficacy data are important considerations for compound selection.[29,30]

BOVINE VIRAL DIARRHEA VIRUS PERSISTENT INFECTION TESTING

Despite the large volume of scientific literature on the subject, the role of BVDV persistent infection (PI) testing at arrival to operations that manage high-risk cattle is not universally agreed upon by professionals, perhaps owing to the lack of conclusive evidence in all production models.[31] Measuring the impact of the continually improving technology for PI testing is relatively straightforward with regard to the immediate measurable metrics traditionally used to evaluate arrival health[32]; however, it is important for veterinarians and producers to understand from a systems perspective the implications of PI testing, which is much more difficult to study and measure. Key questions include the following.

- What are the long-term health risks associated with the presence of BVDV PI animals in the population, and what is the risk tolerance of the business model?
- Can the variation and unpredictability of health outcomes inherent to high-risk cattle operations be reduced or mitigated by BVDV PI testing, and is there value in understanding the limitations for the business model?
- For stocker operations, is there a risk of damage to industry reputation by not testing?
- Are there unique areas within the business model where BVDV PI testing is applicable?
- Is there the potential for disrupting other important components of the cattle business model?

PARASITE CONTROL

Internal and external parasite control are important considerations in high-risk cattle from a disease and productivity standpoint. Parasite management programs should be designed with the details of the production model in mind. Parasite burdens have been linked to alteration in immune responses and other negative health outcomes and thus need to be corrected[33,34]; however, recent work suggests internal parasite control strategies at arrival can be delayed a period of time without negative impacts.[3] Parasite control should be considered both regionally and seasonally. Horn flies (*Haemotobia irratans*) and stable flies (*Stomoxys calcitrans*) have important production impacts especially in grazing models and should be addressed appropriately.[35]

SURGICAL PROCEDURES AT ARRIVAL

Routine surgical and management-related procedures such as castration and dehorning/tipping have measurable impacts on health and performance outcome.[36] The timing of procedures and the techniques used should be managed not only as tools to add value to the cattle, but also as important risk factors for disease. Many business models of operations handling high-risk cattle hinge on the ability to move cattle through the operation quickly, and management is often reluctant to implement changes that delay the cattle flow. Progressive operations have developed multiple options regarding these procedures and apply them in prescribed ways that optimizes their business model and the health of the cattle in the rapidly changing economic structure of the cattle industry.

Other arrival options include the following.

- DNA Immunostimulants: an innovative, nonantibiotic technology that enhances the animal's natural defenses against BRD. This technology is particularly applicable in production models that limit and restrict antibiotic use and may gain importance as the beef industry evolves away from antibiotic use in general.[37]
- Ancillary injectable and oral compounds designed to correct mineral, vitamin, and microbiome imbalances and deficiencies. Many products are currently being marketed that are designed to improve the health of high-risk calves at arrival. Although the supporting data for some products can be limited, there are opportunities to investigate their value with field-based clinical trials at most operations, particularly when there are clinical manifestations of deficiencies and imbalances.[38]
- Growth implants: these products are heavily used in conventional productions system as a means to increase operational efficiency. Most studies show no impact on health outcomes.[39]

EMERGING AND FUTURE TECHNOLOGIES FOR USE AT ARRIVAL

New technologies to efficiently and effectively screen incoming cattle populations for BRD are developing and show promise in the ability to more precisely diagnose and manage BRD in high-risk cattle operations. Examples include the following.

- WHISPER (Merck Animal Health USA, Kenilworth, NJ) Veterinary Stethoscope is designed to facilitate more targeted and controlled use of antibiotics.[40]
- Thoracic ultrasound examination is currently being applied in dairy productions systems as a tool to understand the disease dynamics of BRD and to identify clinical and subclinical BRD cases earlier in the disease process.[41]
- Biomarker assays are noninvasive and minimally invasive diagnostics technologies that use metabolomics (proteomics) to study the primary and secondary metabolites of a biological system and their response to disease conditions.[42] Research into the metabolic signatures associated with BRD may lead to more accurate and precise diagnosis of disease processes.

NUTRITIONAL CONSIDERATIONS

Cattle businesses that purchase high-risk feeder cattle do not always have access to unbiased nutritional expertise. Many production units are geographically located in areas not served or underserved by independent qualified nutritionists. Further complicating the nutritional component of management is that many business models rely on the ability to purchase many nontraditional, byproduct, and co-product feedstuffs in volatile markets, which can lead to increased variability in available feed ingredients.[43] Many veterinarians develop skills to play critical roles in this arena.

Conventional wisdom has been to feed high roughage diets containing long-stem grass hay during the receiving period. Owing to the price competitiveness of fiber containing feedstuffs that are byproducts of grain milling and other industries, as well as the mechanization of feed delivery equipment, ration balancing decisions are more complex.[43] High-risk calves tend to be dehydrated and in catabolic states when they reach their destinations. Diets too high in roughage often fail to meet dietary requirements successfully. Furthermore, high-risk calves are usually not adapted to diets high in energy.[18] Frequently, calves overconsume diets with rapidly fermentable carbohydrates, and the health issues are complicated by metabolic acidosis.[43] As energy levels in receiving rations go up, so does the BRD risk. Finding the optimum balance of energy and roughage can be challenging, especially as feed ingredients and incoming weights change over time, but is requisite for effectively managing health in high-risk cattle.

MONITORING FOR SICKNESS AND BOVINE RESPIRATORY DISEASE TREATMENT IN HIGH-RISK CATTLE

Although it is standard practice for cattle feeding and finishing operations located on the High Plains to use established and experienced pen riders to monitor the health status of the cattle on feed, this is not the case for many operations in the Midwest and Southeast that manage high-risk cattle. Many times, these operations are family managed, and job responsibilities are overlapping, poorly defined, and multiple. These challenges are especially true for large diverse operations that contract out the care and feeding of much of their cattle inventory. Veterinarians in these operations have an opportunity to play a key role in helping animal caretakers develop skills needed to identify sick cattle early. Examples include the following.

- Use and apply principles of low-stress handling. The nature of high-risk cattle is to be stoic and to hide clinical signs of disease effectively when not handled correctly,[44] and this nature can delay diagnosis and treatment of disease, leading to poorer outcomes.
- Train caretakers about the characteristics and behaviors associated with health. Departures from those characteristics and behaviors lie at the foundation of what sickness looks like and is essential to finding illness early.[45,46]
- Develop disciplined routines and habits when evaluating the health status of cattle populations. It is not unusual for high-priority issues to supplant time designated to observe cattle for sickness at busy operations that do not have workers dedicated to riding pens.
- From an epidemiologic and biocontainment standpoint, the value of detecting and treating early in the disease process cannot be overemphasized.

Hospital pen use and management should be critically evaluated on operations that manage high-risk cattle. If mismanaged, hospital facilities quickly become a point source of pathogen spread for the entire operation. From a biocontainment standpoint, it is not logical to commingle BRD cases from multiple pens. Populations with elevated BRD treatment rates can be especially prone to overwhelming the design capacity of the hospital pens. Some innovative and experienced producers and veterinarians have developed penning strategies that dedicate a supplementary treatment recovery pen for each pen of high-risk cattle received. These strategies can be very effective in enhancing biocontainment efforts and limiting pathogen spread and show tremendous benefit in the long term, but they are big financial and logistical commitments for management.[8]

Antimicrobials are the primary treatment modality for BRD in high-risk cattle. Veterinarians in North America have access to many compounds from multiple classes of antimicrobials approved for the treatment of BRD. Product choice decisions have traditionally been made by practitioners and consultants based on the literature, clinical observations, analysis of treatment records, and interpretations of diagnostic results. Much scientific literature has been published and is available for review regarding the comparative efficacy of available products. Increasing the complexity of developing treatment protocols is the increased societal concern for antibiotic use in food animal production systems, as well as advances in our understanding of the mechanisms responsible for the emergence of antimicrobial resistance.

EMPLOYEE MORALE

Some metrics affecting animal health are difficult to measure. To the inexperienced, it is difficult to appreciate how mentally taxing it can be to work with high-risk cattle over long periods of time. Failures of one sort or the other are frequent and paths to improvement are often difficult to find. When caretakers are asked to be engaged, invested, and work hard, repeated failures can be disheartening; thus, burnout is an issue. Mental attitude could be the number one factor associated with successfully managing high-risk cattle over the long term. Workers who are not motivated to do a good job invariably produce poorer health outcomes. High leverage actions to deal with deteriorating morale among owners, managers, and caretakers are an often overlooked issue and are important to the long-term success of the operation.

BOVINE RESPIRATORY DISEASE TUNNEL VISION

High-risk cattle often have disease problems unrelated to BRD. Although not the topic of this article, it is important for animal health professionals to be diligent in monitoring high-risk cattle populations for all disease conditions.

SUMMARY

The management of high-risk cattle is a complicated, dynamic, and challenging process that exists within the complex adaptive system of beef production in North America. In addition to traditional veterinary interventions, high leverage opportunities exist at a systems level to impact health outcomes and productivity. Systems thinking and system dynamics provide a means to more deeply understand and study the interrelationships and behaviors inherent to functioning systems. Sustainable long-term fundamental solutions to the problems that plague the high-risk cattle sector, most assuredly, will arise from a greater systems-level understanding the beef production models and an industry-wide willingness to adapt the structure of the system to improve outcomes.

DISCLOSURE

The author has nothing to disclose.

REFERENCES

1. Peel DS. Beef cattle growing and backgrounding programs. Vet Clin North Am Food Anim Pract 2003;19:365–85.
2. Sweiger SH, Nichols MD. Control methods for bovine respiratory disease in stocker cattle. Vet Clin North Am Food Anim Pract 2010;26:261–71.
3. Griffin CM, Scott JA, Karisch BB, et al. A randomized controlled trial to test the effect of on-arrival vaccination and deworming on stocker cattle health and growth performance. Bov Pract (Stillwater) 2018;52:26–33.
4. Peel DS. Economics of stocker production. Vet Clin North Am Food Anim Pract 2006;22:271–96.

5. Goodman M, John B. Armstrong lectureship on systems thinking. Kingsville (TX): King Ranch Institute for Ranch Management; 2015.

6. Woolums AR, Berghaus RD, Smith DR, et al. Case-control study to determine herd-level risk factors for bovine respiratory disease in nursing beef calves on cow-calf operations. J Am Vet Med Assoc 2018;252:989–94.

7. Hubbard KJ, Woolums AR, Karisch BB, et al. Case report: analysis of risk factors and production effects following an outbreak of bovine respiratory disease in stocker cattle. Bov Pract (Stillwater) 2018;52:146–53.

8. Falkner TR. Biocontainment in high-risk commingled cattle: understanding and managing diseases likely to be present. Proceedings Annual Meeting of the Missouri Veterinary Medical Association Proceedings. Osage Beach, Missouri, December 2004; 96–113.

9. Larson RL. A new look at reducing infectious disease in feedlot cattle. Proceedings, Plains Nutrition Council Spring Conference. San Antonio, Texas, April 14-15, 2005;9–18.

10. Gonzalez LA, Schwartzkopf-Genswein KS, Bryan M, et al. Relationship between transport conditions and welfare outcomes during commercial long haul transport of cattle in North America. J Anim Sci 2012;90:3640–51.

11. Gonzalez LA, Schwartzkopf-Genswein KS, Bryan M, et al. Benchmarking study of industry practices during long haul transport of cattle in Alberta, Canada. J Anim Sci 2012;90:3606–17.

12. Gonzalez LA, Schwartzkopf-Genswein KS, Bryan M, et al. Factors affecting body weight loss during commercial long haul transport of cattle in North America. J Anim Sci 2012;90:3630–9.

13. Grooms DL, Brock KV, Bolin SR, et al. Effect of constant exposure to cattle persistently infected with bovine viral diarrhea virus on morbidity and mortality rates and performance in feedlot cattle. J Am Vet Med Assoc 2014;244:212–24.

14. Mars MH, Bruschke CJM, van Oirschot JT. Airborne transmission of BHV1, BRSV, and BVDV among cattle is possible under experimental conditions. Vet Microbiol 1999;66:197–207.

15. Mader TL, Davis MS, Brown-Brandl T. Environmental factors influencing heat stress in feedlot cattle. J Anim Sci 2006;84:712–9.

16. Brown-Brandl TM. Understanding heat stress in beef cattle. Braz J Anim Sci 2018;47:1–9.

17. Mader TL. Mud effects on feedlot cattle. Nebraska Beef Cattle Reports 2011; 613:82–3.

18. Tomczak DJ, Samuelson KL, Jennings JS, et al. Oral hydration therapy with water and bovine respiratory disease incidence affects rumination behavior, rumen pH, and rumen temperature in high-risk, newly received beef calves. J Anim Sci 2019; 97:2015–24.

19. Tomczak DJ, Samuelson KL, Jennings JS, et al. Oral hydration therapy with water affects health and performance of high-risk, newly received feedlot cattle. Applied Animal Science 2019;35:30–8.

20. Rogers KC, Miles DG, Renter DG, et al. Effects of delayed respiratory viral vaccine and/or inclusion of an immunostimulant on feedlot health, performance, and carcass merits of auction-market derived feeder heifers. Bov Pract (Stillwater) 2016;50:154–62.

21. Hughes HD, Carroll JA, Burdick Sanchez NC, et al. Effects of dexamethasone treatment and respiratory vaccination on rectal temperature, complete blood count, and functional capacities of neutrophils in beef steers. J Anim Sci 2017; 95:1502–11.

22. Richeson JT, Carroll JA, Burdick Snachez NC, et al. Dexamethasone treatment differentially alters viral shedding and the antibody and acute phase protein response after multivalent respiratory vaccination in beet steers. J Anim Sci 2016;94:3501–9.

23. Richeson JT, Hughes HD, Broadway PR, et al. Vaccination management of beef cattle delayed vaccination and endotoxin stacking. Vet Clin North Am Food Anim Pract 2019;35:575–92.

24. Ellis JA, Yong C. Systemic adverse reactions in young Simmental calves following administration of a combination vaccine. Can Vet J 1997;38:45–7.

25. U.S. Department of Agriculture, Grain Inspection, Packers and Stockyards Administration. Feedlot 2011 part IV: health and health management on U.S. feedlots with a capacity of 1,000 of more head. United Stated Department of Agriculture; 2013.

26. Vander Ley B. Understanding the mechanism of metaphylaxis form an epidemiologic perspective. Proceeding, 52nd Annual Conference American Association of Bovine Practitioners. St. Louis, Missouri, September 11-14, 2019.

27. Soulsby L. Antimicrobials and animal health: a fascinating nexus. J Antimicrob Chemother 2007;60:i77–8.

28. Dennis EJ, Schroeder TC, Renter DG, et al. Value of arrival metaphylaxis in the U.S. cattle industry. J Agric Resour Econ 2018;43:233–50.

29. Step DL, Engelken TJ, Romano C, et al. Evaluation of three antimicrobial regimens used as metaphylaxis in stocker calves at high risk of developing bovine respiratory disease. Vet Ther 2007;8:136–47.

30. Abell KM, Theurer ME, Larson RL, et al. A mixed treatment comparison meta-analysis of metaphylaxis treatments for bovine respiratory disease in beef cattle. J Anim Sci 2017;95:626–35.

31. Richeson JT, Kegley JG, Powell PA, et al. Weaning management of newly received beef calves with or without continuous exposure to a persistently infected bovine viral diarrhea virus pen mate: effects on health, performance, bovine viral diarrhea virus titers, and peripheral blood leukocytes. J Anim Sci 2012;90:1972–85.

32. Hessman BE, Fulton RW, Sjeklocha DB, et al. Evaluation of economic effects and the health and performance of the general cattle population after exposure to cattle persistently infected with bovine viral diarrhea virus in a starter feedlot. Am J Vet Res 2009;70:73–85.

33. Ballweber LR, Smith LL, Stuedemann TA, et al. The effectiveness of a single treatment with doramectin or ivermectin in the control of gastrointestinal nematodes in grazing yearling stocker cattle. Vet Parasitol 1997;72:53–68.

34. Schutz JS, Carroll JA, Gasbarre LC, et al. Effects of gastrointestinal parasites on parasite burden, rectal temperature, and antibody titer response to vaccination and infectious bovine rhinotracheitis virus challenge. J Anim Sci 2012;90:1948–54.

35. Boxler DJ. External and internal parasites. Proceedings, State of Beef Conference. North Platte, Nebraska, November 7-8, 2018;31–8.

36. Richeson JT, Pinedo PJ, Kegley EB, et al. Association of hematologic variables and castration status at the time of arrival at a research facility with the risk of bovine respiratory disease in beef calves. J Am Vet Med Assoc 2013;243:1035–41.

37. Nickell JS, Keil DJ, Settle TL, et al. Efficacy and safety of a novel DNA immunostimulant in cattle. Bov Pract (Stillwater) 2016;50:9–20.

38. Wilson BK, Step DL, Maxwell CL, et al. Evaluation of multiple ancillary therapies used in combination with an antimicrobial in newly received high-risk calves treated to respiratory disease. J Anim Sci 2015;93:3661–74.

39. Richeson JT, Beck PA, Hughes HD, et al. Effect of growth implant regimen on health, performance, and immunity of high-risk, newly received stocker cattle. J Anim Sci 2015;93:4089–97.

40. Mang AV, Buczinski S, Booker CW, et al. Evaluation of a computer-aided lung auscultation system for diagnosis of bovine respiratory disease in feedlot cattle. J Vet Intern Med 2015;29:1112–6.

41. Ollivet TL, Burton AJ, Bicalho RC, et al. Use of rapid thoracic ultrasonography for detection of subclinical and clinical pneumonia in dairy calves. Proceeding, 44th Annual Conference American Association of Bovine Practitioners. St. Louis, Missouri, September 22-24, 2011;44:148.

42. Maurer DL, Koziel JA, Engelken TJ, et al. Detection of volatile compounds emitted form nasal secretions and serum: towards non-invasive identification of diseased cattle biomarkers. Separations 2018;5:18.

43. Richeson JT, Samuelson KL, Tomczak DJ. Energy and roughage levels in cattle receiving diets and impacts on health, performance, and immune responses. J Anim Sci 2019;97:3596–604.

44. Gill R. Can cattle handling affect morbidity. In: 3rd Annual TVMDL Amarillo Bovine Respiratory Disease Conference Proceedings. West Texas A&M University, Canyon, Texas, July 7, 2018.

45. White BJ, Goehl DR, Amrine DE. Comparison of a remote early disease identification (REDI) system to visual observations to identify cattle with bovine respiratory disease. Intern J Appl Res Vet Med 2015;13:23–30.

46. Pillen JL, Pinedo PJ, Ives SE, et al. Alteration of activity variables relative to clinical diagnosis of bovine respiratory disease in newly received feedlot cattle. Bov Pract (Stillwater) 2016;50:1–8.

Bovine Respiratory Disease Vaccination Against Viral Pathogens

Modified-Live Versus Inactivated Antigen Vaccines, Intranasal Versus Parenteral, What Is the Evidence?

Manuel F. Chamorro, DVM, MS, PhD[a],*,
Roberto A. Palomares, DVM, MS, PhD[b]

KEYWORDS

- Calves • BRD • Vaccine • Modified-live viral (MLV) • Inactivated ("killed") viral (KV)
- Parenteral • IN

KEY POINTS

- Vaccination of beef calves around the time of weaning with multivalent modified-live viral (MLV) vaccines alone or in combination with *Mannheimia haemolytica/Pasteurella multocida* bacterins reduces bovine respiratory disease (BRD) morbidity and mortality after weaning.
- It is uncertain if vaccination of young beef calves reduces BRD morbidity and mortality before weaning age.
- There is conflicting evidence of the efficacy of vaccination of young dairy calves with MLV vaccines alone or in combination with *M haemolytica/P multocida* bacterins on the reduction of BRD morbidity and mortality.
- The level of specific maternal antibodies from colostrum, the ecosystem of respiratory viruses in each farm, and the degree of homology of field versus vaccine virus strains affect efficacy of BRD vaccination in young beef and dairy calves.

INTRODUCTION

The bovine respiratory disease (BRD) complex is the most important cause of morbidity and mortality in beef and dairy cattle operations.[1] Although respiratory

[a] Department of Clinical Sciences, College of Veterinary Medicine, Auburn University, Large Animal Teaching Hospital, 2020 J.T. Vaughn, Auburn, AL 36849, USA; [b] Department of Population Medicine, College of Veterinary Medicine, University of Georgia, 501 D.W. Brooks Drive, Athens, GA 30602, USA
* Corresponding author.
E-mail address: mfc0003@auburn.edu

Vet Clin Food Anim 36 (2020) 461–472
https://doi.org/10.1016/j.cvfa.2020.03.006
0749-0720/20/© 2020 Elsevier Inc. All rights reserved.

disease can affect cattle of any age and stage of production, economic losses associated with BRD occur most commonly in the following calf populations:

1. Beef calves around the time of weaning, between 5 and 8 months of age
2. Preweaning beef calves younger than 5 months of age
3. Dairy calves younger than 3 months of age.

Stress and immunosuppression are important risk factors for the development of BRD in any of these population groups; however, different factors play a role in the presentation of clinical disease in each group. Failure in the transfer of passive immunity, the level and decay of maternal antibodies (MA), commingling, transport/shipping, dietary changes, and biosecurity breaches can influence the presentation of BRD in calves.[2,3] The impact of these factors on individual operations introduce variation in the clinical presentation of BRD in each calf group. Despite this variation, whole-herd vaccination against BRD pathogens is a common practice among producers and veterinarians to minimize calf losses associated with morbidity and mortality.[4,5] Modified-live (MLV) and killed virus (KV) vaccines with different label specifications are commercially available.[6,7] Recently, a meta-analysis of the efficacy of BRD vaccines demonstrated inconsistency of the reduction of morbidity and mortality in calves.[6,7] The lack of evidence of efficacy of vaccination against BRD pathogens may affect the practitioner's decision-making process when developing vaccination protocols for cattle operations. The objective of this article is to perform an assessment of the quality of evidence on whether MLV and inactivated antigen vaccines administered parenterally or intranasally provide similar clinical protection against BRD in different calf groups. "High-quality evidence" was defined as an outcome reported by 3 or more naturally occurring or experimentally induced BRD vaccine efficacy studies that fulfilled all of the following requirements: clear definition of study population, random and clear allocation of treatment groups, clear definition of disease (morbidity and mortality) outcomes, and blinding of evaluators. "Moderate-quality evidence" was defined as an outcome reported by at least one vaccine efficacy study that fulfilled all the previously mentioned requirements, and "low-quality evidence" was defined as failure to fulfill any of the requirements.

Modified-Live Versus Inactivated Virus Vaccination Against Bovine Respiratory Disease. What Is the Evidence?

In general, MLV vaccines induce complete humoral and cell-mediated long-lasting immunity, and fewer doses are required to provide clinical protection.[8–11] In contrast, KV vaccines induce strong humoral responses but less robust cell-mediated immunity and require at least 2 doses 21 days apart to provide protection.[12] Several studies have evaluated the effect of MLV and KV vaccines on the prevention of BRD in calves of different ages, immune status, and production settings.[13–17] Among practitioners, it is thought that MLV vaccines provide better clinical protection against BRD compared with KV[4]; however, selection of vaccination protocols should be based on field (naturally occurring) BRD vaccine-efficacy trials that provide strong evidence on vaccine selection for BRD prevention.[6,7]

Are modified-live virus and killed virus respiratory vaccines similarly effective for providing clinical protection against bovine respiratory disease in weaned beef calves?

The highest economic impact of BRD on the beef industry is associated with morbidity and mortality of calves shortly after weaning.[1] Therefore, a fundamental goal of vaccination of this group of cattle is to reduce the incidence of BRD after arrival to stocker/

feedlot operations. Nine studies evaluated the effect of vaccination with MLV (8 studies) and KV (1 study) vaccines on the natural occurrence of BRD in beef calves after conventional (5–8 months) weaning age.[13,15,16,18–22] MLV and KV vaccines included at least one of the following agents: bovine herpes virus 1 (BHV-1), bovine viral diarrhea virus 1 (BVDV 1), BVDV 2, bovine respiratory syncytial virus (BRSV), bovine coronavirus (BCV), and parainfluenza-3 virus (PI3V). In all studies, vaccination occurred in the transition from weaning to arrival at the stocker/feedlot operation. Significant reduction of morbidity was reported in 75% (6/8) of the studies using MLV vaccination. Further, significant reduction of mortality was observed in 67% (4/6) of studies using MLV vaccination that reported mortality rates. Only one study evaluating the efficacy of KV vaccines reported significant reduction of BRD-associated morbidity and mortality.[21] The introduction of BVDV-2, BCV, *Mannheimia haemolytica* and *Pasteurella multocida* in combination with MLV, and early vaccination (before weaning, before arrival) increased vaccination efficacy.[22] *There is strong and high-quality evidence that vaccination of beef calves around the time of weaning with MLV vaccines alone or in combination with M haemolytica/P multocida bacterin/toxoids is superior to vaccination with KV vaccines in reducing naturally occurring BRD morbidity and mortality after weaning.*

Thirteen studies evaluated the effect of vaccination of beef calves around the time of weaning with MLV or KV vaccines on BRD-associated morbidity and mortality after experimental challenge with respiratory viruses.[12,23–34] In all studies, calves were vaccinated between 5 and 12 months of age, and experimental inoculation/exposure occurred between 3 and 230 days after vaccination. In 11 studies calves were challenged with BVDV; one study used BHV-1 and one study used BRSV as challenge agents. Eleven studies evaluated MLV vaccines and 2 studies evaluated KV vaccines. Significant reduction of BRD morbidity was reported in 82% (9/11) of studies using MLV vaccines. Significant reduction of mortality was reported in 100% (5/5) of MLV vaccination studies that reported mortality rates. In both of the 2 studies using KV vaccines, there was a significant reduction of BRD morbidity but none reported mortality. One study compared the effect of MLV versus KV vaccination in recently weaned beef calves and reported no significant differences on BRD morbidity after challenge with BVDV.[35] A recent study compared the effect of vaccination of beef calves at birth and again at 2 months of age, with 1 of 3 vaccine-combination protocols, MLV/MLV, MLV/KV, or no-vacc/MLV, on clinical protection of calves after experimental challenge with BRSV at weaning. No differences on BRD morbidity and mortality were reported among vaccinated groups.[36] *There is strong and high-quality evidence that vaccination of beef calves with vaccines containing MLV alone or in combination with M haemolytica/P multocida bacterins is superior to KV vaccination for reducing BRD-associated morbidity and mortality after experimental challenge with BVDV, BHV-1, or BRSV.*

Are modified-live virus and killed virus respiratory vaccines similarly effective for providing clinical protection against bovine respiratory disease in preweaning beef calves?

Respiratory disease is the leading cause of death of beef calves between 3 weeks of age and weaning.[37] The proportion of preweaning beef calves affected by BRD is variable among cow-calf operations, with some farms reporting a very high incidence of the disease (~20%) and other farms with no calf-BRD issues at all.[38,39] The goal of vaccination is to reduce the risk of BRD before weaning; however, in this case the presence and level of colostrum-derived immunity at the time of vaccination can play a role in clinical protection as well as interfere with vaccine efficacy. Two studies reported no effect of vaccination on the natural occurrence of BRD after 4 months of age in calves previously vaccinated with 2 doses of an inactivated BRSV vaccine between 2 and 4 months of age.[14,34] One study reported increased BRD-associated morbidity and mortality on vaccinated calves.[14] The investigators suggested that detrimental priming induced by the inactivated BRSV vaccine could have been responsible for inducing a hypersensitivity reaction after natural exposure to field virus in vaccinated calves. *There is very limited evidence of moderate quality indicating deleterious or no effect of KV BRSV vaccination in reducing naturally occurring BRD morbidity and mortality of young beef calves.*

Three studies evaluated the effect of vaccination (2 studies using MLV vaccines and 1 study using a KV vaccine) of 2.5- to 4-month-old beef calves on BRD-associated morbidity and mortality after experimental challenge/exposure to BVDV.[40–42] Experimental challenge/exposure occurred between 30 and 45 days after vaccination in all studies. No effect of vaccination on reduction of BRD-associated morbidity and mortality was reported in the 2 studies that vaccinated calves with a multivalent MLV vaccine 45 days before BVDV challenge.[40,41] In these studies, MA against BVDV 1 and BVDV 2 at the time of challenge provided protection against respiratory signs in unvaccinated calves. In contrast, the high level of BVDV-specific antibodies observed before challenge in vaccinated calves not only protected against clinical disease but also resulted in greater protection against viremia and BVDV shedding. Results from the third study using a KV vaccine demonstrated reduction of clinical signs associated with acute BVDV infection in calves vaccinated with 2 doses of an inactivated BVDV vaccine 30 days before challenge.[42] *There is limited evidence of moderate quality indicating no effect of MLV vaccination or positive effects of KV vaccination for reducing BRD-associated morbidity and mortality after experimental challenge with BVDV of young beef calves.*

Are modified-live virus and killed virus respiratory vaccines similarly effective for providing clinical protection against bovine respiratory disease in young dairy calves?

BVD is a common cause of morbidity and mortality of young dairy heifers before and after weaning.[5] In contrast to the lower prevalence of preweaning calf pneumonia reported in young beef calves, results from a recent report indicated that overall preweaning dairy heifer BRD-associated morbidity is 22.8%. Similarly, overall preweaning dairy heifer BRD-associated mortality is 19%.[43] The level of interference of colostrum-derived immunity at the time of vaccination can similarly affect clinical protection and efficacy of vaccination in dairy calves. Two studies evaluated the effect of vaccination of dairy calves between 3 days and 6 weeks of age, with single or 2 doses of a multivalent MLV vaccine on the natural occurrence of BRD between 1 and 3 months of age.[17,44,45] Vaccination did not result in significant reduction of naturally occurring BRD morbidity and mortality in any of the studies. One study reported that 21% of the risk of BRD in young dairy calves was the result of failure in the transfer of passive immunity.[46] Calves with a higher colostrum-derived BRSV and IBR antibodies had lower odds of developing signs of BRD compared with calves with lower titers. In another study, calves vaccinated with 2 doses of an intranasal (IN) multivalent MLV vaccine between 3 to 6 days and at 6 weeks of age demonstrated no difference in BRD signs but had less lung consolidation compared with calves vaccinated at 6 weeks, with a single dose of a subcutaneous (SC) MLV vaccine or unvaccinated calves.[45] *There is limited moderate quality evidence indicating that vaccination of young dairy calves with multivalent MLV vaccines is ineffective for reducing naturally occurring BRD morbidity and mortality.*

Seventeen studies evaluated the effect of vaccination of young dairy calves in the presence of different levels of MA with MLV (14 studies) or KV vaccines (3 studies) on reduction of BRD-associated morbidity and mortality after experimental inoculation with respiratory viruses.[9–11,47–63] In all studies, calves were vaccinated between 3 days and 4.5 months of age. Experimental inoculation with respiratory viruses occurred between 5 days and 9 months after vaccination. Six studies used BVDV as the experimental challenge agent; 10 studies used BRSV, and 1 study used BHV-1. Significant reduction of BRD morbidity was reported in 86% (12/14) of studies using MLV vaccines. Significant reduction of mortality was reported in 57% (4/7) of MLV vaccine studies that reported mortality rates. Vaccination in the face of maternal antibodies (IFOMA) and experimental challenge with a homologous BVDV strain provided clinical protection up to 7 months after vaccination in one study.[11] In contrast, in another study vaccination IFOMA and experimental challenge with a heterologous BVDV strain 4.5 months after vaccination did not prevent clinical disease.[50] Colostrum-deprived or seronegative dairy calves vaccinated with a MLV vaccine were clinically protected after experimental challenge with BVDV, BRSV, or BHV-1.[10,50,53]

Significant reduction of BRD-associated morbidity and mortality was reported in only 1 of 3 (33.3%) studies where a KV BRSV vaccine was used to vaccinate calves subsequently challenged with BRSV. *There is robust, moderate-quality evidence that vaccination of young dairy calves with multivalent MLV vaccines is superior to vaccination with KV vaccines for reducing BRD-associated morbidity and mortality after experimental challenge with respiratory viruses. Clinical protection may depend on the level of colostrum-derived immunity at the time of vaccination (seronegative vs seropositive), homology between the vaccine and experimental challenge strains, and time between vaccination and challenge.*

Intranasal Versus Parenteral Vaccination Against Bovine Respiratory Disease. What Is the Evidence?

Numerous studies have demonstrated the inhibitory effects of passive immunity on vaccine-induced immune responses and complete protection against respiratory viruses after parenteral administration of BRD vaccines.[50,64,65] Young calves prime-vaccinated with parenteral MLV vaccines IFOMA do not usually seroconvert. However, there is evidence that they can mount specific T- and B-cell–mediated immune responses that provide variable clinical protection later in life when MA have decayed.[9,11,50,62] Because variability in the transfer of specific passive immunity has been reported in young calves,[66] it becomes challenging to estimate the timing when parenteral vaccination would provide the highest efficacy on protection against respiratory pathogens. Intranasal vaccination is an effective mechanism to induce local mucosal immune priming and immunoglobulin A production IFOMA.[67] Greater mucosal (nasal secretions) and systemic-specific immunity has been reported in calves vaccinated IFOMA intranasally with a MLV BRSV and/or BHV-1 vaccine versus parenteral vaccination.[68] Several studies have demonstrated efficacy of IN vaccination of calves IFOMA on protection against respiratory viruses[53,58,68]; however, few field and experimental challenge studies have compared their efficacy to parenteral vaccines for reducing BRD morbidity or mortality.

Are modified-live virus intranasal and parenteral vaccines similarly effective for providing clinical protection against bovine respiratory disease in young dairy calves?

Only one field study using 468 dairy calves compared the effects of 2 MLV vaccination protocols using IN or SC vaccination on the risk of BRD from 8 to 12 weeks of age.[45]

The vaccination protocol (IN vs SC) did not have an effect on the natural occurrence of BRD. The IN vaccine demonstrated potential to reduce lung consolidation based on ultrasound examination findings and improve growth of calves. *There is very limited moderate quality evidence indicating that vaccination of young dairy calves with neither multivalent MLV IN nor parenteral vaccines is effective in reducing naturally occurring BRD morbidity and mortality.*

Fifteen studies evaluated the efficacy of vaccination of young dairy calves with a multivalent MLV vaccine containing all or some of the following agents: BVDV 1, BVDV 2, BHV-1, BRSV, and PI3V on clinical protection against experimental viral challenge. Six studies used IN MLV vaccines[10,49,52,53,58,60] and 9 used parenteral MLV vaccines (see previous sections in this article). Significant reduction of BRD-associated morbidity after challenge was reported in 83.3% of IN vaccination studies and in 67% of parenteral vaccination studies. Significant reduction of BRD-associated mortality was reported in 75% of both IN and parenteral vaccination studies that reported mortality rates. Maternally derived antibodies affected immune response and clinical protection offered by parenteral MLV vaccination in calves subsequently challenged with BRSV in one study[9]; in contrast, maternal immunity had no effect in calves vaccinated parenterally with an adjuvanted MLV BRSV vaccine and subsequently challenged with BRSV in another study.[63] Similarly, calves vaccinated IFOMA with a parenteral MLV BVDV vaccine and subsequently challenged with a homologous BVDV strain were protected against clinical disease.[9,56,62] Regardless of the level of MA, IN and parenteral vaccination of dairy calves against BRSV resulted in clinical protection when experimental challenge occurred less than 4 months of vaccination.[52,53,63] *There is strong, high-quality evidence that both intranasal and parenteral vaccination of young dairy calves with MLV vaccines result in similar reduction of BRD-associated morbidity and mortality after experimental challenge with respiratory viruses.*

Are modified-live virus intranasal and parenteral vaccines similarly effective for providing clinical protection against bovine respiratory disease in beef calves?

Intranasal or parenteral vaccination of beef calves from cow-calf or feedlot operations with MLV vaccines containing some or all of the following viruses—BVDV 1, BVDV 2, BHV-1, BRSV, BCV, and PI3V—for BRD prevention usually occurs at branding (~2 months of age), around weaning, or at stocker/feedlot arrival. Only 25% of studies (1/4) evaluating MLV IN vaccines reported significant reduction of naturally occurring BRD morbidity in vaccinated calves.[13,19,20,69] In contrast, significant reduction of naturally occurring BRD morbidity in calves vaccinated with a parenteral MLV vaccine was reported in 75% (3/4) of studies (see previous sections in this article).[15,16,18,22] Significant reduction of naturally occurring BRD mortality was reported in 50% (2/4) of parenteral vaccination studies and in 25% (1/4) of IN vaccination studies that reported mortality rates. One study reported a greater reduction of BRD in recently weaned beef calves vaccinated with 2 doses of a parenteral MLV vaccine versus calves vaccinated with a single dose of an IN MLV vaccine.[19] Another study reported no impact on clinical health or mortality of feedlot calves that received a single dose of a MLV IN vaccine when treated the first time for BRD.[69] *There is strong, high-quality evidence that parenteral vaccination of beef calves before or shortly after weaning with MLV vaccines is superior to IN vaccination for reducing naturally occurring BRD-associated morbidity and mortality after arrival to stocker/feedlot operations.*

Fourteen studies evaluated MLV vaccines on the reduction of BRD-associated morbidity and mortality of beef calves after experimental challenge with respiratory viruses (see previous sections of this article). Only 2 studies[36,70] (14.3%) evaluated intranasal vaccines alone or in a combination protocol with parenteral vaccines. In one study, calves were vaccinated with an IN vaccine containing BHV-1, BRSV, and PI3V and subsequently challenged with BRSV. In the other study, calves were vaccinated with an IN vaccine containing BVDV 1, BVDV 2, BHV-1, BRSV, and PI3V and subsequently challenged with BHV-1. Significant reduction of BRD-associated morbidity and mortality was reported in the BHV-1 challenge study but not in the BRSV challenge study. Significant reduction of BRD morbidity and mortality was reported in 67% and 57% of studies, respectively that used parenteral MLV vaccines in calves that were subsequently challenged with BVDV, BRSV, or BHV-1.[24–29,31–33,35,40,41] Intranasal vaccination of beef calves at 3 to 6 weeks of age and again at 6 months of age with an IN or SC vaccine was associated with reduced BRD morbidity after BHV-1 challenge.[70] Moreover, in this study, the vaccination protocol based on IN priming and IN booster resulted in reduced BHV1 shedding. In addition, vaccination with a single dose of the IN vaccine at 3 to 6 weeks or at 6 months of age with no additional booster was associated with reduction of mortality but not BRD morbidity. In another study, IN MLV vaccination at birth in addition to SC MLV or KV booster at 2 months of age was not different from SC MLV vaccination at 2 months for reducing BRD morbidity after BRSV challenge at weaning.[36] *There is limited, moderate-quality evidence that vaccination of beef calves with parenteral multivalent MLV vaccines is superior to IN MLV vaccines on reducing BRD-associated morbidity and mortality after experimental challenge with BVDV, BHV-1, or BRSV.*

SUMMARY

Assessment of the evidence of efficacy of vaccination of different calf populations with MLV and KV vaccines on the reduction of BRD-associated morbidity and mortality produced the following conclusions:

- There is strong high-quality evidence that vaccination of beef calves at or shortly after weaning with parenteral multivalent MLV vaccines alone or in combination with *M haemolytica/P multocida* bacterins is effective for reducing naturally occurring and experimentally induced BRD morbidity and mortality after weaning. The presence of BVDV 1 and BVDV 2 antigens in parenteral multivalent MLV vaccines plays an important role in providing clinical protection against BRD.
- There is limited evidence of efficacy of vaccination of young beef calves (preweaning) with parenteral or IN MLVor KV vaccines in reducing naturally occurring or experimentally induced BRD morbidity and mortality before weaning age. There is an evident need for additional research to determine true effects of vaccination, type of vaccines, and routes of administration in this group of cattle.
- With respect to vaccination of dairy calves for the prevention of BRD, there is a lack of connection between results from naturally occurring and experimentally induced BRD vaccine-efficacy studies. There is limited moderate-quality evidence that vaccination of young dairy calves with parenteral or IN MLV vaccines is ineffective for reducing naturally occurring BRD. In contrast, there is strong evidence that vaccination of young dairy calves with parenteral or IN MLV vaccines is effective providing clinical protection against BRD after experimental challenge with respiratory viruses.
- The level and duration of specific MA against respiratory viruses of calves from individual cow-calf and dairy operations play an important role in providing clinical protection as well as in affecting vaccine efficacy against BRD.

DISCLOSURE

The authors have nothing to disclose.

REFERENCES

1. USDA. National Agricultural Statistics Service.Cattle death loss. 2011. Available at:usda.mannlib.cornell.edu/usda/current/CattDeath/CattDeath-05-12-2011.pdf.   . Accessed December 3, 2019.
2. Fulton RW. Bovine respiratory disease research (1983-2009). AnimHealth Res Rev 2009;10(2):131–9.
3. Smith DR. Field epidemiology to manage BRD risk in beef cattle production systems. AnimHealth Res Rev 2014;15(2):180–3.
4. Wilson BK, Richards CJ, Step DL, et al. Best management practices for newly weaned calves for improved health and well-being. J Anim Sci 2017;95(5):2170–82.
5. Windeyer MC, Timsit E, Barkema H. Bovine respiratory disease in pre-weaned dairy calves: Are current preventative strategies good enough? Vet J 2017;224:16–7.
6. Larson RL, Step DL. Evidence-based effectiveness of vaccination against Mannheimiahaemolytica, Pasteurellamultocida, and Histophilussomni in feedlot cattle for mitigating the incidence and effect of bovine respiratory disease complex. Vet Clin North Am FoodAnimPract 2012;28(1):97–106, 106e101-107, ix.
7. Theurer ME, Larson RL, White BJ. Systematic review and meta-analysis of the effectiveness of commercially available vaccines against bovine herpesvirus, bovine viral diarrhea virus, bovine respiratory syncytial virus, and parainfluenza type 3 virus for mitigation of bovine respiratory disease complex in cattle. J Am Vet Med Assoc 2015;246(1):126–42.
8. Endsley JJ, Ridpath JF, Neill JD, et al. Induction of T lymphocytes specific for bovine viral diarrhea virus in calves with maternal antibody. ViralImmunol 2004;17(1):13–23.
9. Ellis J, Gow S, Bolton M, et al. Inhibition of priming for bovine respiratory syncytial virus-specific protective immune responses following parenteral vaccination of passively immune calves. Can Vet J 2014;55(12):1180–5.
10. Mahan SM, Sobecki B, Johnson J, et al. Efficacy of intranasal vaccination with a multivalent vaccine containing temperature-sensitive modified-live bovine herpesvirus type 1 for protection of seronegative and seropositive calves against respiratory disease. J Am Vet Med Assoc 2016;248(11):1280–6.
11. Stevens ET, Michael BS, Burdett WW, et al. Efficacy of a non-adjuvanted, modified-live virus vaccine in calves with maternal ntibodies against a virulent bovine viral diarrhea virus type 2a challenge seven months following vaccination. Bovine Pract 2011;45(1):23–31.
12. Ridpath JF, Dominowski P, Mannan R, et al. Evaluation of three experimental bovine viral diarrhea virus killed vaccines adjuvanted with combinations of Quil A cholesterol and dimethyldioctadecylammonium (DDA) bromide. Vet Res Commun 2010;34(8):691–702.
13. Martin W, Willson P, Curtis R, et al. A field trial, of preshipment vaccination, with intranasal infectious bovine rhinotracheitis-parainfluenza-3 vaccines. Can J Comp Med 1983;47(3):245–9.
14. Schreiber P, Matheise JP, Dessy F, et al. High mortality rate associated with bovine respiratory syncytial virus (BRSV) infection in Belgian white blue calves

previously vaccinated with an inactivated BRSV vaccine. J Vet Med B Infect Dis Vet PublicHealth 2000;47(7):535–50.

15. Schumaher TF, Cooke RF, Brandao AP, et al. Effects of vaccination timing against respiratory pathogens on performance, antibody response, and health in feedlot cattle. J Anim Sci 2019;97(2):620–30.

16. Step DL, Krehbiel CR, Burciaga-Robles LO, et al. Comparison of single vaccination versus revaccination with a modified-live virus vaccine containing bovine herpesvirus-1, bovine viral diarrhea virus (types 1a and 2a), parainfluenza type 3 virus, and bovine respiratory syncytial virus in the prevention of bovine respiratory disease in cattle. J Am Vet Med Assoc 2009;235(5):580–7.

17. Windeyer MC, Leslie KE, Godden SM, et al. The effects of viral vaccination of dairy heifer calves on the incidence of respiratory disease, mortality, and growth. J Dairy Sci 2012;95(11):6731–9.

18. Griffin CM, Scott JA, Karisch BB, et al. A randomized controlled trial to test the effect of on-arrival vaccination and deworming on stocker cattle health and growth performance. BovPract (Stillwater) 2018;52(1):26–33.

19. Hanzlicek GA, White BJ, Renter DG, et al. A field study evaluating health, performance, and behavior differences in crossbred beef calves administered different vaccine-parasiticide product combinations. Vaccine 2010;28(37):5998–6005.

20. Plummer PJ, Rohrbach BW, Daugherty RA, et al. Effect of intranasal vaccination against bovine enteric coronavirus on the occurrence of respiratory tract disease in a commercial backgrounding feedlot. J Am Vet Med Assoc 2004;225(5): 726–31.

21. Stilwell G, Matos M, Carolino N, et al. Effect of a quadrivalent vaccine against respiratory virus on the incidence of respiratory disease in weaned beef calves. Prev Vet Med 2008;85(3–4):151–7.

22. Wildman BK, Perrett T, Abutarbush SM, et al. A comparison of 2 vaccination programs in feedlot calves at ultra-high risk of developing undifferentiated fever/bovine respiratory disease. Can Vet J 2008;49(5):463–72.

23. Beer M, Hehnen HR, Wolfmeyer A, et al. A new inactivated BVDV genotype I and II vaccine. An immunisation and challenge study with BVDV genotype I. Vet Microbiol 2000;77(1–2):195–208.

24. Brock KV, Widel P, Walz P, et al. Onset of protection from experimental infection with type 2 bovine viral diarrhea virus following vaccination with a modified-live vaccine. Vet Ther 2007;8(1):88–96.

25. Dean HJ, Leyh R. Cross-protective efficacy of a bovine viral diarrhea virus (BVDV) type 1 vaccine against BVDV type 2 challenge. Vaccine 1999;17(9–10): 1117–24.

26. Ellis JA, Gow SP, Goji N, et al. Efficacy of a combination viral vaccine for protection of cattle against experimental infection with field isolates of bovine herpesvirus-1. J Am Vet Med Assoc 2009;235(5):563–72.

27. Fairbanks K, Schnackel J, Chase CC. Evaluation of a modified live virus type-1a bovine viral diarrhea virus vaccine (Singer strain) against a type-2 (strain 890) challenge. Vet Ther 2003;4(1):24–34.

28. Fulton RW, Johnson BJ, Briggs RE, et al. Challenge with Bovine viral diarrhea virus by exposure to persistently infected calves: protection by vaccination and negative results of antigen testing in nonvaccinated acutely infected calves. Can J Vet Res 2006;70(2):121–7.

29. Grooms DL, Brock KV, Bolin SR, et al. Effect of constant exposure to cattle persistently infected with bovine viral diarrhea virus on morbidity and mortality rates and performance of feedlot cattle. J Am Vet Med Assoc 2014;244(2):212–24.

30. Hamers C, Couvreur B, Dehan P, et al. Assessment of the clinical and virological protection provided by a commercial inactivated bovine viral diarrhoea virus genotype 1 vaccine against a BVDV genotype 2 challenge. Vet Rec 2003;153(8): 236–40.

31. Kelling CL, Hunsaker BD, Steffen DJ, et al. Characterization of protection from systemic infection and disease by use of a modified-live noncytopathic bovine viral diarrhea virus type 1 vaccine in experimentally infected calves. Am J Vet Res 2005;66(10):1785–91.

32. Kelling CL, Hunsaker BD, Steffen DJ, et al. Characterization of protection against systemic infection and disease from experimental bovine viral diarrhea virus type 2 infection by use of a modified-live noncytopathic type 1 vaccine in calves. Am J Vet Res 2007;68(7):788–96.

33. Palomares RA, Givens MD, Wright JC, et al. Evaluation of the onset of protection induced by a modified-live virus vaccine in calves challenge inoculated with type 1b bovine viral diarrhea virus. Am J Vet Res 2012;73(4):567–74.

34. Larsen LE, Tegtmeier C, Pedersen E. Bovine respiratory syncytial virus (BRSV) pneumonia in beef calf herds despite vaccination. Acta Vet Scand 2001;42(1): 113–21.

35. Fulton RW, Briggs RE, Ridpath JF, et al. Transmission of bovine viral diarrhea virus 1b to susceptible and vaccinated calves by exposure to persistently infected calves. Can J Vet Res 2005;69(3):161–9.

36. Ellis J, Gow S, Berenik A, et al. Comparative efficacy of modified-live and inactivated vaccines in boosting responses to bovine respiratory syncytial virus following neonatal mucosal priming of beef calves. Can Vet J 2018;59(12): 1311–9.

37. USDA. NAHMS.Beef. Part IV: refernce of beef cow-calf management practices in the United States. 2007-08. Available at:aphis.usda.gov/animal_health/nahms/beefcowcalf/downloads/beef0708/Beef0708_dr_PartIV.pdf. . Accessed December 3, 2019.

38. Hanzlicek GA, Renter DR, White BJ, et al. Management practices associated with the rate of respiratory tract disease among preweaned beef calves in cow-calf operations in the United States. J Am Vet Med Assoc 2013;242(9):1271–8.

39. Woolums AR, Berghaus RD, Smith DR, et al. Producer survey of herd-level risk factors for nursing beef calf respiratory disease. J Am Vet Med Assoc 2013; 243(4):538–47.

40. Chamorro MF, Walz PH, Passler T, et al. Efficacy of four commercially available multivalent modified-live virus vaccines against clinical disease, viremia, and viral shedding in early-weaned beef calves exposed simultaneously to cattle persistently infected with bovine viral diarrhea virus and cattle acutely infected with bovine herpesvirus 1. Am J Vet Res 2016;77(1):88–97.

41. Chamorro MF, Walz PH, Passler T, et al. Efficacy of multivalent, modified- live virus (MLV) vaccines administered to early weaned beef calves subsequently challenged with virulent Bovine viral diarrhea virus type 2. BMC Vet Res 2015;11:29.

42. Makoschey B, Janssen MG, Vrijenhoek MP, et al. An inactivated bovine virus diarrhoea virus (BVDV) type 1 vaccine affords clinical protection against BVDV type 2. Vaccine 2001;19(23–24):3261–8.

43. Dubrovsky SA, Van Eenennaam AL, Karle BM, et al. Bovine respiratory disease (BRD) cause-specific and overall mortality in preweaned calves on California dairies: The BRD10K study. J Dairy Sci 2019;102(8):7320–8.

44. Aubry P, Warnick LD, Guard CL, et al. Health and performance of young dairy calves vaccinated with a modified-live Mannheimiahaemolytica and Pasteurella-multocida vaccine. J Am Vet Med Assoc 2001;219(12):1739–42.
45. Ollivett TL, Leslie KE, Duffield TF, et al. Field trial to evaluate the effect of an intra-nasal respiratory vaccine protocol on calf health, ultrasonographic lung consoli-dation, and growth in Holstein dairy calves. J Dairy Sci 2018;101(9):8159–68.
46. Windeyer MC, Leslie KE, Godden SM, et al. Association of bovine respiratory dis-ease or vaccination with serologic response in dairy heifer calves up to three months of age. Am J Vet Res 2015;76(3):239–45.
47. Bowersock TL, Sobecki BE, Terrill SJ, et al. Efficacy of a multivalent modified-live virus vaccine containing a Mannheimiahaemolytica toxoid in calves challenge exposed with Bibersteiniatrehalosi. Am J Vet Res 2014;75(8):770–6.
48. Cortese VS, Grooms DL, Ellis J, et al. Protection of pregnant cattle and their fe-tuses against infection with bovine viral diarrhea virus type 1 by use of a modified-live virus vaccine. Am J Vet Res 1998;59(11):1409–13.
49. Ellis J, Gow S, West K, et al. Response of calves to challenge exposure with viru-lent bovine respiratory syncytial virus following intranasal administration of vac-cines formulated for parenteral administration. J Am Vet Med Assoc 2007;230(2):233–43.
50. Ellis J, West K, Cortese V, et al. Effect of maternal antibodies on induction and persistence of vaccine-induced immune responses against bovine viral diarrhea virus type II in young calves. J Am Vet Med Assoc 2001;219(3):351–6.
51. Ellis J, West K, Konoby C, et al. Efficacy of an inactivated respiratory syncytial vi-rus vaccine in calves. J Am Vet Med Assoc 2001;218(12):1973–80.
52. Ellis JA, Gow SP, Goji N. Response to experimentally induced infection with bovine respiratory syncytial virus following intranasal vaccination of seropositive and seronegative calves. J Am Vet Med Assoc 2010;236(9):991–9.
53. Ellis JA, Gow SP, Mahan S, et al. Duration of immunity to experimental infection with bovine respiratory syncytial virus following intranasal vaccination of young passively immune calves. J Am Vet Med Assoc 2013;243(11):1602–8.
54. Ellis JA, West KH, Waldner C, et al. Efficacy of a saponin-adjuvanted inactivated respiratory syncytial virus vaccine in calves. Can Vet J 2005;46(2):155–62.
55. Patel JR, Didlick SA. Evaluation of efficacy of an inactivated vaccine against bovine respiratory syncytial virus in calves with maternal antibodies. Am J Vet Res 2004;65(4):417–21.
56. Platt R, Widel PW, Kesl LD, et al. Comparison of humoral and cellular immune re-sponses to a pentavalent modified live virus vaccine in three age groups of calves with maternal antibodies, before and after BVDV type 2 challenge. Vac-cine 2009;27(33):4508–19.
57. Ridpath JE, Neill JD, Endsley J, et al. Effect of passive immunity on the develop-ment of a protective immune response against bovine viral diarrhea virus in calves. Am J Vet Res 2003;64(1):65–9.
58. Vangeel I, Antonis AF, Fluess M, et al. Efficacy of a modified live intranasal bovine respiratory syncytial virus vaccine in 3-week-old calves experimentally chal-lenged with BRSV. Vet J 2007;174(3):627–35.
59. West K, Petrie L, Haines DM, et al. The effect of formalin-inactivated vaccine on respiratory disease associated with bovine respiratory syncytial virus infection in calves. Vaccine 1999;17(7–8):809–20.
60. West K, Petrie L, Konoby C, et al. The efficacy of modified-live bovine respiratory syncytial virus vaccines in experimentally infected calves. Vaccine 1999;18(9–10):907–19.

61. Xue W, Mattick D, Smith L, et al. Vaccination with a modified-live bovine viral diarrhea virus (BVDV) type 1a vaccine completely protected calves against challenge with BVDV type 1b strains. Vaccine 2010;29(1):70–6.
62. Zimmerman AD, Boots RE, Valli JL, et al. Evaluation of protection against virulent bovine viral diarrhea virus type 2 in calves that had maternal antibodies and were vaccinated with a modified-live vaccine. J Am Vet Med Assoc 2006;228(11):1757–61.
63. Kolb EA, Buterbaugh RE, Rinehart CL, et al. Protection against bovine respiratory syncytial virus in calves vaccinated with adjuvanted modified live vaccine administered in the face of maternal antibody. Vaccine 2020;38(2):298–308.
64. O'Neill RG, Fitzpatrick JL, Glass EJ, et al. Optimisation of the response to respiratory virus vaccines in cattle. Vet Rec 2007;161(8):269–70.
65. O'Neill RG, Woolliams JA, Glass EJ, et al. Quantitative evaluation of genetic and environmental parameters determining antibody response induced by vaccination against bovine respiratory syncytial virus. Vaccine 2006;24(18):4007–16.
66. Chamorro MF, Walz PH, Haines DM, et al. Comparison of levels and duration of detection of antibodies to bovine viral diarrhea virus 1, bovine viral diarrhea virus 2, bovine respiratory syncytial virus, bovine herpesvirus 1, and bovine parainfluenza virus 3 in calves fed maternal colostrum or a colostrum-replacement product. Can J Vet Res 2014;78(2):81–8.
67. Hill KL, Hunsaker BD, Townsend HG, et al. Mucosal immune response in newborn Holstein calves that had maternally derived antibodies and were vaccinated with an intranasal multivalent modified-live virus vaccine. J Am Vet Med Assoc 2012;240(10):1231–40.
68. Kimman TG, Westenbrink F, Straver PJ. Priming for local and systemic antibody memory responses to bovine respiratory syncytial virus: effect of amount of virus, virus replication, route of administration and maternal antibodies. Vet Immunollmmunopathol 1989;22(2):145–60.
69. Wilson BK, Step DL, Maxwell CL, et al. Evaluation of multiple ancillary therapies used in combination with an antimicrobial in newly received high-risk calves treated for bovine respiratory disease. J Anim Sci 2015;93(7):3661–74.
70. Hill K, Arsic N, Nordstrom S, et al. Immune memory induced by intranasal vaccination with a modified-live viral vaccine delivered to colostrum fed neonatal calves. Vaccine 2019;37(51):7455–62.

Bovine Respiratory Disease Vaccination

What Is the Effect of Timing?

John T. Richeson, PhD[a],*, T. Robin Falkner, DVM[b]

KEYWORDS

- Bovine respiratory disease • Cattle • Delayed vaccination • Vaccine timing

KEY POINTS

- To be effective, vaccination against bovine respiratory disease (BRD) antigen should be administered several weeks before homologous or heterologous infectious challenge.
- Physiologic stress can result in transient immunosuppression, and vaccination during this time can differentially alter the antigenicity of killed virus and modified-live virus vaccine agents.
- If BRD vaccines are administered at inappropriate times, they are capable of being more detrimental than beneficial, and vaccine safety should be considered when designing vaccine regimens at various periods in the beef production system.
- The current USDA biological approval process uses safety and efficacy models that consider ideal vaccine timing relative to infectious challenge, but this model is not always representative of current field application of BRD vaccine timing in cattle.

INTRODUCTION

Bovine respiratory disease (BRD) is arguably the most complicated mammalian disease that exists. It involves stress-induced immunosuppression, infection with one or more viruses, and culminates with bronchopneumonia caused by otherwise commensal bacterial organisms that originate in the nasopharynx. One must recognize the systematic pathogenesis of BRD, host immunologic and epidemiologic interplay, vaccinology, and commercial beef production practices to fully appreciate the importance of timing of vaccination against BRD causative agents. Regarding BRD vaccination, timing is (almost) everything. Sufficient time is required for the act of vaccination to result in desirable immunization against BRD causative agents, and without immunization before pathogen challenge, it is imprudent to expect positive

[a] Department of Agricultural Sciences, West Texas A&M University, WTAMU Box 60998, Canyon, TX 79016, USA; [b] CattleFlow Consulting, 2404 Walnut Grove Road, Christiana, TN 37037, USA
* Corresponding author.
E-mail address: jricheson@wtamu.edu

Vet Clin Food Anim 36 (2020) 473–485
https://doi.org/10.1016/j.cvfa.2020.03.013
0749-0720/20/© 2020 Elsevier Inc. All rights reserved.

health outcomes as a result of vaccination. Moreover, research and empirical evidence suggests that BRD health outcomes may worsen overall if the timing of vaccination occurs in the face of physiologic stress and/or natural BRD outbreak.

Multivalent viral vaccines against bovine herpesvirus 1 (BHV-1), bovine viral diarrhea virus (BVDV) type 1 and 2, bovine respiratory syncytial virus (BRSV), and parainfluenza virus 3 (PI-3V) are commercially available in inactivated (killed) and active (modified-live) forms. Furthermore, bacterin and/or leukotoxoid formulations are available against *Mannheimia haemolytica* (*Mh*; including its leukotoxin), *Pasteurella multocida* (*Pm*), and *Histophilus somni* (*Hs*). All of these vaccines against recognized BRD causative agents require various time to stimulate an active immune response that results in protection. None of the vaccines are expected to provide full protective immunity in every animal in every population. However, the timing of administration of the different BRD antigens is critical for vaccine efficacy and efficiency. Key times of BRD vaccine administration in beef cattle include near birth (neonates), during the management event known as branding (nursing calves 60–120 days of age), at or near weaning (typical age of 205 days), and on arrival at subsequent production sectors such as stocker and/or feedlot facilities. The adoption rate of BRD vaccination is typically increased as beef cattle age and progress through the segments of the beef production system. For example, only 39% of beef calves at their ranch origin were vaccinated against respiratory antigens before sale, yet 96% of cattle arriving at US feedlots are administered a respiratory vaccine.[1] The objective of this review is to summarize pertinent research and discuss BRD vaccination at different times of the North American beef production system.

THE BEEF PRODUCTION SYSTEM AND BOVINE RESPIRATORY DISEASE VACCINE TIMING

There are several key times that vaccination occurs during the segmented and dynamic beef production system.[2] The earliest opportunity to vaccinate beef calves is immediately after birth; however, this can be problematic both logistically and immunologically.[3] Previous doctrine based on antibody titers supposed a lack of vaccine efficacy in the face of acquired maternal antibodies in young beef calves; however, subsequent research has since demonstrated efficacy of modified-live virus (MLV) vaccination during this time. Specifically, cell-mediated immunity can be acquired from MLV vaccination in young calves with significant concentration of maternal antibodies present from colostrum.[4] Also, neonatal calves vaccinated with live-attenuated BVDV antigen were protected from subsequent BVDVchallenge.[5,6] In calves vaccinated at approximately 60 days of age, during the production practice known as "branding," BVDV-specific humoral immunity was conferred even though BVDV antibody from maternal transfer was present at the time of MLV vaccination.[7,8]

Practical considerations of vaccinating during the cow calf, preconditioning (post-weaning at the origin ranch), stocker, and feedlot levels of the beef production system are illustrated previously.[2] Regarding vaccination timing, it seems prudent that a need exists to "shift BRD vaccination upstream" compared with the current timing of BRD vaccine administration. Vaccine use in feedlots is nearly unanimous; more than 93% of feedlots vaccinated cattle against BVDV and BHV-1, with a lesser majority vaccinating against other respiratory viruses (BRSV = 89.5%; PI-3V = 85.1%) or bacteria (*Mh* or *Pm* = 63.8%; *Hs* = 69.7%). Compare that with the much smaller percentage of cow-calf operations that vaccinated against respiratory disease before sale (39% of all cow-calf operations[9]), and one could undoubtedly make the claim that the beef industry has BRD vaccination timing "backwards." Unfortunately, the structure of the cow-calf production and marketing system does not promote widespread adoption of BRD vaccination and is one reason that the BRD vaccine adoption rate within the cow-calf segment has remained relatively low and unchanged. For example, most of the US cow-calf operations have less than 50 head[9] and are less likely to have facilities, expertise, or economic incentive to vaccinate before marketing, and the marketing system may not provide sufficient economic signals needed to promote wider adoption of BRD vaccination at the cow-calf level. Current adoption rates indicate that many calves receive primary vaccination as they transition between segments, under stress and in the face of pathogen exposure. This situation is not ideal for vaccine efficiency and is potentially harmful.

Preconditioning is a longstanding management practice that can be implemented at the ranch origin to improve subsequent health and performance in cattle.[10] Preconditioning requires a series of vaccination and management practices to better prepare beef calves for the transition to subsequent production sectors (ie, stocker and/or feedlot). Yet, there is limited field evidence and understanding of the contribution of acquired BRD resistance afforded by vaccination at birth, branding, and/or weaning, because few studies have attempted to delineate the effects of the individual practices that are implemented during preconditioning, including BRD vaccination. Indeed, the management practices implemented during preconditioning, such as weaning, may be more important than vaccination for providing health subsequent benefit in the feedlot. In a study that compared ranch calves weaned for 45 days, with or without a pentavalent MLV vaccine and Mh leukotoxoid, there was no difference in health or performance attributed to BRD vaccination. However, both weaned groups had improved health and performance compared with cohorts that were not weaned at the ranch origin and shipped directly to the feedlot.[11]

Likewise, stress-induced immunosuppression and the rapid onset of BRD that is common in high-risk, newly received stocker and feedlot cattle should influence thought processes of the veterinary practitioner when recommending and designing vaccine protocols. The recently modified USDA vaccine label guidelines indicate, "This product has been shown to be efficacious in healthy animals. A protective immune response may not be elicited if animals are incubating an infectious disease, are malnourished or parasitized, are stressed due to shipment or environmental conditions, are otherwise immunocompromised, or the vaccine is not administered in accordance with label directions." On arrival, high-risk beef calves are more likely to be incubating an infectious disease, malnourished and parasitized, stressed, and immunocompromised, all of which are cautioned against in the USDA vaccine label indication. Therefore, research has evaluated delayed MLV vaccination to understand if benefits might exist when adequate time postarrival has elapsed such that all or most of the previously stated cautionary conditions are resolved before vaccination.

DELAYED BOVINE RESPIRATORY DISEASE VACCINATION IN HIGH-RISK CATTLE
Vaccine Efficacy

Vaccine efficacy may be simply defined as the ability of a particular vaccine to induce a significant immunologic response in the host. Delayed administration of a pentavalent MLV vaccine in high-risk, auction-derived beef calves was first conceptualized by researchers at the University of Arkansas over a decade ago[12] to improve the efficacy (ie, humoral immune response) of BRD vaccination. Subsequently, the concept of delaying MLV vaccination in high-risk beef calves has been further evaluated, and a recent meta-analysis summarized research on delayed MLV vaccination in high-risk beef cattle.[13] Although the original hypothesis for evaluating delayed administration of MLV antigens in stressed, newly received beef calves was to allow a more desirable immunologic response (efficacy) to the vaccine in the delayed cohort, limited research coupled with systematic immunologic reasoning suggests other justifications (**Figs. 1** and **2**).

In the first published study evaluating the delayed administration of MLV vaccine in high-risk, newly received beef calves, an improvement in BHV-1-specific seroconversion was noted on equivalent days past initial vaccination and at the end of the 42-day receiving period for the delayed MLV group.[12] However, this observation has not been repeatable; subsequent studies evaluating MLV vaccine timing and antibody titer responses in high-risk, newly received beef calves suggest faster and greater overall antibody response for the on-arrival MLV procedure. A subsequent study[14] reported BVDV type 1a–specific antibody to be greater for the on-arrival group 14 and 28 days postpentavalent MLV vaccination, and BVDV-specific antibody titers were similar on day 42. Poe and colleagues[15] (2013) also observed earlier and greater BVDV-specific antibody titer for high-risk calves vaccinated on arrival beginning on day 14, and antibody concentration remained increased for the on-arrival group until at least day 42 postarrival.

An erroneous paradigm exists regarding stress-induced immunosuppression and vaccine response (efficacy) in beef cattle. It is often stated that stress reduces the ability of beef cattle to respond to vaccination, and indeed this concept was the original hypothesis for evaluating delayed MLV vaccination in stressed, high-risk beef calves. However, the interaction of stress and BRD vaccination in high-risk beef calves is extremely complicated and influenced by several factors such as (1) the type of vaccine antigen administered (MLV vs killed virus [KV] vs inactivated bacterin/leukotoxoid), (2) acute infection with wild-type virus in vaccines, and (3) natural and genetic variation of stress impact on the immunocompetence of individual animals within a population.

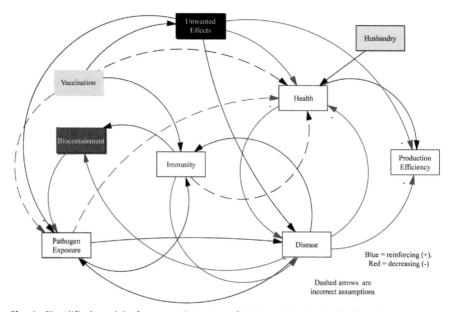

Fig. 1. Simplified model of systems dynamics of MLV vaccination in beef cattle.

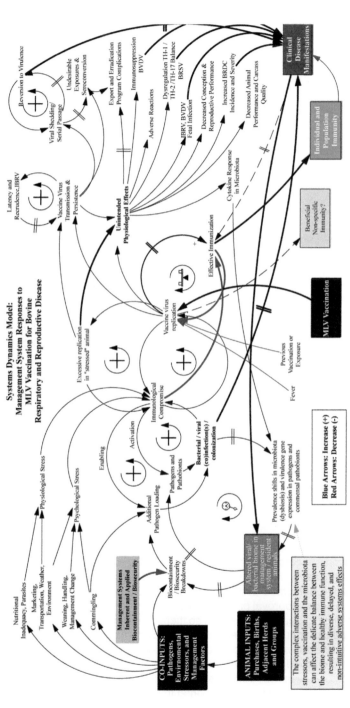

Fig. 2. Systems dynamics model of MLV vaccination in beef cattle.

A previous review of glucocorticoid impacts on the bovine immune system[16] illustrates differences in the humoral immune response to vaccine antigens influenced by the type of vaccine antigen being administered to stressed cattle (MLV vs KV). Indeed, cortisol and other physiologic components of the stress response such as catecholamines may suppress antibody production via plasma cells or increased protein (antibody) catabolism in the bovine. Ultimately, the humoral immune response in high-risk, newly received beef cattle affected by stress-induced immunosuppression is more greatly influenced by the altered antigenicity of MLV (increased antigenicity) or KV (decreased antigenicity) antigens being administered versus direct antibody catabolism or impairment of immunologic products from vaccination. This altered antigenicity is explained by increased cortisol from chronic stress (ie, combination of weaning, handling, transportation, commingling, environment), causing an immunosuppressive state that allows enhanced replication of MLV vaccine antigens in host cells, increased antigenic stimulus toward the hosts immune system, and a subsequently enhanced antibody titer response for immunosuppressed vaccinates. Cattle treated with an acute, chronic, or no dexamethasone challenge and vaccinated with a multivalent, combination respiratory vaccine-bacterin had different antibody titer responses depending on the antigen-specific antibody evaluated.[17] The leukotoxin-specific antibody response from a nonreplicating toxoid was least in the chronically stressed steers, intermediate for acute stress, and greatest for control. Conversely, both the BHV-1- and BVDV-specific antibody response from the MLV component of the vaccine was greatest for chronically stressed steers, intermediate for acute, and least for control. Because antibody titer concentration is used as a proxy for vaccine response and is a major component of vaccine efficacy, researchers and veterinary practitioners should consider the differential response to vaccine antigen type in stressed cattle and recognize that the all-encompassing paradigm of "stress reduces vaccine response in cattle" is false. It is also important to question the safety of enhanced viral replication from an MLV vaccine administered to chronically stressed calves. One should consider that a primary means of achieving safety in current MLV vaccines is reducing the replication rate, balancing it with the ability of the immune system of a healthy animal to respond appropriately and end the acute MLV infection. This balance between (1) sufficient MLV "infectivity" to produce enough antigen exposure for a competent immune response and (2) sufficient MLV "attenuation" to prevent or reduce viremia and diseaselike adverse effects may be misplaced in the stressed or immunocompromised animal.

Vaccine Safety and Efficiency

For a vaccine to be efficient it must also be safe under the conditions of administration, yet a vaccine may be inefficient and also safe. Vaccination that results in net detriment to health and performance outcomes should not be considered safe. *Vaccine efficiency exists when vaccination is clearly demonstrated to result in improved clinical health and performance outcomes compared with nonvaccinated cohort.* Unfortunately, the current biological approval process does not require commercial vaccines to demonstrate efficiency under field conditions so there is little incentive for manufacturers of vaccine products to fund field research that includes a nonvaccinated control, yet a control treatment is required to determine vaccine efficiency.

Research evaluating delayed MLV vaccination has provided insight, albeit perhaps inadvertent, on the efficiency of MLV vaccines in high-risk cattle, because a negative control group exists for the length of the delay period from arrival and typically most of the initial cases of clinical BRD occurs during the first 14 days of the implemented MLV delay period. Relative safety and inefficiency of MLV vaccination is demonstrated in most of the delayed MLV literature. In small-pen research studies evaluating on-arrival versus 14-day delayed MLV administration, health outcomes for the delayed procedure have varied from beneficial[12] to statistically equivocal or numerically detri-mental.[14,15,18] Large-pen (larger sample size) studies have the distinct advantage of evaluating binomial and infrequent (ie, mortality) health outcomes with greater statis-tical power and confidence, albeit at the expense of methodological control. Also noteworthy, the previously discussed small pen studies used a delay period of only 14 days, and a longer delay of 28 days or more is probably more beneficial given the typical pathogenesis of BRD in high-risk, newly received beef calves.[19] Rogers and colleagues (2016)[20] evaluated an MLV delay period of 30 days in 5179 auction-derived feedlot heifers (large pen) and reported health results in periods of day 0 to 60, day 0 to 116, and day 0 to closeout. For the early period (day 0–60), the percentage of heifers requiring 2 BRD treatments was reduced for the delayed groups, and a numerical reduction in third BRD treatment, BRD case fatality percent-age, BRD mortality, and overall mortality rate was noted for heifers administered MLV on day 30 versus on arrival. Retreatment percentage was less, and overall mortality tended to be less through day 116 for the delayed MLV groups with similar numerical improvement for other health variables, whereas during the entire feedlot finishing period (day 0 to closeout), the percentage of heifers requiring 2 BRD treatments was less and a reduction in BRD retreatment risk existed for the 30-day delayed MLV procedure.

In a similar large-pen experiment,[21] delayed (28 days) MLV administration was compared with 2 traditional on-arrival regimens and no statistical differences were noted; however, morbidity was slightly increased and mortality was slightly decreased for the delayed procedure. In response to industry and veterinary practitioner interest in delayed MLV vaccination, a systematic review was recently conducted.[13] Although the number of qualified studies included in the analysis was small, the risk ratio out-comes for morbidity and retreatment risk between delayed and on-arrival MLV vacci-nation was equivocal. However, there was a slight (confidence interval 0.57, 1.10) reduction in BRD mortality risk for delayed MLV. The investigators concluded that there is no benefit to delayed MLV vaccination in high-risk, newly received cattle and that vaccination of high-risk beef cattle in the feedlot is equally ineffective regard-less of timing. In previous reviews of field efficacy of viral respiratory vaccination of feedlot cattle published in 1983,[22] 1997,[23] and 2013[24] the same general conclusions over the decades are evident; the effect of vaccination in feedlot cattle is "equivocal, at best".[23]

Conclusions regarding MLV field efficiency in cattle are wrought with poor confi-dence, because a negative control treatment is rarely used and thus efficiency inter-pretations are often confounded in most of the existing literature. However, a recent study in high-risk stocker calves that used a negative control MLV treatment reported MLV and clostridial vaccination to adversely affect both health and performance.[25] In that study population, calves vaccinated with an MLV vaccine and clostridial bacterin-toxoid were 3.2 times more likely to be treated for BRD and had 8.3 times greater odds of death, with weight gain across the 85-day observation period being 10.3 lb less than nonvaccinated (control) calves. A study comparing the efficacy of MLV on arrival with revaccination on day 14 to that of metaphylaxis with tulathromycin in same population of high-risk feedlot cattle observed clear health and performance benefit for cattle receiving metaphylaxis and no statistical effect of MLV vaccination.[26] Performance was numerically less from day 0 to 28 in MLV vaccinates on receiving vaccine on day 0 and 14, followed by compensatory increase in average daily gain from day 28 to 56, such that the overall gain was not different for cattle administered MLV or not.

Revaccination 14 days following initial MLV has been a common practice in stocker and feedlot cattle; however, the value of this practice is questionable given the additional labor, handling, and immunologic cost. Indeed, revaccination during a preconditioning program resulted in greater BRD morbidity and no differences in performance.[27] In the subsequent feedlot period, no differences in performance or closeout characteristics existed for calves vaccinated, revaccinated, or with or without MLV vaccination on feedlot arrival. Therefore, it is probably redundant to vaccinate against respiratory viruses in well-immunized (preconditioned) cattle on feedlot arrival. Preconditioned calves arriving at a stocker research facility with sufficient antibody titers against BVDV type 1a, 1b, and 2a seemed to be protected against natural BVDV type 1b challenge sans MLV vaccination on arrival.[28] Because existing research rarely demonstrates a benefit to MLV vaccination in either naïve or immunized groups of cattle, why do we continue to implement the practice? If the practice of MLV vaccination postweaning is largely ceased across the stocker and feedlot segments, would epidemic ramifications emerge? Conversely, if we continue extensive use of MLV in stressed, immunosuppressed calves that may harbor acute infection with respiratory virus, has this practice contributed to the frustrating trend of increased BRD mortality rate over time[29]? These are just a few of the vaccination questions that require additional research to better understand.

STRESS-INDUCED IMMUNOSUPPRESSION AND VACCINE TIMING

The impetus for delayed vaccination in high-risk, newly received beef cattle exists primarily because stress-induced immunosuppression significantly alters the outcomes of MLV-influenced immunity in the host. Because immune functions in stressed cattle are compromised,[30] MLV antigens are permitted to replicate in host cells to a much greater degree compared with a nonstressed animal with immunocompetence, resulting in marked increase in the antigenicity of an MLV vaccine administered to the immunosuppressed host. This effect is demonstrated in the bovine model after dexamethasone challenge[17] and adrenocorticotropic hormone challenge[31]; both stress challenge models resulted in immunosuppression and presumably greater replication of MLV antigens in the host. The antigenicity of BVDV and BHV-1 antigens contained in the MLV were enhanced, as illustrated by significantly greater antibody titer and virus presence in nasal swab samples postvaccination in dexamethasone-treated groups.[17] Conversely, antibody against the nonreplicating Mh leukotoxin fraction of the combination vaccine and the concentration of acute phase proteins were reduced after vaccination of dexamethasone-treated animals. Therefore, the authors provide 3 primary reasons why the literature does not clearly support MLV vaccine efficiency in high-risk stocker and feedlot cattle: (1) natural virus exposure during the marketing process and inappropriate timing of vaccination relative to natural challenge with various respiratory pathogens, (2) enhanced MLV replication when administered to cattle influenced by stress-induced immune dysregulation, and (3) negative interactions or synergism with MLV and otherwise commensal host bacteria that cause bronchopneumonia. Delaying MLV vaccination for at least 28 days probably mitigates the risk for adverse effects versus on-arrival MLV when stress and/or natural BRD challenge are most likely present.

Furthermore, because of the latent properties known to exist for BHV-1, whether transmitted naturally or via MLV vaccine, the potential exists for BHV-1 recrudescence during subsequent periods of immunosuppression.[32] Overreplication of live attenuated BVDV vaccine antigen in stressed animals can result in viremia, leukopenia, serial passage, and undesirable replication in respiratory epithelium.[33] Other unwanted

A

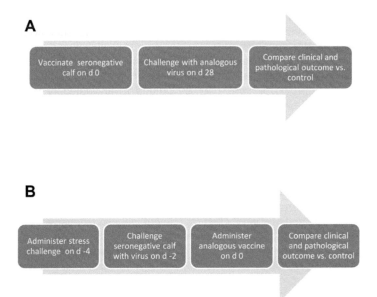

B

Fig. 3. Example of vaccine safety and efficacy models used for USDA approval of biologicals (*A*) and field conditions of vaccine used in high-risk beef calves (*B*).

effects under current study include viral vaccine-induced cytokine signaling for (1) shifts in the microbiome, (2) activating pathobiont virulence, and (3) dysregulation of immune responses to other pathogens. An example is the synergy between BRSV vaccination and *Hs*. In 2 experiments, (1) administration of a commercial MLV BRSV vaccine increased adverse reactions to *Hs* bacterins and (2) clinical bronchopneumonia was greater when the BRSV vaccine was concomitantly administered with an intratracheal *Hs* challenge.[34] Other researchers characterized a synergy between BRSV and *Hs*, demonstrating that sequential intranasal exposure to BRSV before *Hs* produced severe lung immunopathology while neither organism induced such pathology independently.[35] Intranasal MLV vaccines offer the conundrum of slightly faster specific immunity at the likely site of natural exposure and negative consequences for other potential pathogens from vaccine virus replication and cytokine signaling in the respiratory epithelium. Other examples are illustrated with a vaccinal strain of BVDV causing immunosuppression of neutrophils harvested from stressed and unstressed cattle[31] and voluntary withdrawal of an USDA-approved multivalent MLV intranasal vaccine by the manufacturer due to associated adverse events, including increased BRD morbidity and mortality in highly stressed cattle.

Of the 25 USDA-approved *Hs* bacterins, all were licensed before 1985 and neither the manufacturers nor USDA can produce safety and efficacy data for them.[36] A systematic review of the published scientific literature did not find sufficient evidence to conclude that *Hs, Pm,* or *Mh* bacterins in feedlot cattle are effective against BRD.[37] Many bacterins labeled for BRD pathogens use antiquated technology, questionable efficacy models, and were approved before modern safety and efficacy requirements existed.[38]

Further research is necessary to determine the safety and efficacy of different vaccine antigens administered to high-risk or high-stress or chronically stressed cattle. It is thought that current USDA approval and safety studies do not adequately assess the circumstances under which many vaccines are commonly administered, that is, in times of stress, concurrently with other products, and/or in the face of disease challenge (**Fig. 3**). Nor does the current biologics approval process anticipate and measure adverse events that might be expected, given literature showing interactions between vaccine antigens with each other or pathobionts in the microbiome. The incomplete approval process may be confusing to veterinary practitioners, because the development and approval of vaccine products within a narrow set of safety parameters encourages use in circumstances that may cause net harm. Although it is unrealistic to expect manufacturers to demonstrate the safety and efficiency of their products in every possible production setting, the lack of negative control vaccine studies in the circumstances of most frequent use and promotion such as primary or booster vaccination at weaning or during arrival processing in stocker or feedlot production settings is concerning. Veterinarians should carefully develop vaccination protocols for each particular circumstance, evaluating all of the animal, disease, and husbandry factors present including management expectations and constraints. No product or protocol is a "one-size-fits-all or most," and vaccine applications may be based on marketing, company promotion, and habit without sufficient evidence of safety and efficiency. For example, it is unlikely that a single MLV vaccine product could be optimized for a mature cow for fetal protection, duration of immunity, and also arrival vaccination of a naïve, stressed, pathogen-exposed calf, although the same products are widely recommended for both purposes. Little effort has been expended in developing and identifying products optimized for use in stressed cattle despite widespread use of MLV vaccines during stress. Vaccination several weeks before transitioning to the next production segment is preferable to arrival vaccination. Delaying traditional arrival vaccination to a later time may be the best option when animals are stressed and/or exposed to multiple pathogens, regardless of prior vaccination history. Products of questionable efficiency and probable deleterious effects should be abandoned altogether. Most importantly, during postweaning segments prioritization of management strategies in addition to vaccination and antimicrobials, such as stress mitigation, improved husbandry and housing condition, and biocontainment within and between groups are likely to have meaningful impacts on BRD incidence and severity.

SUMMARY

The best time to vaccinate cattle against BRD causative agents is when they are in a state of immunologic homeostasis, free of acute infection, and at least several weeks before natural BRD challenge is expected. Simply put, BRD vaccination should occur before weaning and entering marketing channels to the next production segment. Any arrival vaccination is suboptimal and may be inferior to delayed vaccination or no vaccination at all within a given product and management setting interaction. Historically, these basic principles of appropriate BRD vaccination timing have been overlooked, and cattle vaccine research has consisted of safety and efficacy testing under model conditions for USDA approval, or in postapproval vaccine product comparisons ("marketing studies") under field conditions, without a negative control treatment necessary to truly determine vaccine efficiency. To better understand the effect of BRD vaccine timing and efficiency, biological manufacturers and independent investigators should focus future research efforts on developing and testing antigenic technology, different antigen combinations, and timing of administration to meet the needs of the industry that are appropriate for the animal factors, management constraints, and pathogen challenges that are present. Such research would allow veterinary practitioners to provide better-informed vaccine recommendations through evidence-based decision-making, rather than decision-based evidence making. Currently, unnecessary burden is placed on veterinary practitioners to deduce appropriate vaccination protocols from insufficient evidence of product safety and efficiency in the production scenarios they are presented.

DISCLOSURE

Drs J.T. Richeson and R. Falkner have received financial support from veterinary biologics and pharmaceutical manufacturers for consulting and to conduct research in the area of bovine respiratory disease. Dr R. Falkner is currently employed by Elanco Animal Health, a company that develops and markets products used for the prevention, treatment, and control of bovine respiratory disease.

REFERENCES

1. USDA. Vaccine usage in U.S. feedlots.No. 672.0513. Fort Collins (CO): USDA, Animal and Plant Health Inspection Service, Veterinary Services, Centers for Epidemiology and Animal Health; 2013.
2. Richeson JT, Hughes HD, Broadway PR, et al. Vaccination management of beef cattle: delayed vaccination and endotoxin stacking. Vet Clin North Am Food AnimPract 2019;35:575–92.
3. Windeyer MC, Gamsjager L. Vaccinating calves in the face of maternal antibodies: challenges and opportunities. Vet Clin North Am Food AnimPract 2019; 35:557–73.
4. Platt R, Widel PW, Kesi LD, et al. Comparison of humoral and cellular immune responses to a pentavalent modified live virus vaccine in three age groups of calves with maternal antibodies, before and after BVDV type 2 challenge. Vaccine 2009; 27:4508–19.
5. Zimmerman AD, Buterbaugh RE, Schnackel JA, et al. Efficacy of a modified-live virus vaccine administered to calves with maternal antibodies and challenged seven months later with a virulent bovine viral diarrhea type 2 virus. BovPract (Stillwater) 2009;43:35–43.
6. Stevens ET, Brown MS, Burdett WW, et al. Efficacy of a non-adjuvanated, modified-live virus vaccine in calves with maternal antibodies against a virulent bovine viral diarrhea virus type 2a challenge seven months following vaccination. BovPract (Stillwater) 2011;45:23–31.
7. Kirkpatrick JG, Step DL, Payton ME, et al. Effect of age at the time of vaccination on antibody titers and feedlot performance in beef calves. J Am Vet Med Assoc 2008;233:136–42.
8. Powell JG, Richeson JT, Kegley EB, et al. Immunologic, health, and growth responses of beef calves administered pentavalent modified-live virus respiratory vaccine in the presence of maternal antibody versus a traditional vaccination regimen. BovPract (Stillwater) 2012;46:122–30.
9. USDA. Beef 2007-08. Part IV: reference of beef cow-calf management practices in the United States, 2007-08. #523.0210. Fort Collins (CO): USDA, Animal and Plant Health Inspection Service, Veterinary Sciences, Centers for Epidemiology and Animal Health; 2010.
10. Seeger JT, Grotelueschen DM, Stokka GL, et al. Comparison of feedlot health, nutritional performance, carcass characteristics and economic value of unweaned beef cavles with unknown health history and weaned beef calves

receiving various herd-of-origin health protocols. BovPract (Stillwater) 2008;42: 27–39.

11. Step DL, Krehbiel CR, DePra HA, et al. Effects of commingling beef calves from different sources and weaning protocols during a forty-two-day receiving period on performance and bovine respiratory disease. J AnimSci 2008;86:3146–58.

12. Richeson JT, Beck PA, Gadberry MS, et al. Effects of on-arrival versus delayed modified live virus vaccination on health, performance, and serum infectious bovine rhinotracheitis virus titers of newly received beef calves. J AnimSci 2008;86:999–1005.

13. Snyder ER, Credille BC, Heins BD. Systematic review and meta-analysis comparing arrival versus delayed vaccination of high-risk beef cattle with 5-way modified-live viral vaccines against BHV-1, BRSV, PI3 and BVD types 1 and 2. BovPract (Stillwater) 2019;53:1–7.

14. Richeson JT, Kegley EB, Gadberry MS, et al. Effects of on-arrival versus delayed clostridial or modified live respiratory vaccinations on health, performance, bovine viral diarrhea virus type I titers, and stress and immune measures of newly received beef calves. J AnimSci 2009;87:2409–18.

15. Poe KD, Beck PA, Richeson JT, et al. Effects of respiratory vaccination timing and growth-promoting implant on health, performance, and immunity of high-risk, newly received stocker cattle. Prof Anim Sci 2013;29:413–9.

16. Roth JA. Cortisol as a mediator of stress-associated immunosuppression in cattle. In: Moberg GP, editor. Animal stress. New York: Springer; 1985. p. 225–43.

17. Richeson JT, Carroll JA, Burdick Sanchez NC, et al. Dexamethasone treatment differentially alters viral shedding and the antibody and acute phase protein response after multivalent respiratory vaccination in beef steers. J AnimSci 2016;94:3501–9.

18. Richeson JT, Beck PA, Poe KD, et al. Effects of administration of a modified-live virus respiratory vaccine and timing of vaccination on health and performance of high-risk beef stocker calves. BovPract (Stillwater) 2015;49:37–42.

19. Taylor JD, Fulton RW, Lehenbauer TW, et al. The epidemiology of bovine respiratory disease: what is the evidence for predisposing factors? Can Vet J 2010;51: 1095–102.

20. Rogers KC, Miles DG, Renter DG, et al. Effects of delayed respiratory viral vaccine and/or inclusion of an immunostimulant on feedlot health, performance, and carcass merit of auction-market derived feeder heifers. BovPract (Stillwater) 2016;50:154–62.

21. Hagenmaier JA, Terhaar BL, Blue K, et al. A comparison of three vaccine programs on the health, growth performance, and carcass characteristics of high-risk feedlot heifers procured from auction markets. BovPract (Stillwater) 2018; 52:120–30.

22. Martin SW. Vaccination: is it effective in preventing respiratory disease or influencing weight gains in feedlot calves? Can Vet J 1983;24:1–9.

23. Perino LJ, Hunsaker BD. A review of bovine respiratory disease vaccine field efficacy. BovPract (Stillwater) 1997;31:59–66.

24. Tripp HM, Step DL, Krehbiel CR, et al. Evaluation of outcomes in beef cattle comparing preventative health protocols utilizing viral respiratory vaccines. BovPract (Stillwater) 2013;47:54–64.

25. Griffin CM, Scott JA, Karisch BB, et al. A randomized controlled trial to test the effect of on-arrival vaccination and deworming on stocker cattle health and growth performance. BovPract (Stillwater) 2018;52:26–33.

26. Munoz V, Samuelson K, Tomczak D, et al. Efficacy of metaphylaxis with tulathro-mycin and pentavalent modified-live virus vaccination in high-risk cattle. Conf Res Workers Anim Dis, Chicago, IL, November 2-5, 2019. Abstract 218, p. 135.

27. Step DL, Krehbiel CR, Burciaga-Robles LO, et al. Comparison of single vaccina-tion versus revaccination with a modified-live virus vaccine containing bovine herpesvirus-1, bovine viral diarrhea virus (types 1a and 2a), parainfluenza type 3 virus, and bovine respiratory syncytial virus in the prevention of bovine respira-tory disease. J Am Vet Med Assoc 2009;235:580–7.

28. Richeson JT, Kegley EB, Powell JG, et al. Weaning management of newly received beef calves with or without continuous exposure to a persistently in-fected bovine viral diarrhea virus pen mate: Effects on health, performance, bovine viral diarrhea virus titers, and peripheral blood leukocytes. J AnimSci 2012;90:1972–85.

29. Miles D. Overview of the North American beef cattle industry and the incidence of bovine respiratory disease (BRD). AnimHealth Res Rev 2009;10:101–3.

30. Hughes HD, Carroll JA, Burdick Sanchez NC, et al. Natural variations in the stress and acute phase response of cattle. InnateImmun 2013;20:888–96.

31. Roth JA, Kaeberle ML. Suppression of neutrophil and lymphocyte function induced by a vaccinal strain of bovine viral diarrhea virus with and without the administration of ACTH. Am J Vet Res 1983;44:2366–72.

32. Seiver HA, Samuelson KL, Posey RD, et al. Administration of a DNA immunosti-mulant does not mitigate bovine herpesvirus-1 recrudescence in dexamethasone challenged beef cattle. J AnimSci 2019;97(Suppl 1):16–7.

33. Ridpath JF. Immunology of BVDV vaccines. Biologicals 2013;41:14–9.

34. Ruby KW. Immediate (type-1) hypersensitivity and HaemophilusSomnus. PhD Dissertation. Ames (IA): Iowa State University; 1999.

35. Gershwin LJ, Berghaus LJ, Arnold K, et al. Immune mechanisms of pathoge-netic synergy in concurrent bovine pulmonary infection with Haemophilussom-nus and bovine respiratory syncytial virus. Vet ImmunolImmunopathol 2005; 107:119–30.

36. Ruby KW. Senior Staff Reviewer, USDA-APHIS. Histophilus vaccine research. Proceedings of the Academy of Veterinary Consultants. Denver, CO, August 8-10, 2019.

37. Larson RL, Step DL. Evidence-based effectiveness of vaccination against Man-nheimiahaemolytica, Pasteurellamultocida, and Histophilussomni in feedlot cattle for mitigating the incidence and effect of bovine respiratory disease complex. Vet Clin North Am FoodAnimPract 2012;28:97–106.

38. Confer AW, Ayalew S. Mannheimiahaemolytica in bovine respiratory disease: im-munogens, potential immunogens, and vaccines. AnimHealth Res Rev 2018;19: 79–99.

Bovine Respiratory Disease Treatment Failure
Impact and Potential Causes

Calvin W. Booker, DVM, MVetSc[a], Brian V. Lubbers, DVM, PhD[b],*

KEYWORDS

- Bovine respiratory disease • Antimicrobial • Treatment failure

KEY POINTS

- Treatment failures in bovine respiratory disease (BRD) result from the interactions between the bacterial pathogen, drug, host, drug administrator, and the environment.
- Changing antimicrobial or antimicrobial class has little impact on many of the interactions that result in BRD treatment failures.
- Treatment failures provide an opportunity to evaluate case definition and treatment records for improving diagnosis and therapy for BRD.

INTRODUCTION

There are many ways to define bovine respiratory disease (BRD) treatment failure. In addition, individual veterinarians and producers likely have different thresholds for considering something a failure. However, from a practical perspective, BRD treatment failure occurs when animals receiving a treatment regimen for BRD fail to directly respond and recover after treatment, resulting in BRD relapse therapy, chronic illness, sale for salvage slaughter, and/or euthanasia/death. When BRD treatment failure occurs, it has both direct impacts (costs associated with BRD relapse treatment, management of chronically ill animals, reduced proceeds received for animals sent for salvage slaughter, the original purchase of the feeder animal and accumulated feed/production expenses to death, and carcass disposal) and indirect impacts (effects on infrastructure, morale of employees, animal welfare, and antimicrobial exposure). This article discusses the impacts of BRD treatment failures and explores the interactions between the host, pathogen, environment, drug, and drug administrator that contribute to BRD treatment failure.

[a] Feedlot Health Management Services, Box 140, Okotoks, Alberta T1S 2A2, Canada; [b] Clinical Sciences, College of Veterinary Medicine, Kansas State University, 1800 Denison Avenue, Manhattan, KS 66506, USA
* Corresponding author.
E-mail address: blubbers@vet.k-state.edu

Vet Clin Food Anim 36 (2020) 487–496
https://doi.org/10.1016/j.cvfa.2020.03.007
0749-0720/20/© 2020 Elsevier Inc. All rights reserved.

vetfood.theclinics.com

IMPACTS OF BOVINE RESPIRATORY DISEASE TREATMENT FAILURES
Direct Impacts

Bovine respiratory disease relapse treatment

When animals receiving a treatment regimen for BRD fail to directly respond and recover after treatment, it may be necessary to provide additional treatment of BRD. In the feedlot, this generally requires identifying and separating the affected animals from pen-mates, moving the animals through an animal handling facility, making a diagnosis of BRD relapse, administering an antimicrobial drug plus or minus ancillary or supportive therapeutic products, recording what was done in the medical record, and returning the animals to the pens of origin directly after treatment or after spending 1 or more days in a hospital/convalescent pen. The direct impact is the sum of the drug product, personnel, and handling costs associated with each of these activities.

Management of chronically ill animals

Although most animals treated for BRD respond directly after initial BRD treatment or after 1 or more additional BRD treatments, some animals develop chronic BRD that is deemed nonresponsive to additional antimicrobial, ancillary, or supportive therapy. In the feedlot, animals with chronic illness, including chronic BRD, are generally housed in pens designated for animals with chronic disease (known as chronic pens). Ideally, these pens are equipped and managed to provide a comfortable environment with easier access and less competition for feed/water than a regular production pen. In addition, animals should be evaluated on a daily and weekly basis to assess/monitor the clinical progression of each animal so that recovered animals can be returned to a regular production pen. Cattle that are chronically ill but suitable for salvage slaughter and have fulfilled all pharmaceutical withdrawal times can be shipped, moribund or suffering animals can be euthanized, and animals requiring additional time in the chronic pen can be maintained there for a defined time period. This approach generally works well in most feedlots when the number of chronically ill animals is small and relatively constant, and the personnel assigned to assess/monitor the clinical progression of each animal are well trained and have enough time and support to attend to their job duties. However, whenever the occurrence of BRD peaks (generally in the fall of the year in the United States and Canada), it is followed by an increase in chronically ill animals, resulting in overcrowded chronic pens and insufficient time/support for personnel to adequately assess/monitor the clinical progression of each animal. When this occurs, it generally requires direct intervention by a veterinarian and/or supervisor/manager to prioritize the management of chronically ill animals. The direct impact is the sum of the costs associated with managing chronically ill animals. The indirect impact of managing chronically ill animals is the effect on morale of employees and animal welfare.

Sale for salvage slaughter

Animals with chronic BRD that do not recover and have fulfilled all pharmaceutical withdrawal times may be deemed suitable for salvage slaughter. Compared with euthanasia or death, sale for salvage slaughter may seem like a substantially better economic outcome of BRD treatment failure cases. However, in many cases, especially in lighter animals, the proceeds received from salvage slaughter of animals with chronic BRD is only 25% to 50% (or less) of the original purchase cost of the feeder animal and does not account for the accumulated feed/production expenses from arrival at the feedlot to shipment. As a result, the direct impact of sale for salvage slaughter is a substantial loss on each affected animal.

Euthanasia/death

The most definitive form of BRD treatment failure is death. Death may occur naturally (ie, without human intervention), caused by rapid pathophysiologic processes that occur in acute BRD, or it can occur through euthanasia of animals with chronic disease or animals that are moribund or suffering. When death occurs, the direct impacts include the original purchase cost of the feeder animal, accumulated feed/production expenses to death (including processing, treatment, bedding, and yardage), and carcass removal/disposal cost. In addition, there is a so-called opportunity cost to the cattle owner of not marketing the animal when cattle ownership is profitable and loss of daily margin for the feedlot until a replacement animal is able to fill the same pen space. The magnitude of these costs varies depending on the underlying value of feeder cattle and feed/production expenses.

Indirect Impacts

Infrastructure

In terms of BRD treatment failure, the biggest impacts on infrastructure are pens to house animals with chronic BRD. In most cases, these are designated pens associated with hospital/treatment facilities. However, in instances where there are large numbers of animals with chronic BRD, it can be necessary to temporarily use a regular production pen as a chronic pen. In addition to pens for chronically ill animals, it is necessary to have access to appropriate infrastructure to ship animals for salvage slaughter and carcass disposal/removal.

Morale of employees

Managing sick animals, including animals with BRD, is a serious responsibility. Trained animal personnel diagnose and treat animals in the feedlot daily. From the employee perspective, successful treatment of sick or injured animals is a rewarding experience. However, whenever treatment failure occurs, it usually has negative impacts on employee morale and the magnitude of the impact is usually greater the more severe the treatment failure. For example, the negative impact on employee morale of having a treatment failure that results in an animal with chronic BRD or death is much more severe than a treatment failure requiring 1 or 2 additional treatment regimens for BRD. However, managing animals with chronic BRD seems to have a greater impact on employee morale than coping or dealing with animals that die acutely from BRD. This revelation is not surprising, but it bears significant consideration when working with animal health personnel that have to deal with large numbers of chronically ill animals on an ongoing basis to make sure that there are adequate protocols, systems, management support, and other resources in place to maintain animal welfare, as well as maintain/promote positive worker morale.

Animal welfare

Animal welfare is a priority throughout the beef production system, including identification and initial treatment of sick animals. When treatment failure occurs for any disease, including BRD, the probability of an adverse outcome (relapse, chronic disease, or death) goes up and animals with a higher probability of an adverse outcome require closer assessment/monitoring to maintain appropriate animal welfare. As noted earlier, this assessment is particularly relevant and important in animals with chronic disease to make sure that adequate protocols, systems, management support, and other resources are in place to maintain animal welfare.

Antimicrobial exposure

Although clinicians do not fully understand the specific impacts of each antimicrobial exposure in cattle on the development of antimicrobial resistance or the spread of resistance elements in bacteria of importance to animal or human health, it is generally thought that lower antimicrobial exposure is a good thing from an antimicrobial stewardship perspective. From a veterinary perspective, this approach makes sense if efforts to reduce antimicrobial exposure do not have significant negative repercussions for animal health and welfare. In terms of BRD treatment failure, the impacts on animal health and welfare were discussed earlier. However, when BRD treatment failure occurs, it may be necessary to provide additional treatment of BRD, which usually includes administration of an antimicrobial. In addition, the antimicrobial used is likely to be of a different antimicrobial class than has been used previously in the same animal. As a result, an indirect impact of BRD treatment failure is increased antimicrobial exposure (compared with animals that respond to therapy). Although the impact, if any, of this increased antimicrobial exposure on the development of antimicrobial resistance or the spread of resistance elements in bacteria of importance to animal or human health is unknown, it is one more thing to keep in mind as the veterinary profession works to develop and validate more effective BRD prevention, control, and treatment strategies.

FACTORS THAT CONTRIBUTE TO BOVINE RESPIRATORY DISEASE TREATMENT FAILURES

BRD is often attributed to complex interactions between the host, pathogen, and the environment.[1] Likewise, many BRD treatment failures result from interactions between the host, pathogen, environment, drug, and drug administrator (**Fig. 1**). Investigating and addressing the underlying causes of BRD treatment failures can improve clinical outcomes and animal welfare in future cases, improve morale of employees, reduce direct costs of dealing with BRD treatment failures, refine antimicrobial prescribing practices, and advance antimicrobial stewardship.

Drug-Pathogen Factors that Contribute to Bovine Respiratory Disease Treatment Failures

In BRD treatment failures, poor clinical response is often attributed to the ability of a bacterial pathogen to survive in the presence of the selected antimicrobial (ie, antimicrobial resistance). Recent literature reports support concerns of antimicrobial resistance among the primary BRD pathogens.[2–4] A thorough review of the literature on antimicrobial resistance in BRD pathogens is provided by DeDonder and Apley.[5]

However, antimicrobial resistance, through acquisition of specific resistance genes or mutation, is not the only way by which bacterial organisms adapt to survive in the presence of an antimicrobial. For example, biofilms are communities of bacteria living in a matrix of extracellular proteins, polysaccharides, and nucleic acids that attach to device surfaces or damaged tissues, can withstand host immune responses, and are less susceptible to the activity of antimicrobial agents than nonattached, free-living bacterial cells.[6] Because antimicrobial effects depend on sufficient concentrations of the drug at the site of infection, bacteria present in a biofilm may be less susceptible to antimicrobial activity through several mechanisms. The physical makeup of biofilms retards the diffusion of some antimicrobials so that they do not reach the bacterial targets within the biofilm.[7] In addition, bacteria in a biofilm exist in varying states of metabolic activity and the dormant cells are more resistant to the activity of antimicrobials.[8] In humans, infections associated with bacterial biofilms often present as chronic or

Environment

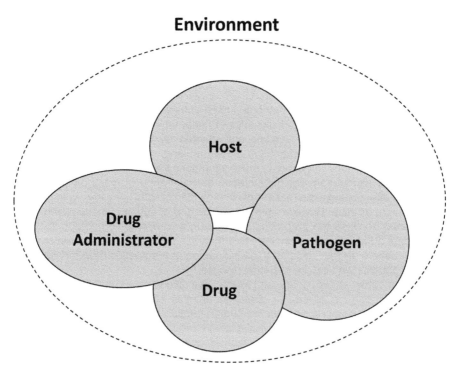

Fig. 1. Interaction of contributing factors that potentially result in BRD treatment failure.

persistent infections. Previous research has shown that *Mannheimia haemolytica* and *Histophilus somni* form biofilms in vitro; therefore, it is possible that biofilms could contribute to treatment failures and relapses of BRD.[9]

Host-Pathogen Factors that Contribute to Bovine Respiratory Disease Treatment Failures

When BRD treatment failure occurs, focusing on 1 drug-pathogen factor (ie, antimicrobial resistance) is easy to do and provides an acceptable reason for the failure and an obvious option for a solution (change the antimicrobial). However, host-pathogen factors may also play a role in BRD treatment failure. For example, delayed onset of treatment (or advanced state of disease) can result in BRD treatment failure even if a pathogen is susceptible to a drug. The most obvious examples of this type of situation are BRD deaths that occur in animals that have never been treated for BRD. In these untreated cases, an animal's immune system is not able to mount a sufficient response to contain the infection. In theory, this inadequate response could be caused by the specific virulence of the pathogens involved, overwhelming bacterial challenge, poor immune system function and general health of the host, or a combination of all of these. Variation in BRD pathogen virulence has been previously described and could include ability to colonize, speed of replication, ability to produce leukotoxin, and ability to resist immune system defenses.[10,11] On the host side, an animal's immune system could be naive to the specific pathogens involved or incapable of mounting a sufficient response to infection because of a compromised state caused by nutritional deficiency or excess, health status (preexisting or concomitant disease), environmental exposure (hot or cold), body condition, physiologic state (pregnancy, lactation, growth), or other stressors (weaning, commingling, shipping, dehorning, castration, or other management procedures). Any combination of these host-pathogen factors could contribute to BRD treatment failure.

Drug-Host Factors that Contribute to Bovine Respiratory Disease Treatment Failures

Another factor that potentially contributes to BRD treatment failures is the impact of the disease state on the pharmacokinetics of the antimicrobial. In critically ill human patients, antimicrobial concentrations are affected by pathophysiologic changes, such as leaky capillaries, alterations in protein binding, changes in renal clearance, and organ dysfunction.[12] In general, these alterations in host physiology (1) increase the volume of distribution, and (2) increase the clearance of many antimicrobials, with the net effect being a decrease in plasma concentrations compared with persons without severe disease. However, the magnitude and direction of these changes are not universal because the properties of the drug (hydrophilic vs hydrophobic) and concomitant administration of ancillary treatments may influence the plasma concentrations in severe disease, leading to consideration of therapeutic drug monitoring in individual patients with severe systemic disease.[13]

Studies in cattle, sheep, goats, and swine have also shown that the disposition of antimicrobials can be altered in diseased animals compared with healthy animals.[14–16] As has been reported in the human medical literature, the effects of disease on pharmacokinetics of antimicrobials in veterinary species may depend on the drug, disease process, or other factors. Gorden and colleagues[17] and Day and colleagues[18] reported increases in volume of distribution (Vd) and clearance (Cl) in mastitic cows and porcine reproductive and respiratory syndrome virus–*Streptococcus suis* coinfected pigs, respectively, compared with healthy animals treated with ceftiofur. The physiologic alterations reported in these studies are likely to result in lower than expected plasma concentrations of the antimicrobial in diseased animals and could contribute to treatment failures. Studies evaluating the effects of lipopolysaccharide challenge on florfenicol disposition in sheep[19] and enrofloxacin in swine[20] showed that endotoxemia reduced the clearance of these antimicrobials, with a resulting increase in drug exposure (area under the curve). Taken together, these studies show that although severe disease can affect the pharmacokinetics of an antimicrobial, the net impact is virtually unpredictable in individual animals. This situation presents a considerable challenge in production medicine settings where therapeutic monitoring of individual patients is not feasible because of logistics of animal handling, test availability, and diagnostic result turnaround times.

Drug-Drug Administrator Factors that Contribute to Bovine Respiratory Disease Treatment Failures

In human medicine, the term medication error is a broad concept defined as "any preventable event that may cause or lead to inappropriate medication use or patient harm while the medication is in the control of the health care professional, patient, or consumer."[21] Medication errors occur at every stage from prescribing to dispensing to administration, with consequences of inappropriate therapy ranging from innocuous to serious morbidity and mortality. In human medicine, medication errors occur in approximately 5% of all medication orders, with the most frequent errors being in the dose, route, or frequency of administration.[22,23]

The overall incidence of medication errors in veterinary settings remains largely unknown.[24,25] Adverse drug events are voluntarily reported to the US Food and Drug

Administration (FDA).[26] However, these reports are not a good estimate of the medication error rate because adverse events represent a small percentage of medication errors (errors that did not result in an adverse event are not included) and adverse events are correlated to product usage; commonly used products are likely to have more reported adverse events. Case examples from the FDA Web site highlight many of the common causes of medication errors in veterinary medicine, including drug names that look or sound alike, drug labeling issues (lack of background contrast, inconsistent presentation of drug strength, and so forth), error-prone abbreviations on written prescriptions, and illegible handwriting.[27]

Improper handling and storage of antimicrobials can also contribute to lack of efficacy. Ondrak and colleagues[28] conducted a study to determine compliance with drug manufacturers' recommended storage temperatures. In this study, temperature loggers were placed in 9 different practice vehicles during the summer months. Temperatures more than 25°C were recorded for 63% of readings in Nebraska and 95% of total readings for Texas. Although the impact of increased storage temperatures on drug effectiveness is likely variable based on the specific product, as well as the magnitude and duration of temperature exposures, it is prudent to adhere to manufacturer recommendations for optimal effectiveness of the product.

Host-Drug Administrator Factors that Contribute to Bovine Respiratory Disease Treatment Failures

The relationship between the host animal and the drug administrator and the impact on outcome of BRD therapy is, beyond points already discussed, largely a reflection of case definition and the ability to accurately detect disease in individual animals. Therapeutic failure rates would potentially increase if the case definition results in poor sensitivity for disease detection, leading to diagnosis in only the most severe BRD cases. Poor sensitivity for diagnosing BRD could also result in a high treatment failure rate if the case definition does not distinguish between BRD and other (noninfectious) clinical syndromes that are not expected to respond to antimicrobial therapy. A discussion of case definitions and BRD diagnostic testing can be found in the article by Buczinski, in this issue.

Evaluating treatment protocols

Although most animals treated for BRD respond directly after initial BRD treatment or after 1 or more additional BRD treatments, some animals develop chronic BRD that is deemed nonresponsive to additional antimicrobial, ancillary, or supportive therapy, whereas other animals die/are euthanized because of severe BRD. As part of assessing the outcome of BRD treatment protocols, it is important to consider first treatment success rates (percentage of initial patients with BRD that recover after 1 treatment), relapse rates (percentage of initial patients with BRD that relapse with BRD and require 1 or more subsequent treatments for BRD), chronicity rates (percentage of initial patients with BRD that develop chronic disease), and case fatality rates (percentage of initial patients with BRD that die). For example, if all animals respond directly to initial BRD treatment and there are no failures, it is highly likely that treated animals did not have BRD requiring antimicrobial therapy, and efforts should be made to reduce the number of treatments that occur by refining the case definition for BRD. In contrast, if the first treatment success rate is low and the case fatality rate and/or chronicity rate in treated animals is high, it is highly likely that 1 or more of the interactive factors described earlier is affecting the outcome. In these cases, a systematic review of these factors is warranted to identify which factors are involved in each situation. This evaluation should include a thorough review and summary of individual animal treatment records, postmortem findings, and diagnostic laboratory results, if available, to determine when and how treatment failure is occurring and which inter-actions between the host, the infecting bacteria, the drug, and the drug administrator are likely having the greatest impact in a given clinical situation.

SUMMARY

Although BRD treatment failures are generally only a small percentage of the animals in a specific production system, the impact of failures can be substantial and include both direct and indirect effects. In many cases, simply changing antimicrobial thera-pies has minimal impact on outcomes. These clinical failures provide an opportunity to combine clinical observations, treatment records, and diagnostic results, when available, to investigate and address the many potential underlying factors that resulted in poor clinical response.

DISCLOSURE

C.W. Booker has received consulting and/or speaking honoraria from Bayer Animal Health, Boehringer Ingelheim Animal Health, Elanco Animal Health, Merck Animal Health, Phibro Animal Health, Vetoquinol, and Zoetis. B.V. Lubbers has received consulting and/or speaking honoraria from Merck Animal Health, Boehringer Ingel-heim Vetmedica, Bayer Animal Health, and Zoetis.

REFERENCES

1. Avra T, Abell K, Shane D, et al. A retrospective analysis of risk factors associated with bovine respiratory disease treatment failure in feedlot cattle. J Anim Sci 2017;95:1521–7.
2. Portis E, Lindeman C, Johansen L, et al. A ten-year (2000-2009) study of antimi-crobial susceptibility of bacteria that cause bovine respiratory disease complex – *Mannheimia haemolytica, Pasteurella multocida,* and *Histophilus somni* – in the United States and Canada. J Vet Diagn Invest 2012;24:932–44.
3. Synder E, Credille B, Berghaus R, et al. Prevalence of multi drug antimicrobial resistance in *Mannheimia haemolytica* isolated from high-risk stocker cattle at arrival and two weeks after processing. J Anim Sci 2017;95:1124–31.
4. Timsit E, Hallewell J, Booker C, et al. Prevalence and antimicrobial susceptibility of *Mannheimia haemolytica, Pasteurella multocida,* and *Histophilus somni* iso-lated from the lower respiratory tract of healthy feedlot cattle and those diag-nosed with bovine respiratory disease. Vet Microbiol 2017;208:118–25.
5. DeDonder K, Apley M. A literature review of antimicrobial resistance in pathogens associated with bovine respiratory disease. Anim Health Res Rev 2015;16: 125–34.
6. Costerton J, Stewart P, Greenberg E. Bacterial biofilms: A common cause of persistent infections. Science 1999;284:1318–22.
7. Shigeta M, Tanaka G, Komatsuzawa H, et al. Permeation of antimicrobial agents through *Pseudomonas aeruginosa* biofilms: a simple method. Chemotherapy 1997;43:340–5.
8. Anwar H, van Biesen T, Dasgupta M, et al. Interaction of biofilm bacteria with an-tibiotics in a novel in vitro chemostat system. Antimicrob Agents Chemother 1989; 33:1824–6.

9. Boukahil I, Czuprynski C. *Mannheimia haemolytica* biofilm formation on bovine respiratory epithelial cells. Vet Microbiol 2016;197:129–36.

10. Singh K, Ritchey JW, Confer AW. *Mannheimia haemolytica*: Bacterial-host interactions in bovine pneumonia. Vet Pathol 2010;48:338–48.

11. Klima CL, Cook SR, Zaheer R, et al. Comparative genomic analysis of *Mannheimia haemolytica* from bovine sources. PLoS One 2016;11:e0149520.

12. Shah S, Barton G, Fischer A. Pharmacokinetic considerations and dosing strategies of antibiotics in the critically ill patient. J Intensive Care Soc 2015;16: 147–53.

13. McKinnon PS, Davis SL. Pharmacokinetic and pharmacodynamics issues in the treatment of bacterial infectious diseases. Eur J Clin Microbiol Infect Dis 2004;23: 271–88.

14. Ismail M, El-Kattan YA. Comparative pharmacokinetics of marbofloxacin in healthy and *Mannheimia haemolytica* infected calves. Res Vet Sci 2007;82: 398–404.

15. Waxman S, San Andres MD, Gonzalez F, et al. Influence of *Escherichia coli* endotoxin-induced fever on the pharmacokinetic behavior of marbofloxacin after intravenous administration in goats. J Vet Pharmacol Ther 2003;26:65–9.

16. Tantituvanont A, Yimprasert W, Werawatganone P, et al. Pharmacokinetics of ceftiofur hydrochloride in pigs infected with porcine reproductive and respiratory syndrome virus. J Antimicrob Chemother 2009;63:369–73.

17. Gorden PJ, Kleinhenz MD, Wulf LW, et al. Altered plasma pharmacokinetics of ceftiofur hydrochloride in cows affected with severe clinical mastitis. J Dairy Sci 2016;99:505–14.

18. Day DN, Sparks JW, Karriker LA, et al. Impact of an experimental PRRSV and *Streptococcus suis* coinfection on the pharmacokinetics of ceftiofur hydrochloride after intramuscular injection in pigs. J Vet Pharmacol Ther 2015;38: 475–81.

19. Perez R, Palma C, Drapela C, et al. Pharmacokinetics of florfenicol after intravenous administration in Escherichia coli lipopolysaccharide-induced endotoxaemic sheep. J Vet Pharmacol Ther 2015;38:144–9.

20. Post LO, Farrell DE, Cope CV, et al. The effect of endotoxin and dexamethasone on enrofloxacin pharmacokinetic parameters in swine. J Pharmacol Exp Ther 2003;304:889–95.

21. National Coordinating Council for Medication Error Reporting and Prevention (NCCMERP). About medication errors: what is a medication error?. Available at: https://www.nccmerp.org/about-medication-errors. Accessed November 1st, 2019.

22. Kaushal R, Bates DW, Landrigan C, et al. Medication errors and adverse drug events in pediatric inpatients. JAMA 2001;285:2114–20.

23. Bates DW, Boyle DL, Vander Vliet MB, et al. Relationship between medication errors and adverse drug events. J Gen Intern Med 1995;10:199–205.

24. Wallis J, Fletcher D, Bentley A, et al. Medical errors cause harm in veterinary hospitals. Front Vet Sci 2019;6:12.

25. Oxtoby C, Ferguson E, White K, et al. We need to talk about error: causes and types of error in veterinary practice. Vet Rec 2015;177:438.

26. Food and Drug Administration. Adverse event reports for animal drugs and devices. Available at: https://www.fda.gov/animal-veterinary/product-safety-information/adverse-event-reports-animal-drugs-and-devices. Accessed November 14th 2019.

27. Food and Drug Administration [b]. Veterinary medication errors. Available at: https://www.fda.gov/animal-veterinary/product-safety-information/veterinary-medication-errors. Accessed November 14th 2019.

28. Ondrak JD, Jones ML, Fajt VR. Temperatures of storage areas in large animal veterinary practice vehicles in the summer and comparison with drug manufacturers' storage recommendations. BMC Vet Res 2015;11:248.

The Effect of Market Forces on Bovine Respiratory Disease

Derrell S. Peel, PhD

KEYWORDS

- Bovine respiratory disease • Respiratory disease • Economics • Market failure

KEY POINTS

- The inability to enhance BRD control is caused partly by market failure.
- The complex economic structure of the cattle industry results in misalignment of costs and benefits across production sectors and suboptimal investment in BRD control.
- Better BRD control requires an industry-wide effort to focus on lifetime animal health.

INTRODUCTION

Bovine respiratory disease (BRD) is the costliest disease affecting the cattle industry, persisting despite efforts to reduce the disease and resulting economic losses. The continued and, arguably, growing impacts of BRD have frustrated animal health professionals and members of the cattle industry, who have been unable to improve BRD control and reduce its economic impact. This article discusses the economic impacts of BRD, some economic considerations for BRD control, and reasons for slow progress in improving BRD control.

WHAT IS BOVINE RESPIRATORY DISEASE?

BRD is caused by a complex of viral and bacterial infection, linked to stressors related to management and environmental conditions. Weaning, crowding, sorting, commingling, processing, and shipping often trigger BRD. For this reason, BRD is commonly referred to as "shipping fever" because many of these stressors are associated with movement between production sectors. Environmental conditions, such as temperature (high or low), wet conditions, exhaust fumes, and dust, also contribute. The interaction and timing between these factors is complex and adds significantly to the challenge in understanding BRD. Although the end-result is typically the same, the sequence and timing of events that lead to BRD varies by case.

Oklahoma State University, 519 Ag Hall, Stillwater, OK 74078, USA
E-mail address: derrell.peel@okstate.edu

Vet Clin Food Anim 36 (2020) 497–508
https://doi.org/10.1016/j.cvfa.2020.03.008   **vetfood.theclinics.com**

BOVINE RESPIRATORY DISEASE AND THE BEEF CATTLE INDUSTRY

The US cattle industry is complex and this adds to the challenge of understanding and controlling BRD. The industry consists of multiple production sectors that are separated by space and time. The biology of cattle production is slow, and this subjects cattle to prolonged opportunity for exposure to pathogens and conditions that contribute to BRD. Depending on the specific production system, cattle production typically covers 24 to 28 months including 9 months of gestation, 7 to 8 months of suckling before weaning, 4 to 6 months in stocker/backgrounding, and 5 to 8 months for finishing.

Cow-calf production is the most widespread sector of the beef cattle industry, occurring over most of the country in climates ranging from subtropical to subalpine. There are 13 states with more than 900,000 head of beef cows, spread from Florida and Kentucky in the east and from Texas to Montana and North Dakota in the west. These 13 states account for 67.1% of the total beef cowherd with another seven states each having more than 500,000 beef cows.[1] The 2017 Census of Agriculture shows that beef cow-calf production occurs on 729,046 farms with an average herd size of 44 head (**Table 1**). Beef cowherds are widely distributed in size with 27.2% of cows in herds of less than 50 cows, 55.6% in herds from 50 to 500 cows, and 17.2% in herds greater than 500 head.[2]

Most beef and dairy steers and feeder and cull heifers are finished in feedlots. Feedlot production is highly concentrated in size and location. The 2017 Census of Agriculture shows that 700 feeding operations of 2500 head or greater account for 70.7% of cattle in feedlots with an average inventory of 15,181 head.[2] These 700 feedlots represent just 2.7% of all feedlots. On January 1, 2020, the top five cattle feeding states of Nebraska, Texas, Kansas, Iowa, and Colorado accounted for 72.1% of total

Table 1
Beef cow, dairy cow, and feedlot inventory by herd size, December 31, 2017

	Beef Cows	Milk Cows	Feedlots
Inventory, head	31,722,039	9,539,631	15,025,052
Farms, n	729,046	54,599	25,776
Average herd size, head	44	175	582
	Cows by herd size, %		By herd size, %
1–9	3.52	0.41	
10–19	6.30	0.36	0.34[a]
20–49	17.34	3.27	1.33
50–99	16.94	8.65	2.34
100–199	17.82	9.35	3.48
200–499	20.84	12.00	6.86
500–999	9.26	10.73	8.44
1000–2499	5.18	20.32	6.48
2500–4999	1.50	18.53	70.72[b]
5000 or more	1.30	16.39	

[a] 1–19 head.
[b] 2500 or more head.
   Data from USDA-NASS. 2017 Census of Agriculture United States Summary and State Data, Volume 1, Geographic Area Series, Part 51. AC-17-A-51, National Agricultural Statistics Service, April 2019.

feedlot inventories.[1] The movement of cattle from small herds of geographically widespread cow-calf production to large, geographically concentrated feedlots implies much assembly, sorting, commingling, and shipping of cattle. Thus, the stressors associated with BRD are an integral and inevitable component of beef cattle production.

Between the cow-calf and feedlot sectors, many cattle pass through stocker or backgrounding operations. These are often grazing-based postweaning growing programs, although they may be confined or semiconfined growing/backgrounding operations.[3] These operations add an additional layer of assembly, handling, commingling, sorting, and shipping that increase exposure to pathogens and stresses that increase BRD risk.

Compared with other sectors, there is little published information describing the size and location of stocker/backgrounding production. Cattle inventory estimates on January 1st allow the calculation of estimated feeder supplies outside of feedlots. This is the best estimate of stocker inventories on that date, but it also includes unweaned calves. Winter stockers are heavily concentrated on cool-season cereal forages and each year 25% to 30% of feeder cattle are located in the states of Kansas, Oklahoma, and Texas, based on the January 1st cattle inventory. Summer stockers are even less well documented but large concentrations are found regionally, including the Flint Hills and Osage regions of Kansas and Oklahoma.

In summary, the geographic concentration of cattle begins as calves move from dispersed cow-calf production to stocker/backgrounding production and is complete as animals are placed in feedlots for finishing. Cattle move through a complex marketing and transportation system that often involves movement through multiple auctions or other sale facilities. Moreover, many calves begin this process leaving primary cow-calf production unweaned and with naive and immature immune systems.

BOVINE RESPIRATORY DISEASE AND THE DAIRY INDUSTRY

The dairy industry is focused on milk production and much of the emphasis on BRD has been in replacement heifers.[4,5] Dairy calves are typically removed from cows shortly after birth and reared separately. Neonatal dairy calves are raised in separate hutches before commingling to grow in calf farms. Dairy steers often move into feeding facilities as lightweight calves and may finish on feed for a year before harvest. Dairy heifers are grown in heifer development facilities. More recently, the use of sexed semen and the production of more valuable beef-dairy crossbreed steer calves, increase the motivation to manage these calves for increased survivability.

IMPACTS OF BOVINE RESPIRATORY DISEASE

BRD affects all sectors of the cattle industry and all classes of animal to varying degrees. Some impacts are general across all classes and some are specific to certain animals/production sectors. The general list of BRD impacts includes

Feedlot/stocker (backgrounding):
- Mortality (value of death loss)
- Reduced weight gain
- Reduced feed efficiency
- Reduced salvage value of chronic animals
- Treatment costs
- Vaccination costs
- Metaphylaxis costs

Cow-calf (beef and dairy):
- Mortality (value of death loss, cows and preweaning calves)
- Reduced weaning weights
- Treatment costs (cows and calves)
- Reduced productivity (eg, milk production)
- Reduced pregnancy percentage (failure to breed or early embryonic death caused by bovine viral diarrhea virus [BVDV])
- Reduced calving percentage (abortion, stillborn, or perinatal mortality caused by BVDV)
- Vaccination costs

BOVINE RESPIRATORY DISEASE MORTALITY

Total nonpredator death loss in all cattle was reported by US Department of Agriculture (USDA) in 2017 at 3.21%.[6] This includes 2.17% death loss among cattle (>500 pounds) and 5.55% among calves. Death loss in cattle caused by respiratory disease accounted for 23.9% of nonpredator death loss or 0.52% of total nonpredator cattle death loss. Among calves, respiratory disease accounts for 26.9% of nonpredator death loss, which is 1.5% of total nonpredator calf death loss. The total value of nonpredator death loss in cattle and calves was reported at $3.69 billion, with $907.8 million, or 24.6%, because of respiratory disease.

Among beef cow operations, respiratory disease accounts for 15.9% of cattle death and 23.0% of calf death with a total value of $370.8 million.[6] Among feedlot and stocker/backgrounding operations, respiratory disease accounts for 55.0% of nonpredator death loss in cattle and 36.3% among calves with a total value of $274.84 million. (The USDA reports cattle operations as beef cattle, dairy cattle, mixed [beef and dairy] and other. Data reported here are for "other," which includes primarily stocker and feedlot operations[6]). In dairy operations, respiratory disease accounts for 16.0% of nonpredator cattle death loss and 32.7% of calf losses with a total value of $197.89 million.

BOVINE RESPIRATORY DISEASE MORBIDITY AND TREATMENT

Respiratory disease is reported to affect 16.2% of all feedlot cattle with 96.9% of feedlots reporting incidence of respiratory disease (100% of large feedlots).[7] All feedlots (100%) reported treating cattle affected with respiratory disease with 87.5% of affected cattle receiving treatment. Most common treatments for respiratory disease include injectable antibiotic (100% of cattle treatments) and respiratory vaccination (48.5%), with other treatments given less frequently. Over all feedlot cattle, 13.4% receive an injectable antibiotic, and 6.5% receive a respiratory vaccine. Average BRD treatment cost was reported at $23.60/head for treated cattle, indicating that feedlots were spending in excess of $75 million annually on BRD treatments at the time of this study. The cost of respiratory treatment has nearly doubled between 1999 and 2011 (from $12.59 to $23.60 per case) suggesting that the direct cost is higher today.[7]

Among feedlot cattle treated for respiratory disease, 81.7% of those placed weighing less than 700 pounds responded, with 14.9% retreated, 4.0% mortality, and 2.3% marketed as chronics.[7] Of those cattle placed weighing less than 700 pounds and treated a second time, 63.1% responded, with 12.0% treated a third time, 13.3% mortality, and 6.1% marketed as chronics. For cattle placed weighing more than 700 pounds, 86.5% responded, 12.4% were retreated, 3.6% mortality, and 1.9% marketed as chronics. Among cattle placed weighing more than 700 pounds and treated a second time, 69.5% responded, with 17.1% treated a third time, 13.2% mortality, and 8.2% marketed as chronics.

The stocker/backgrounding sector likely experiences BRD impact similar to feedlots, although little data are available. In fact, it is possible that stocker morbidity caused by BRD is higher than for feedlots because weaning and other processes associated with movement into stocker or feedlot production lead to substantial stress.

There is little information on BRD in cow-calf production. The 2007 to 2008 NAHMS beef cow-calf report indicates that of 1.5% of breeding animal death loss, just 3.4% of breeding cattle mortality, or 0.05% of total death loss, was attributable to BRD, indicating that respiratory morbidity is low among mature animals.[8] However, the same report indicated of the 3.6% of preweaning calf mortality, 31.4% of mortality among calves older than 3 weeks of age was caused by respiratory disease.

Respiratory disease was reported by 60.5% of dairy operations, affecting 2.8% of dairy cows.[9] Of cows affected by BRD, 62.0% remained in the herd, whereas 27.5% were permanently removed and another 10.5% died. Most of these cows likely received some treatment. Dairy cows are permanently removed from the herd generally as a result of a serious health issue and/or low production. Respiratory disease accounts for 24.0% of mortality in preweaned dairy heifers and 58.9% of weaned dairy heifer mortality.

LOST PRODUCTIVITY CAUSED BY BOVINE RESPIRATORY DISEASE

The costs of BRD include a wide variety of negative impacts on productivity. Animals lose productivity during active BRD infections and, in many cases, those that survive have compromised productivity for the remainder of their lives.

Feedlot and stocker cattle that have BRD experience reduced gains, reduced feed efficiency, and degraded carcass quality. The impacts of BRD on productivity are not well measured because BRD animals are averaged into pen level data at feedlots. An extreme example from a commercial feedlot illustrates the likely impacts of BRD on feedlot production. Production parameters from a "wreck" pen are compared with average metrics for similar cattle.[10] The wreck pen had 37.04% death loss (2.05% average), 7.66% sick head days (0.7% average), 0.66 pounds/day average daily gain (3.78 average daily gain average), 221 days on feed (166 days average), and a feed/gain ratio of 27.48 (5.88 average). It is likely, although unconfirmed, that the example wreck pen was primarily impacted by respiratory disease. Chronic animals represent about 2.1% of feedlot animals treated for respiratory disease that never recover to perform well. These animals are marketed for minimal salvage value.

BRD has a variety of impacts on beef cow-calf productivity. In addition to mortality, calves that survive summer pneumonia typically have reduced weaning weights. BVDV, one component of the BRD complex, results in unique impacts on cow-calf production and in all other cattle production sectors.

THE UNIQUE ROLE OF BOVINE VIRAL DIARRHEA VIRUS

BVDV is an immunosuppressive agent that significantly increases the likelihood of concurrent or subsequent viral and bacterial infections. BVDV has two other unique characteristics: it causes reproductive disease in cows, and it results in persistently infected (PI) animals. Cows can acquire BVDV infections that lead to inapparent or mild signs. However, these infections can cause various reproductive problems that result in lower calving rates. Calves may be born with congenital deformities, or weak, leading to neonatal or preweaning mortality. Cows infected with BVDV during the first trimester of gestation may produce calves that are PI. These calves may seem normal or may be weak or deformed. Many die before weaning but some survive, and may be marketed as feeder or breeding cattle, or be retained in the herd for breeding. Although these PI animals may never develop signs of disease, they constantly shed BVDV and expose all other animals as long as they remain in the herd. PI cows always give birth to PI calves. PI calves that enter the feeder cattle supply expose all cattle with direct or fence line contact. These PI animals are a reservoir of BVDV that spreads across the entire cattle industry through marketing facilities, transportation systems, and in stocker and feedlot operations.

BRD would still occur in the absence of BVDV. It is not known how much controlling or eliminating BVDV would reduce BRD impacts in the cattle industry. However, BVDV is deserving of particular attention because PI cattle clearly represent a known reservoir of a pathogen that impacts the industry, and the source of PI calves is at the cow-calf level. Better control or elimination of BVDV must necessarily be directed at the cow-calf sector.

BOVINE RESPIRATORY DISEASE PREVENTION

Vaccines are available to help prepare cattle for the challenge of BRD. However, among beef cattle operations, 60.6% do not vaccinate calves for respiratory disease. Small herds (<50 cows) were least likely to vaccinate for BRD with 73.7% of operations not vaccinating.[8] Among herds of 200 or more cows, only 18.0% gave no BRD vaccinations. Overall, 69.1% of calves are vaccinated for BRD, which means that 30.9% are not vaccinated. Among small herds, 63.9% of calves received no BRD vaccinations, in contrast to herds with more than 200 cows, in which just 11.9% received no BRD vaccination. Roughly 25% of beef cow operations vaccinate cows for each of the common BRD viruses (infectious bovine rhinotracheitis virus [IBRV], 24.6%; BVDV, 28.1%; parainfluenza type-3 virus [PI3V], 22.6%; bovine respiratory syncytial virus [BRSV], 21.1%). However only 7.9% of operations vaccinate for *Histophilus somni* and 4.5% vaccinate for *Pasteurella/Mannheimia*.

More than 85% of all feedlot operations vaccinate for the major viral respiratory viruses (IBRV, BVDV, PI3V, and BRSV), with more than 90% vaccinating for IBRV and BVDV.[7] Thus, more than 90% of feedlot cattle receive some respiratory vaccinations. However, fewer cattle receive other respiratory vaccinations: only 61.4% of cattle receive BRSV vaccination, and only 55.1% receive PI3V vaccination. Some 60% to 70% of all feedlot operations vaccinate for some bacterial pathogens.

Feedlots can also use metaphylaxis to prevent respiratory disease. Metaphylaxis, or mass medication of incoming feedlot cattle, is a costly practice and is only applied under certain conditions and with specific managerial consideration. Overall, 59.3% of feedlot operations use metaphylaxis on any cattle; with 59.3% of operations using metaphylaxis on 39.2% of cattle weighing less than 700 pounds on arrival and 29.6% of operations using metaphylaxis on 5.2% of all cattle weighing more than 700 pounds on arrival.[7]

In dairy operations, more operations vaccinate cows than pregnant heifers or pre-weaned heifers for respiratory disease. Some 55% to nearly 70% of dairy operations vaccinated cows for various viral pathogens, with the highest at 68% of operations vaccinating for BVDV.[9] The percent of operations vaccinating is lower for IBRV (60.2%), PI3V (55.8%), and BRSV (54.8%). Less than 10% of dairy operations vaccinate for bacterial pathogens, such as *Histophilus* and *Mannheimia*. The levels of vaccination is lower for pregnant heifers, with roughly 45% to 50% of operations using viral vaccines, and lower still for preweaned heifers, with about 20% to 35% of operations using viral vaccines.

In general, vaccines for viral respiratory pathogens are more widely used than those for bacterial pathogens. Efficacy of vaccines for bacterial respiratory pathogens (*Pasteurella*, *Mannheimia*, *Histophilus*, and *Mycoplasma*) is lower and this is likely the reason that these vaccines are less widely used in beef cow-calf, feedlot, and dairy operations.[11]

THE ECONOMICS OF BOVINE RESPIRATORY DISEASE CONTROL

BRD is clearly a huge challenge in the beef and dairy industries with large economic impact on all sectors. The cost of BRD has led to significant research by public and private sectors and vast private sector development and marketing of technologies for detection, prevention, and treatment of BRD. Despite continued improvement and effectiveness of vaccines and other technologies, BRD persists as the most economically significant disease affecting the cattle industry. In fact, BRD may be getting worse instead of better. **Fig. 1** shows feedlot death loss (12-month moving average) as reported from monthly surveys of Kansas feedlots. Death loss has generally trended up over the data period from 1994 to present. Although the specific contribution of BRD to this trend is uncertain, it is believed to be a significant component.

Industry participants and animal health professionals are increasingly frustrated by the inability to make significant progress in reducing the impact of BRD. This situation raises the question of whether limitations or factors that extend beyond animal health, narrowly focused, contribute to the failure to make progress in controlling BRD. The following sections discuss several considerations that may be important to enhanced control of BRD.

IMPROVED BOVINE RESPIRATORY DISEASE AWARENESS

As noted previously, 60.9% of all cow-calf operations gave zero vaccinations for respiratory disease, including 73.7% of small operations. Failure to be aware of the disease or failure to understand the impact of BRD is surely part of the problem. For cow-calf producers, the direct impacts may be unrecognized or underrecognized.

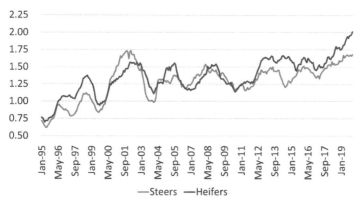

Fig. 1. Feedlot death loss. (*Data from* Focus on Feedlots Monthly Reports. Kansas State University Animal Sciences and Industry Website. https://www.asi.k-state.edu/about/newsletters/focus-on-feedlots/monthly-reports.html. Updated March 5, 2020. Accessed March 16, 2020.)

Producers who experience an outbreak of summer pneumonia perhaps become more aware, but operations that experience, for example, low levels of BVDV infections may fail to notice the reductions in reproductive productivity that occur. USDA surveys showed that although 64% of cow-calf producers were fairly knowledgeable or knew some basics about BVDV, 36% either had not heard of it or had heard the name but knew nothing about the disease.[12]

Stocker and feedlot operations are keenly aware of the impacts of BRD. Frustration is high and mounting because, despite better (and more expensive) pharmaceuticals, cattle morbidity and mortality continues. Although the problems are well recognized among stocker and feedlot producers, it is possible that there is only now a growing recognition that the problems are coming to them from the cow-calf level. It has long been recognized that the stressors involved in weaning and shipping cattle trigger respiratory disease (ie, shipping fever), but there is growing recognition that the calf health situation before weaning determines much of the impact later.

The evolution of preconditioning programs illustrates this changing sentiment. Originally, many preconditioning programs started as VAC-30 or VAC-35 programs, which meant that the preconditioning protocol included weaning calves a minimum of 30 or 35 days. Within a few years most programs changed to VAC-45 protocols, requiring a minimum of 45 days of weaning along with vaccinations and other management. Although most programs still require the 45-day weaning protocol, feeder cattle buyers are increasingly emphasizing longer weaning periods and buyers are paying additional premiums for 60 to 90 days of weaning.

The dairy sector is more aware of BRD because the focus of the industry is the growth of heifers into milk-producing cows. However, smaller percentages of dairy operations vaccinate pregnant heifers for respiratory disease and fewer still vaccinate preweaned heifers. Only 20% to 35% of preweaned heifers are vaccinated for viral respiratory pathogen and less than 5% of operations vaccinate for *Histophilus* and *Mannheimia*.[9]

Continued and enhanced education is clearly a vital component of any strategy to better control BRD. Until producers at all levels recognize and understand the impacts of BRD, make better use of the pharmaceutical technology, and make some changes in management, progress in controlling BRD will be slow. Among beef cow-calf producers and dairies, in particular, smaller operations tend to be less aware of BRD and its impacts, and generally vaccinate less. Lack of awareness is less the case for feedlots where the differences in vaccine use between small and large operations is less pronounced. However, smaller feedlots are less likely to use metaphylaxis than larger feedlots.[7]

Producers at all levels of the industry use animal health inputs (eg, vaccines, treatments, testing), like any other input into production, so long as expected returns exceed the cost of the input. However, the complex production structure of the industry increases the difficulty of recognizing and understanding the impacts of BRD as animals move through multiple production stages with different ownership. Additionally, the complexity of the disease makes it extremely challenging to evaluate the costs and benefits of BRD control on an individual level. Moreover, awareness and understanding of the disease and the impacts on an individual level may not be enough.

A COMPREHENSIVE APPROACH IS NEEDED

Historically, most BRD control has been focused on individual production sectors. In particular, stocker and feedlot operations, which face the most BRD impacts and costs, have attempted to deal with BRD as best they can with the animals that come to them. There is little communication across sectors, and even fewer attempts to coordinate animal health management comprehensively in the industry. Feedlots routinely maintain records of sources of cattle and, in many cases, are aware of the health history of those sources. That information is often reflected in prices paid, which does send information back to the producer, but the information is more likely used to plan treatment and management of the cattle. Initiatives, such as certified preconditioning programs, have had a positive impact but have limited adoption across the industry.[13] The growing emphasis on long-weaned calves noted previously provides incentives for cow-calf producers, but is not widely recognized or adopted at this time. In general, the cattle industry has focused more on treatment instead of immunity and prevention of BRD. An industry-wide shift to focus more on immunity and prevention implies education; improved communication; more coordination; and, critically, improved economic signals across industry sectors to improve incentives for changing health and management practices.

Quantifying the costs of BRD and the benefits of enhanced control is a challenge. The figure of $800 to $900 million annually caused by feedlot mortality, reduced feed efficiency, and treatment cost from Chirase and Greene[14] has been widely quoted. A wide range of estimates have been offered for various aspects of BRD including mortality, treatment cost, reduced productivity, and reduced value of chronics. Most of the estimates have focused on feedlot production. Brooks and colleagues[15] also looked at the impact of BRD on backgrounding heifers. Little information is available on the cost of BRD at the cow-calf level, although Hurt[16] did provide estimates of the value of BVDV control for cow-calf producers. The impact of BRD in the dairy industry is similarly difficult to estimate and is likely underestimated.

THE ECONOMICS OF DISEASE CONTROL

Despite the difficulties in comprehensively quantifying the costs of BRD, the value to the industry of improving BRD control probably exceeds the cost of improved control. This situation leads to the question of why the industry is underinvesting in BRD control. The answer is most likely because of economics rather than animal health limitations. Markets are efficient when individual participants make decisions for their own interest that ultimately results in a socially optimal allocation of resources. If all producers in cattle and dairy industries had the correct incentives to control BRD at an optimal level, the entire industry would be better off. The use of the word "optimal" highlights that striving for 100% control or eradication is probably not economic even if it were achievable.

There are several reasons why markets may not be efficient. One has already been discussed: when producers do not fully understand BRD and its impacts, and thus do not use optimal levels of disease detection, prevention and/or treatment. In this situation, producers can make themselves better off by reducing the direct impacts of the disease with additional investment in health technology and/or management. Enhanced education to improve BRD awareness and adoption of detection, prevention, and treatment technology may be beneficial.

The more challenging economic problem is market failure. Market failure occurs when the full costs and/or benefits are not recognized by the decision-maker and the resulting decision is not socially optimal. Although markets are generally efficient, market failure can occur in several ways. For example, the broader public value of education likely exceeds the value that individuals realize from better education, and thus results in a suboptimal level of investment in education. This example is the argument for public support of education. In another example, a manufacturing firm that is able to dump wastes into air or water will not take the negative social costs of pollution into account and would thus produce more of a product than is socially optimal. With market failure, individual firms make entirely economical decisions based on the costs and benefits they realize, and yet the overall outcome to society is suboptimal, and results in an incorrect allocation of resources.

In the case of BRD, the stocker and feedlot sectors experience most of the treatment costs, lost productivity, and death loss from the disease and would benefit the most from enhanced BRD control. However, evidence is growing that the health of stocker and feedlot cattle is largely determined at the cow-calf level, who currently receive little economic incentive to manage cattle for better lifetime health and immunity. This market failure results in less than optimal efforts and investment in BRD control in the cattle industry. Riley and colleagues[17] discuss market failure in the context of BVDV control. Johnson and Pendell[18] note that improved BRD control would have short-run market impacts because of changing the supply of cattle and beef with reduced BRD morbidity and mortality.

Research on fetal (developmental) programming suggests that nutrition and management of the cow in gestation is a principal determinant of lifetime productivity and health of the calf, whether for feedlot finishing or replacement heifers.[19] At birth, the health of the calf is greatly influenced by the availability of colostrum and the passive immunity it provides. The incidence of BVDV in the herd may determine whether the calf is PI or exposed, which increase the probability of disease. Appropriate vaccinations at the proper time, good calf management, and low-stress weaning all impact health in the stocker and feedlot phases. One example is castration of bulls. Despite that bull calves are discounted, many bull calves are still marketed. These feeder bulls will suffer productivity losses because of later castration and are three times more likely to get BRD in the feedlot.[20]

The beef industry will benefit from more emphasis on immunity and keeping cattle healthy than from better treatment technology for management of sick cattle. The cow-calf sector is key to this, but currently have no incentive to enhance efforts to ensure healthy, immune calves leaving the ranch. It will require some way to realign the benefits and costs of enhanced BRD control to see significant progress. The complex, multisector structure of the cattle industry means that stresses that contribute to BRD cannot be eliminated but they can be managed and minimized. Weather and other environmental factors cannot be controlled, they can only be managed for or around to a limited degree.

However, one of the biggest factors impacting BRD is simply that too little is known about calves that arrive at auction or the feedlot. Visual appraisal and the limited information that passes from sellers to buyers is insufficient to reveal the true health status (and therefore the value) of calves when ownership is transferred from cow-calf to stocker or feedlot. The buyer would have to know the answer to a long list of questions to properly value calves and provide better incentives to the cow-calf producers. The list of questions includes

- Did the dam receive adequate and proper nutrition during gestation?
- Was the dam properly vaccinated and not exposed to disease during gestation?
- Did the calf receive ample, high-quality colostrum after birth?
- Is the calf persistently infected with BVDV?
- Was the calf exposed to BVDV after birth?
- Did the calf have BRD (summer pneumonia) before weaning?
- Was the calf properly managed before weaning (eg, castration, dehorning, worming)?

- Did the calf receive appropriate vaccinations in the correct amount and at the proper time?
- Was the calf weaned (low stress) for at least 45 days before marketing?

At the current time, cow-calf producers likely do not know the answer to some of these questions, in part because they do not currently have any incentive to know those answers.

The challenge of increasing cattle health and immunity to prevent BRD rather than focusing on treatment likely requires an increased emphasis on health management at the cow-calf level. This in turn implies that the industry must consider economic mechanisms to realign costs and benefits to provide additional incentives for cow-calf producers to provide healthier calves for the rest of the industry. This might involve industry-designed and managed programs to provide incentives in the form of premiums for adoption of desired health practices, or indemnity to test for and eliminate PI BVDV animals and so forth. It could also be accomplished as a government-administered program of testing, vaccination, and eradication similar to brucellosis or tuberculosis programs.

SUMMARY

BRD continues to be a persistent negative economic impact on the beef and dairy industries, and the inability to show any progress in controlling BRD is a source of increasing frustration among animal health professionals and producers. Although there is a continuing need for more and better animal health testing, prevention, and treatment technology, the challenges of enhancing BRD control likely extend beyond veterinary science. The complex economic structure of the cattle industry leads to market failures in which producers, particularly at the cow-calf level, do not have sufficient economic incentive to invest in better BRD control, which leads to higher costs for stocker and feedlot sectors. An industry-wide comprehensive effort is needed to coordinate and motivate enhanced BRD control focusing on producing calves with better immunity and less morbidity rather than treatment.

DISCLOSURE

No disclosure or conflict of interest.

REFERENCES

1. USDA-NASS. Cattle. National Agricultural Statistics Service; 2020. Available at: https://downloads.usda.library.cornell.edu/usda-esmis/files/h702q636h/rb68xv24k/76537h73d/catl0120.pdf.
2. USDA-NASS. 2017 Census of agriculture United States summary and state data, Vol. 1, Geographic area series, Part 51. AC-17-A-51. National Agricultural Statistics Service; 2019. Available at: https://www.nass.usda.gov/Publications/AgCensus/2017/Full_Report/Volume_1,_Chapter_1_US/usv1.pdf.
3. Peel DS. Beef cattle growing and backgrounding programs. Vet Clin North Am Food Anim Pract 2003;19:365–85.
4. Jenny BF, Gramling GE, Glaze TM. Management factors associated with calf mortality in South Carolina dairy herds. J Dairy Sci 1981;64:2284–9.
5. Wells SJ, Dargatz DA, Ott SL. Factors associated with mortality to 21 days of life in dairy heifers in the United States. Prev Vet Med 1996;29:9–19.
6. USDA. Death loss in U.S. cattle and calves due to predator and nonpredator causes, 2015. USDA-APHIS-VS-CEAH-NAHMS; 2017. Available at:

https://www.aphis.usda.gov/animal_health/nahms/general/downloads/cattle_calves_deathloss_2015.pdf.

7. USDA. Feedlot 2011 Part IV: health and health management on U.S. feedlots with a capacity of 1,000 or more head. USDA-APHIS-VS-CEAH-NAHMS; 2013. Available at: https://www.aphis.usda.gov/animal_health/nahms/feedlot/downloads/feedlot2011/Feed11_dr_PartIV_1.pdf.

8. USDA. Beef 2007-08 Part IV: reference of beef cow-calf management practices in the United States, 2007-08. USDA-APHIS-VS-CEAH-NAHMS; 2010. Available at: https://www.aphis.usda.gov/animal_health/nahms/beefcowcalf/downloads/beef0708/Beef0708_dr_PartIV_1.pdf.

9. USDA. Dairy 2014 health and management practices on U.S. dairy operations, 2014. USDA-APHIS-VS-CEAH-NAHMS; 2018. Report 3. Available at: https://www.aphis.usda.gov/animal_health/nahms/dairy/downloads/dairy14/Dairy14_dr_PartIII.pdf.

10. Stehle A, Peel DS, Riley JM. A profile of cattle feeding: beyond the averages. West Econ Forum 2018;16-2:62–77.

11. Larsen RL, Step DL. Step. Evidence-based effectiveness of vaccination against *Mannheimia haemolitica*, *Pasteurella multocida* and *Histophilis somni* in feedlot cattle for mitigating the incidence and effect of bovine respiratory disease complex. Vet Clin North Am Food Anim Pract 2012;28:97–106.

12. USDA. Beef 2007-08 Part II: reference of beef cow-calf management practices in the United States, 2007-08. USDA-APHIS-VS-CEAH-NAHMS; 2009. Available at: https://www.aphis.usda.gov/animal_health/nahms/beefcowcalf/downloads/beef0708/Beef0708_dr_PartII_1.pdf.

13. Williams GS, Raper KC, DeVuyst EA, et al. Determinants of price differentials in Oklahoma value-added feeder cattle auctions. J Ag & Res Econ 2012;37-1:115–28.

14. Chirase, NK, LW Greene. Dietary zinc and manganese administered from the fetal stage onward affect immune response of transit stressed and virus infected offspring steer calves. Anim Sci Feed Tech 2001;93:217.

15. Brooks KR, Raper KC, Ward CE, et al. Economic effects of bovine respiratory disease on feedlot cattle during backgrounding and finishing phases. The Professional Animal Scientist 2011;27(27):195–203.

16. Hurt C. Market failure in disease control: bovine viral diarrhea virus (BVDV) and the economic feasibility of enhanced control in the beef cattle industry. Unpublished M.S. Thesis, Dept of Ag Econ, Oklahoma State Univ; 2018. Available at: https://shareok.org/bitstream/handle/11244/317801/Hurt_okstate_0664M_15723.pdf?sequence=1&isAllowed=y.

17. Riley JM, Peel DS, Raper KC, et al. Economic consequences of cow-calf disease mismanagement: bovine viral diarrhea virus. Appl Anim Sci 2019;35(6). https://doi.org/10.15232/aas.2019-01861.

18. Johnson KK, Pendell DL. Market impacts of reducing the prevalence of bovine respiratory disease in United States beef cattle feedlots. Front Vet Sci 2017;4:189.

19. Summers AF, Funston RN. Fetal programming: implications for beef cattle production. Range Beef Cow Symposium. 2013. Available at: http://digitalcommons.unl.edu/rangebeefcowsymp/319. Accessed April 16, 2020.

20. Richeson JT, Pinedo PJ, Kegley EB, et al. Association of hematologic variables and castration status at the time of arrival at a research facility with the risk of bovine respiratory disease in beef calves. J Am Vet Med Assoc 2013;243(7):1035–41.

Moving?

Make sure your subscription moves with you!

To notify us of your new address, find your **Clinics Account Number** (located on your mailing label above your name), and contact customer service at:

Email: journalscustomerservice-usa@elsevier.com

800-654-2452 (subscribers in the U.S. & Canada)
314-447-8871 (subscribers outside of the U.S. & Canada)

Fax number: 314-447-8029

Elsevier Health Sciences Division
Subscription Customer Service
3251 Riverport Lane
Maryland Heights, MO 63043

*To ensure uninterrupted delivery of your subscription, please notify us at least 4 weeks in advance of move.

Printed and bound by CPI Group (UK) Ltd, Croydon, CR0 4YY

03/10/2024

01040400-0005